Juvenile Offenders
With
Mental Health Disorders:

Who Are They and What Do We Do With Them?

By Lisa Melanie Boesky, Ph.D.

a publication of the
AMERICAN CORRECTIONAL ASSOCIATION
Professional Development Department
4380 Forbes Boulevard
Lanham, MD 20706
1-800-222-5646
http://www.aca.org

ISBN 1-56991-154-1

© American Correctional Association

Dedications

To the juvenile offenders and juvenile justice professionals who have shared their lives with me. I have been amazed and humbled by their courage, strength, wisdom, and love.

To my mother. I would not be who I am today without her love, support, and spirit. May she rest in peace.

Acknowledgments

First, I would like to thank those psychologists, psychiatrists, and psychiatric nurses, who have shared their knowledge and experience with me throughout my years of school and work. Our discussions were valuable on many levels.

Second, I would like to thank the members of the committee who reviewed the finished manuscript: Kathy Black-Dennis; Nancy Cunningham, Psy.D.; Steven Fadoir, Ph.D.; Norris Gregoire; Jack McCllellan, M.D.; and Jim Maxwell. Their time and assistance is so very appreciated.

Finally, I would like to thank my friends and family for understanding my time limitations. They graciously and generously provided me with the space and support I needed to complete this book. I am truly blessed.

L.M.B.

All of the artwork in this book was created by juvenile offenders. Some of the drawings were created by youth on probation through the Snohomish County Juvenile Court in Washington State. Some of the drawings were created through The Enchanted Way, an art therapy program that uses the fundamentals of mythology and Chinese philosophy. For more information on this program, please go to http://www.enchantedway.com.

Foreword

As Dr. Lisa Boesky notes, our nation's juvenile justice system is encountering more and more juveniles with mental health disorders. While we do not know the exact number of juvenile offenders with mental health disorders, we do know that the rate is higher than that of their peers in society. A significant number of these mentally ill juvenile offenders are incarcerated in facilities, which causes complex and challenging problems for staff. Many of these juveniles can be difficult for staff to manage—especially those staff who already are dealing with issues related to crowding, budgetary constraints, and limited mental health training.

Juvenile Offenders with Mental Health Disorders: Who Are They and What Do We Do With Them? is designed to help juvenile justice staff who "supervise, manage, teach, or treat juvenile offenders with mental health disorders." Dr. Lisa Boesky explains in simple language how to identify and manage mentally ill youth. She provides practical, effective management strategies that can help staff defuse situations and avoid problems. Perhaps more important, Dr. Boesky's strategies will help staff learn how to "make a difference" in the lives of many of these troubled youth.

We hope that this book helps you expand your skills for managing juvenile offenders with mental health disorders.

James A. Gondles, Jr. C.A.E.
Executive Director
American Correctional Association

Preface

If you picked up this book, you are probably— like many individuals working with juvenile offenders who have mental health disorders— confused, frustrated, and searching for answers about this complex and difficult-to-manage group of youngsters.

You came to the right place.

An increasing number of youths with mental health disorders continue to enter and remain involved with the juvenile justice system. The exact number of mentally ill juvenile offenders is currently unknown. But it is clear that the rate of mental health disorders is higher among youth involved with juvenile justice versus their peers in the general population. A significant number of these mentally ill youths are currently incarcerated in juvenile justice facilities, and the management of this population is fraught with challenges and complexities.

Many juvenile justice facilities:

- Are overcrowded

- Are underfunded

- Have limited or no mental health resources

- Provide little to no training on mental health issues to juvenile justice professionals

This book was written as a guide to assist a variety of professionals who supervise, manage, teach, or treat juvenile offenders with mental health disorders. The following individuals require information about mental health issues in order to make strategic decisions, as well as interact more effectively with mentally ill juveniles:

- Juvenile careworkers/juvenile service workers/correctional officers/youth specialists/line staff

- Security staff

- Supervisors

- Program managers

- Administrators

- Probation officers/probation counselors

- Parole officers/parole counselors

- Mental health counselors

- Substance abuse treatment counselors

- Teachers

- Nurses

- Physicians

- Clergy

- Vocational program supervisors

- Recreation staff

- Mentors

- Volunteers

- Interns

- Attorneys

- Judges

- Law enforcement officials

The content of this book is primarily focused on juvenile offenders with mental health disorders who reside in residential facilities (*e.g.,* detention centers, training schools, diagnostic/reception centers, ranches, work camps, boot camps, group homes, treatment facilities). However, the information is just as relevant and applicable to juvenile offenders on community supervision (*e.g.,* probation, parole). It is also pertinent to youths who engage in delinquent or antisocial behavior but who may not yet have come into contact with the legal system.

The information contained in this book is not designed to train juvenile justice professionals to function as if they were mental health professionals. The following chapters provide essential information regarding the *identification* and *management* of juvenile offenders with mental health disorders. However, they do not provide the necessary and extensive education, training, and clinical experience required to assign a psychiatric diagnosis to juveniles or to conduct psychotherapy with youth.

Juvenile justice professionals need to have basic information related to the most common psychiatric disorders seen among juvenile offenders. This knowledge can assist them in accurately identifying and referring mentally ill youth to appropriate mental health professionals for evaluation and treatment.

Most juvenile justice professionals interact with youth who have mental health disorders on a regular basis. Therefore, they also require practical, "user-friendly," and effective management strategies to use during these interactions. Every interaction juvenile justice professionals have with youth can reinforce appropriate behavior or reinforce inappropriate behavior among these juveniles. These continual interactions between staff and youth make effective behavior management critical.

The more educated juvenile justice professionals are about mental health disorders, the more strategic they can be when supervising and managing mentally ill youth. With a greater understanding of how mental health symptoms can play a role in juveniles' behavior, staff can take the necessary steps to help diminish youths' distress versus inadvertently escalating it. An increased understanding of mental health also results in a less stressed workforce, smoother and safer-running juvenile justice facilities, and mentally ill juvenile offenders who are able to function more successfully in the activities of daily living.

A significant factor related to job satisfaction is feeling successful regarding the job one is doing and believing one's actions make a difference. It is easy to become burned out when

working with juvenile offenders if one feels that he or she is not effective or that one's efforts are not meaningful in some way. Many juvenile justice professionals feel frustrated and hopeless about some of the mentally ill offenders with whom they work. This typically occurs when staff do not understand these youths' unusual (and sometimes frightening) behavior. It also commonly occurs when mentally ill youth are unable to participate successfully in standard programs or services—or when usual sanctions have little to no effect in modifying youth behavior. Increased knowledge about how mental health symptoms are manifested among adolescents, particularly adolescent offenders, can decrease staff confusion and fear. It can also increase juvenile justice professionals' ability to design and implement creative management and programming strategies that are beneficial to mentally ill youth.

The following chapters focus on some of the most important issues related to the identification and management of juvenile offenders with mental health disorders. After a brief introduction to the topic of mentally ill juveniles, there is discussion about the complexity of providing mental health diagnoses to this unique population of youth. The majority of the book provides descriptions of the most common psychiatric disorders seen among juvenile offenders:

- Conduct Disorder
- Oppositional Defiant Disorder
- Major Depression
- Dysthymic Disorder
- Bipolar Disorder
- Attention-Deficit/Hyperactivity Disorder
- Posttraumatic Stress Disorder
- Mental Retardation
- Learning Disorders
- Fetal Alcohol Syndrome

And suggestions regarding the effective management of youth with these disorders are provided. The identification and management of juveniles with the following disorders and behavior are also discussed:

- Substance use disorders
- Co-occurring mental health and substance use disorders
- Suicidal behavior
- Self-injurious behavior

Relevant issues related to the following key areas are covered:

- Screening and assessment of mentally ill juveniles
- Treatment of mentally ill juveniles

Finally, there is a brief review of additional issues that should be considered when working with this distinct group of juveniles:

- Minority issues
- Female offenders
- Homosexual youth
- Head trauma
- Violence and mental illness
- Seclusion and restraint
- Malingering
- Staff training

Some may wonder why a discussion of the various personality disorder diagnoses (*e.g.*, Antisocial Personality Disorder, Borderline Personality Disorder, Narcissistic Personality Disorder) is not included. There are definitely some youth in the juvenile justice system who suffer from a personality disorder (*e.g.*, Borderline Personality Disorder, Antisocial Personality Disorder, Narcissistic Personality Disorder).

However, a discussion about this type of disorder is beyond the scope of this book. The discussion is complicated by the clinical complexity of personality disorder. The discussion is also complicated because the validity of personality disorder diagnoses in adolescents has still not been definitively established (Myers, Burket, & Otto, 1993). Many juvenile offenders with mental health disorders exhibit *traits* of a person-

ality disorder. But it is often difficult to determine when these youth are truly suffering from one of the full-blown *disorders*. Diagnosing personality disorders among *juvenile offenders* is particularly complicated because many of these youth:

- Are at an age/developmental level in which they are still developing their personalities
- Have been exposed to significant trauma during their childhood and/or teen years
- Have experienced head injuries/neuropsychological trauma as infants, children, or adolescents
- Have been severely abused (emotionally, physically, and/or sexually)
- Have been severely neglected
- Have low I.Q.'s
- Use significant amounts of drugs and alcohol
- Have experienced high levels of stress related to incarceration
- Suffer from psychiatric disorders such as Major Depression, Posttraumatic Stress Disorder, Bipolar Disorder, etc.

Each of these factors can significantly impact juveniles' functioning. And youths' resulting behavior may be misinterpreted as reflecting a personality disorder when one is not fully present. Individuals diagnosed with personality disorders are often perceived by the mental health and juvenile justice systems as difficult to treat and unlikely to improve. Until more information is known about personality disorders among adolescents (especially among juvenile offenders), these diagnoses can unnecessarily stigmatize an already-shunned group of youngsters in need of services.

Whenever possible, the information and recommendations included in the following chapters are based on the research literature. There is a great deal of variation regarding the amount of research available on each of the mental health disorders. We know a great deal about some mental health issues but little about others. The material chosen reflects what is currently known in the field of mental health. However, the field continues to develop and expand as additional studies are conducted and new information is discovered. Unfortunately, there is almost a complete absence of studies regarding *juvenile offenders* who have mental health disorders. With regard to topics where research is lacking, information and suggestions are based on years of clinical experience and best practice in the fields of juvenile justice and mental health.

In order for the material to be applicable to a wide range of settings and professionals, the information and recommendations in this book are provided as a general guide. There are no hard-and-fast rules with regard to working with juvenile offenders with mental health disorders. Each young person is different and has his or her own unique set of beliefs, experiences, behaviors, and characteristics. Juvenile justice agencies have their own philosophies, policies, and procedures. They also differ in availability (or lack thereof) of mental health resources.

Juvenile justice professionals can have a profound impact on the lives of the juvenile offenders with whom they work. In fact, it is not unusual for these staff members to be viewed by some youth as greater parental figures than the juveniles' own parents/caretakers. When working with these youth, juvenile justice professionals often need to find a balance between serving as:

- Authority figures
- Rule makers
- Disciplinarians
- Trusted confidants
- Supporters
- Nurturers

However, walking this fine line is also one of the challenges of effective parenting. And some juvenile offenders with mental health disorders need to be re-parented. Juvenile justice professionals may be the most consistent adults in a young offender's life, particularly for those youth who have remained in the system for many years. The educational, mental health, substance abuse, and child welfare systems have deemed some of these juveniles untreatable and hopeless. Characteristics of some juvenile offenders (*e.g.*, anger, aggression, antisocial behavior) can make it difficult for various professionals to remain committed to helping these youth or to advocate for their needs over an extended period of time.

Yet, many professionals within juvenile justice have seen a significant number of juvenile offenders turn their lives around. Many youth who dropped out of school eventually received their GEDs or high school diplomas. Some juveniles who used to sell drugs to support themselves learned a trade and obtained reputable jobs. These changes are often related to adults believing in and consistently supporting juvenile offenders. Juvenile justice professionals often play this role in young offenders' lives, particularly when youth are not supported within their families.

It is the combination of expertise from juvenile justice professionals *and* mental health professionals that results in effective treatment for juvenile offenders with mental health disorders. Mental health professionals rely on juvenile justice staff to provide the empathy, support, and positive role modeling necessary for mentally ill youth to be successful.

There are a variety of vocations more prestigious and less dangerous than working with juvenile offenders. The majority of juvenile justice professionals could find other employment in which they could work fewer hours, make more money, and have less physical and emotional demands placed on them. Juvenile justice is a tough field for anyone working with today's juvenile offenders. There are not many people outside of the system who can truly "understand" and "relate to" what is required of juvenile justice professionals on a daily (sometimes hourly) basis. Despite the challenges, most professionals working within the juvenile justice courts, residential programs, community supervision programs, classrooms, etc., are committed to their jobs and consciously choose to remain in their positions. Making a difference in the lives of adolescents is likely a powerful motivating factor for many of them. Juvenile justice professionals may not make a difference in the life of each and every offender with whom they come into contact. But they make a difference in the lives of a significant number of youth. I believe this is one of the main reasons most individuals enter the field and why they keep coming back. All juvenile justice professionals have developed their own expertise regarding the juveniles with whom they work. Hopefully, they will view the information and recommendations contained in this book as additional tools to use when working with juvenile offenders who suffer from mental health disorders.

To the world, you might be one person
But to one person, you might be the world

Brandon, 16

Table of Contents

CHAPTER 1

Youth with Mental Health Disorders in the Juvenile Justice System

"When did this detention facility become a psychiatric hospital? And why didn't anyone tell me?"

A Juvenile Careworker

Michael is a 13-year-old male who has repeatedly been arrested for breaking into his school on the weekends. Michael was sent to a minimum-security group home. However, staff are considering transferring him to a more secure facility. The group home is not staff-intensive, and there is concern that the program does not have the resources necessary to manage Michael.

Staff members refer to Michael as the "needy one" because he constantly asks them the same questions over and over. Although the daily schedule remains unchanged, Michael continuously asks, "When is lunch?" "When is lunch?" "When is lunch?" Or he asks, "When do we get to go outside?" "Is it time to go outside?" "Is it my time to go outside yet?" Michael repeatedly misplaces his belongings and cannot keep track of his written assignments. He also forgets to complete the chores for which he is responsible. Michael bangs on the door, hits the wall, jumps on his bed, or tries to disassemble his desk whenever the boys are placed in their rooms. The other youth in the group home find Michael immature, intrusive, and annoying. He continuously interrupts their conversations. And he becomes loud and demanding when they do not include him in activities. Most treatment in the facility takes place within a group format. But Michael has been unable to sit still for more than one-third of his 90-minute groups. This has resulted in numerous sanctions—including being removed from five of the seven treatment groups he is required to attend.

Kelvin is a 16-year-old male detained at a local juvenile detention center on assault charges. From the moment he arrived at the facility, he has been angry, hostile, and intimidating. He refuses to follow staff directions, stating that detention staff are "working with the devil in a conspiracy against him." Nighttime is particularly troublesome for Kelvin. He becomes increasingly upset and refuses to go into his room when it is time for bed. Staff have had to physically restrain him twice. Kelvin has been confined to his room during much of his short stay at the facility, due to his hostile attitude and behaviors. Peers have told staff that Kelvin has been making suicidal statements about hanging himself on the weekend. Half of the unit staff think Kelvin is being manipulative and is just trying to get out of spending time in his room. The other half are worried that something is wrong with him and are fearful that he may truly be a danger to himself.

Amy is a 15-year-old female with a history of shoplifting and running away from home. She has been at a juvenile justice facility for girls for six months and has had intense mood changes much of that time. One minute Amy is happily engaged with staff and peers—often to the point of singing aloud and dancing in the dayroom. However, her mood can change quickly in response to negative interpersonal interactions. Amy often feels that the other girls are "ganging up" on her, and she accuses staff of "hating" her and trying to "ruin" her life. When she is upset, she isolates herself from others and superficially scratches her arm with staples or paper clips. Because Amy is verbal, articulate, and friendly much of the time, both staff and peers genuinely like to interact with her. They also try to be supportive when she is distressed. Nevertheless, Amy's intense mood changes are increasingly irritating everyone in the unit, and they are starting to reduce their involvement with her. This is intensifying Amy's belief that no one likes her.

Marshall is a 17-year-old male committed to a state training school for a sexual offense. He has had little success in the program. After 12 weeks at the facility, he is still on the first level of a four-level token economy program. This has resulted in his having minimal access to privileges and incentives in comparison to his peers. Michael has been unable to accomplish the basic living tasks (e.g., keeping his room clean, making his bed, showering daily, arriving to meals on time) required to move to the next level of the token economy program. He has also had difficulty with his academic assignments in school and becomes disruptive when frustrated. Although Marshall is over 6 feet tall and weighs more than 240 pounds, his behavior is childlike and suggestive of a much younger youth. He is preoccupied with dinosaurs and enjoys repeatedly looking at the same picture book related to the prehistoric era. He has seen the movie *Jurassic Park* more than 12 times and takes pleasure in showing staff how he can recite his favorite lines from it. Marshall is typically easy-going and fairly quiet, but he can become oppositional and angry. He often does not follow staff directions. However, it is unclear as to whether he is doing this purposely or whether he does not understand what is expected of him. Marshall has had some brief successes in the program when staff have provided him with individualized attention and made minor modifications in his treatment plan. However, given the current staff-to-youth ratio, this is becoming increasingly difficult to provide.

2

Juvenile Offenders with Mental Health Disorders: Who Are They and What Do We Do With Them?

Juvenile crime and violence is of national concern. The media continue to broadcast images of high profile cases of teenagers involved in murder, rape and burglary. Based on media portrayals, one could easily get the impression that most adolescents steal, carry weapons, and are involved in gang activity. Although the number of teenagers engaging in these activities is of concern, juvenile violence and crime have actually decreased since the mid-1990's (Snyder & Sickmund, 1999).

There is much variation among youth involved with the juvenile justice system. The majority of youth in the general population engage in some type of delinquent activity by the time they graduate from high school. However, most of these young people will not come into contact with juvenile justice. Of the minority of youth who do, approximately half of the adolescent males and three-quarters of the adolescent females will not return (Snyder & Sickmund, 1999). For the youth who continue their juvenile justice involvement, some will return a few times; others may become serious and chronic offenders. A small number of juveniles are responsible for the majority of serious and violent crimes.

Most people are unaware of the significant numbers of mentally ill youth involved with the juvenile justice system. Much of society views juvenile offenders as "bad kids in need of punishment." In truth, there are large numbers of juvenile offenders who are "ill kids in need of treatment." Anyone who has worked in a juvenile justice facility has come into contact with youth who have mental health disorders. Some of these youth are mildly disturbed, some of them significantly disturbed. Juvenile detention facilities and training schools—as well as juvenile justice ranches, camps, and group homes—across the nation, are filled with a sizable number of juveniles suffering from a variety of psychiatric disorders. These youths' ability to function in a juvenile justice setting may be compromised by:

- Severe attention and concentration problems
- Serious mood disorders
- Histories filled with traumatic events
- Thought processes that are unusual and bizarre
- Low intellectual functioning
- Issues related to using drugs and alcohol

Currently, the study of mentally ill juvenile offenders is in its infancy. We have little information regarding how mental health disorders and juvenile crime are related. And we have few solutions for effectively intervening with this complex and clinically complicated group of youth. This is unfortunate, given the high financial cost to society in relation to responding to juvenile criminal behavior (*e.g.*, law enforcement, juvenile courts, probation/parole, incarceration). This is in addition to the emotional and financial costs to youths' victims, as well as to youths' families. Only within recent years has attention been paid to the issue of juvenile offenders with mental health disorders, and it is long overdue. This chapter will provide an overview of this important issue.

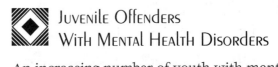 Juvenile Offenders With Mental Health Disorders

An increasing number of youth with mental health disorders continue to enter, and remain involved with, the juvenile justice system. The exact number of mentally ill juvenile offenders is currently unknown. However, it is clear that the rate of mental health disorders is higher among youth involved with juvenile justice versus their peers in the general population. Although no national statistics are currently available regarding the rate of mentally ill juvenile offenders, several small studies have attempted to obtain this information. Some of these studies have been conducted with incarcerated youth; some have been conducted with juveniles under community supervision. Many of these studies have methodological problems (*e.g.*, small numbers of youth, lack of comprehensive assessments, biased selection of youth interviewed), which limit the usefulness of the findings. Therefore, the following incidence rates should be viewed only as an estimate, until larger and more scientific investigations are conducted.

In addition, many of the studies evaluated incarcerated male juveniles. Thus, they may not generalize to juvenile offenders who have not been placed in residential juvenile justice facilities and/or to young female offenders. Most of the diagnostic categories listed below are associated with a range of percentages. This is because some of the studies used different assessment tools, assessed youth during different periods of juvenile justice involvement, and defined the same mental health disorder in a different manner. Not surprisingly, the various studies often found different rates of disorders among youth.

THE NEED IS GREAT FOR LARGE-SCALE STUDIES ON MENTAL HEALTH DISORDERS WITHIN THE JUVENILE JUSTICE SYSTEM IN ORDER TO DETERMINE HOW MANY YOUTH SUFFER FROM PSYCHIATRIC DISORDERS—AS WELL AS THE NATURE OF THEIR DISORDERS.

The need is great for large-scale studies on mental health disorders within the juvenile justice system in order to determine how many youth suffer from psychiatric disorders—as well as the nature of their disorders. Unfortunately, national studies are very expensive, time-consuming, and require a significant amount of coordination and collaboration between several systems (*e.g.*, mental health and juvenile justice). Until these types of studies are conducted, the following information can only serve as a rough approximation concerning the rate of mental health disorders among juvenile offend-

ers. One should not rely upon the particular numbers in the table below, but should take to heart the general message represented by the numbers: youth involved with the juvenile justice system have significantly more mental health disorders than youth in the general population. And the mental health disorders from which these youth suffer are often serious and debilitating.

	General Population	Juvenile Justice (in percentage)
Mood Disorders	5–9	10–88
Attention Deficit Hyperactivity Disorder	3–7	2–76
Learning Disorders	4–9	36–53
Mental Retardation	1	13
Posttraumatic Stress Disorder	6	5–49
Conduct Disorder	1–10	32–100
Psychotic Disorders	.05–5	1–16
Substance Abuse/ Dependence	5.5–9	46–88

(American Psychiatric Association, 2000; Burrell & Warboys, 2000; Casey & Keilitz, 1990; Cauffman, Feldman, Waterman, & Steiner, 1998; Davis, Bean, Shumaker, & Stringer, 1991; Fergussson, Horwood, & Lynskey, 1993; Giaconia, Reinherz, Silverman, Bilge, Frost, & Cohen, 1995; Kashani, *et al.*, 1987; Regier, *et al.*, 1984; Smykla, & Willis, 1981; Steiner, Garcia, & Matthews, 1997; Timmons-Mitchell, *et al.*, 1997; Ulloa, *et al.*, 2000; Wasserman, *et al.*, 2002)

Adolescents suffering from mental health disorders often suffer from more than one disorder at the same time. This is most commonly known as *co-morbidity* and is often the rule versus the exception among juvenile offenders. For example, it is not uncommon for youth to be simultaneously diagnosed with Conduct Disorder, a Learning Disorder and Major Depression or Attention-Deficit/Hyperactivity Disorder. Many of these youth suffer from a *co-occurring* substance abuse disorder as well. Issues related to co-morbidity and co-occurring disorders increase the complexity of screening, assessing, and intervening with this population of youth.

In addition to having a mental health disorder, a significant number of juvenile offenders have other issues that complicate their clinical picture. Suicide threats and actual suicide attempts are not uncommon among juvenile offenders and occur at much higher rates in comparison to youth in the general population. Cutting, carving, or burning themselves without the intent to die (self-injury/self-mutilation) is also not unusual; neither are extreme levels of irritability and aggression. Many juvenile offenders have experienced physical abuse, sexual abuse, and parental neglect. Their homes are often characterized by family conflict, low income, domestic violence, parental drug/alcohol use, and parental mental illness. Many juvenile offenders have been exposed to serious, sometimes life-threatening, traumatic events during their childhood and adolescent years. A considerable number of youth involved with juvenile justice have received some form of outpatient mental health treatment. Close to one-fifth have been hospitalized in inpatient psychiatric facilities, with some youth requiring multiple hospitalizations (Davis *et al.*, 1991).

A small subset of juvenile justice professionals remain unconvinced about the large numbers of juvenile offenders who are truly mentally ill. These individuals often assume that youths with mental health disorders reside in psychiatric hospitals, and youths who engage in delinquent/criminal behavior reside in juvenile justice facilities. This assumption is reasonable and consistent with common sense.

In truth, however, the population of youths residing within in-patient psychiatric hospitals and youth incarcerated within juvenile justice facilities often share more similarities than differences. One study compared the emotional and behavioral characteristics of youth in a state-operated psychiatric hospital for children and adolescents to youth admitted to a state juvenile justice facility. Youth were assessed on "Total Behavior Problems," which included separate measures of "Internalizing" problems (*e.g.*, sadness, anxiety, somaticizing) and "Exter-

nalizing" problems (*e.g.*, fighting, delinquency, swearing), as well as "Social Competence." Extreme behavior problems were noted for both groups, with no difference between the types of behavior problems exhibited by youth in the psychiatric hospital versus the juvenile justice facility (Cohen, *et al.*, 1990). In addition, more than one-third of the hospitalized youth had records of criminal charges or convictions. Race was the only factor that predicted the facility in which youth resided. African-American youth were more likely to be placed in the juvenile justice facility, and Caucasian youth were more likely to be placed in the psychiatric hospital. Although some professionals working in juvenile justice facilities may find these results difficult to believe, many would not be at all surprised. In fact, a number of juvenile justice professionals have recently reported feeling like they work on an inpatient psychiatric unit—given the emotional and behavioral difficulties among the juveniles in their care. This is particularly true among professionals working in facilities with female offenders.

It is unclear whether there has been an actual increase in the number of youth with mental health disorders becoming involved with juvenile justice. The perception of an increase may be due to juvenile justice professionals becoming more skillful at recognizing these youth. Recognition of juveniles with mental health disorders is definitely on the rise. More attention has been paid to issues related to mentally ill juvenile offenders during the past few years than has occurred in the past few decades. New mental health screening tools have been developed to better identify these youth. And staff training in identifying and managing juvenile offenders with mental health disorders has become available to juvenile justice professionals in all settings.

The perception of an increase in the number of youth with mental health disorders may also be due to the severity of mental health problems exhibited by juveniles currently entering the system. Working with severely mentally ill juveniles can make it seem like there are more of them because these youth are particularly difficult to manage and control in juvenile justice settings —as well as on probation/parole. Although juvenile offenders with mental health disorders have always existed, the extreme nature of some of today's youths' emotional and behavioral problems is a new phenomenon. There appear to be an increasing number of mentally ill juveniles for whom standard mental health interventions (*e.g.*, psychotropic medication, effective behavior management, cognitive-behavioral therapy) have minimal effect. Usual management strategies that are effective with the majority of offenders can sometimes escalate the emotions and behaviors of some mentally ill youth. Further, some juvenile offenders with mental health disorders find negative sanctions rewarding (*e.g.*, room confinement, increased monitoring, removal from school).

It is also likely that there has been an actual increase in the number of mentally ill youth becoming involved with juvenile justice.

In addition to the above factors, it is also likely that there has been an actual increase in the number of mentally ill youth becoming involved with juvenile justice. This rise may be due to a variety of factors. For example, recent changes in the mental health system have had considerable effects on juvenile justice. Accessing intensive quality mental health care has become increasingly difficult for adolescents. Across the country, many states report a significant reduction in the number of residential treatment options for youth with serious mental health disorders. Many adolescent treatment programs have closed or have restricted the number of beds available to mentally ill youth. Among the inpatient mental health treatment programs that remain in operation, many are

hesitant to accept youth with a criminal and/or aggressive history; some refuse outright to admit youth with these characteristics into their programs. Reasons for this cautiousness often include: needing to protect other youth (particularly those who are more vulnerable) in their programs from being victimized, and/or not possessing the level of resources necessary to manage youth with aggressive, criminal, and/or escape tendencies.

Even if juveniles are accepted into a residential mental health treatment program, they are not likely to remain there for a significant period of time. Years ago, youth with mental health disorders could remain in an inpatient treatment program for several months or even a year or more. Current changes in health care have resulted in much shorter lengths of stay. Most adolescents who are hospitalized in psychiatric facilities are released within a couple of weeks to several months.

Moreover, if juveniles become angry and aggressive while residing in a mental health treatment program, law enforcement may be contacted. This situation often results in youth being transferred to the juvenile justice system for assaultive behavior. Changes in health care have affected outpatient mental health services as well. Juvenile offenders with mental health disorders often encounter long waiting lists for treatment—even when their behavior is significantly problematic. In addition, limits have been placed on the types of mental health evaluations and interventions youth are eligible to receive. Even when juveniles are eligible for mental health services, the number of visits with mental health professionals is often limited.

When mentally ill youth are not appropriately evaluated and provided effective treatment services, their mental health is likely to deteriorate—resulting in a worsening of emotional and behavioral problems. When these youth are in the community (in our neighborhoods and schools), they often engage in behaviors or actions that bring them to the

6

Juvenile Offenders with Mental Health Disorders: Who Are They and What Do We Do With Them?

attention of law enforcement. Sometimes these behaviors are minor; sometimes they are serious. These youths' troublesome behaviors may or may not be related to the juveniles' mental health disorder. Youth involved with the mental health system have little difficulty transferring into the juvenile justice system. Unfortunately, once youth are involved with the juvenile justice system, accessing the mental health system can be difficult. Unlike the mental health system, juvenile justice has little say regarding which youth it accepts or does not accept into its care. **The juvenile justice system has become the default placement for many youth with mental health disorders who are not receiving appropriate psychological and psychiatric treatment in the community.**

Certain patterns of drug and alcohol use may also play a role in the increasing numbers of mentally ill youth involved with juvenile justice. A considerable number of juvenile offenders are consuming alcohol and illegal drugs on a daily basis, which can result in harm to their developing brains. In addition, some youth are inhaling toxic chemicals ("huffing"), dipping marijuana cigarettes in formaldehyde, known more commonly as embalming fluid ("wet"), and regularly using substances with hallucinogenic properties (*e.g.*, LSD, PCP, Ecstasy). These drugs can negatively affect youths' cognitive, emotional, and behavioral development.

The growing number of females entering the juvenile justice system also adds to the increasing number of juvenile offenders with mental health disorders. Female juvenile offenders typically demonstrate a higher need for mental health services than their male counterparts (Timmons-Mitchell, *et al.*, 1997).

The result of each of these above factors (and there are likely additional factors as well) is that the juvenile justice system continues to house and manage increasingly higher numbers of youth with mental health disorders. This situation would not be especially detrimental if:

- Juvenile justice facilities were equipped to handle the multitude of needs of mentally ill juveniles
- Current juvenile justice policy were geared more toward treatment versus accountability and sanctions.

Currently, this is not the case.

 Differences Between the Mental Health and Juvenile Justice Systems

Juvenile justice facilities are not psychiatric hospitals, and should not be expected to function in that capacity. Psychiatric facilities typically employ a number of full-time licensed professionals formally trained in mental health (*e.g.*, psychiatrists, psychologists, psychiatric nurses, social workers). Mental health professionals are usually on the premises daily for a significant period of time and are available by telephone when they are off-site. The average youth-to-line staff ratio on a typical mental health unit ranges from 4:1 to 6:1. The general philosophy of a mental health residential facility emphasizes treatment, and efforts are made to create a therapeutic environment. Youth are seen as having problems and in need of assistance. Intervention services are provided in a variety of modalities: individual, group and family. Trained mental health or medical professionals typically:

- Meet individually with youth on a regular basis

- Run daily or weekly treatment groups with four to eight youth at a time

- Meet with youths' families on several occasions

In residential mental health treatment programs, youth often have access to "talk" therapy, recreational therapy, and other modes of therapeutic services conducted by trained professionals. Psychotropic medication is routinely prescribed to youth who have emotional and/or behavioral problems, and medical professionals monitor potential side effects of these medications. Most youth have their own rooms or are assigned one roommate. Mental health facilities typically have special rooms in which agitated or suicidal youth can safely spend time, calm themselves down, or recover from an upsetting incident. When applying for their job at a psychiatric facility, staff members consciously choose to work with children and adolescents with mental health disorders.

The mental health resources in a juvenile justice facility are typically different than those in a psychiatric facility. There are usually fewer professionals formally trained in mental health, and not all of them are licensed. Many of these professionals work on less than a full-time basis. Depending on the size of a particular juvenile justice facility, there may never be a mental health professional on-site. In these cases, juvenile justice professionals may need to:

- Manage acutely mentally ill youth without the help of a mental health professional

- Attempt to have a mental health professional drive to the facility to evaluate acutely mentally ill youth

- Transport acutely mentally ill youth to another location where a mental health professional is available (*e.g.*, hospital emergency room, psychiatric hospital, juvenile justice facility with mental health resources)

Therapeutic modalities tend to be limited in justice facilities, and there is usually minimal access to individual or family therapy. Most treatment occurs in a group format, and many treatment groups are run by juvenile justice professionals with little to no training in mental health. Depending on the facility, some groups may include as many as 12 to 20 young offenders at a time. Recreational and art therapy services are becoming more common in juvenile justice facilities but are still only currently available at a minority of facilities. Although psychotropic medication is often prescribed to

youth in juvenile justice facilities, far fewer medical professionals are usually available to monitor the side effects of these medications. Additionally, due to the limited availability of medical personnel in some facilities (particularly small and/or rural facilities), juvenile justice professionals may be required to physically administer psychotropic medication to youth.

The environment of juvenile justice facilities is often different than that of mental health treatment programs. For example, in most facilities the youth-to-line staff ratio ranges anywhere from 8:1 to 40:1. Even when none of the youth are mentally ill, managing this number of *juvenile offenders* can be challenging for any one adult. Having one juvenile with mental health disorders can make supervision of a group this large significantly more difficult. Mentally ill youth can be disruptive to group dynamics due to symptoms of their mental health disorder (*e.g.*, monopolizing group time, interrupting others, needing all attention on them, not having empathy for others, not understanding material that others understand, not respecting personal boundaries of others).

And most juvenile justice professionals report that one-third or more of the youth under their supervision display symptoms of mental illness! The use of strategic and effective interventions becomes less likely as the youth-to-line staff ratio increases. Although most facilities assign one or two youth to a room, some juvenile justice facilities place three or four youth in the same room. Some facilities do not have individual rooms at all; they are designed as dormitory-style settings. Youth may be required to sleep in one large room with 20, 40 or even 80 other youth. Not surprisingly, managing mentally ill juveniles in this type of setting can be particularly challenging. Most juvenile justice facilities have designated rooms in which an agitated or suicidal youth may reside. These rooms may be located on the youths' living unit or youth may need to be transferred to another unit (typically a more restrictive maximum security unit designed to manage juveniles with

8

Juvenile Offenders with Mental Health Disorders: Who Are They and What Do We Do With Them?

severe behavior problems). However, some facilities do not have special rooms where a suicidal or aggressive youth can be placed. This can sometimes result in serious management problems when youth are experiencing significant distress.

Although rehabilitation and treatment are important goals of the juvenile justice system, safety and security issues must be held at the forefront. To protect the safety of youth and the staff, the behavior of juveniles is closely supervised, scrutinized, and evaluated. Room confinement may be relied upon—appropriately or inappropriately—as a sanction for negative behaviors. To protect the community at large, tall fences (sometimes with barbed wire) often surround the perimeter of juvenile facilities. And locks are placed on most, if not all, internal and external doors. Not surprisingly, the focus on custody, security and control of juvenile justice facilities can interfere with the development of a therapeutic environment. Although some juvenile justice programs are more "therapeutic" in nature, they are typically the exception rather than the rule. In addition, most individuals who seek employment within juvenile justice facilities do not consciously choose to work with mentally ill youth. In fact, many are completely surprised by the number of youth with mental health disorders under their supervision.

As stated earlier, large numbers of mentally ill youth continue to be detained or committed to short- and long-term juvenile justice facilities. Most juvenile justice professionals, however, receive little to no training about mental illness. In fact, most professionals who interact with juvenile offenders have not been formally trained in how to identify or effectively manage this complex population. These individuals quickly discover that standard programs and management strategies, which work with non-mentally ill juveniles, do not always work with juveniles who have mental health disorders (e.g., low IQ, psychotic thought processes, severe attention problems). Unfortunately, if

youth are not accurately recognized as having a mental illness, their inability to function successfully in a generic juvenile justice program can be viewed as a conscious—and purposeful—choice. This situation often results in sanctions for mentally ill youth and a delay in referral to appropriate intervention services.

Additionally, juvenile justice professionals are responsible for supervising a significant number of juveniles who are taking psychotropic medication. Most professionals in juvenile justice facilities have not received training in the various types of psychotropic medications prescribed to these youth. This type of training is critical because facility staff are often the first to observe behaviors that may indicate negative side effects of medication. Juvenile justice professionals also play a key role in referring youth to medical/mental health professionals for evaluation. Without proper training in how to identify juveniles with mental health disorders, staffs' ability to appropriately refer youth for proper assessment is severely compromised.

Moreover, for juvenile justice professionals without an understanding of mental illness, working with juvenile offenders who have mental health disorders can result in significant frustration, confusion, and exhaustion. The feelings of ineffectiveness often experienced by those trying to manage mentally ill juveniles can lead to staff burnout and hopelessness regarding particular youth. Once professionals have lost hope, they are less effective with juveniles. Gaining an understanding of how mental health disorders manifest in adolescents, particularly adolescent offenders, can help decrease this dynamic. Juvenile justice professionals can be more strategic when developing and implementing supervision and management strategies once they have a better understanding of the thinking and behavior of youth with mental health disorders.

Young offenders with mental health disorders also become frustrated and confused when juvenile justice professionals do not have knowledge or training related to mental illness.

For example, many juvenile justice professionals are trained to treat all youth equally in the name of fairness. However, this practice can put some youth with mental health disorders, particularly those with severe emotional and behavioral disorders, at a disadvantage. These juveniles may be putting forth as much effort as they possibly can within a facility. But they may still receive sanctions from staff because they do not have the capacity to meet the generic expectations of a particular living unit.

Juveniles with mental health disorders are typically aware when they are not progressing as quickly as their peers. Yet they often do not understand why they keep getting into trouble. When mentally ill youth have difficulty successfully meeting behavioral expectations, they may be denied certain privileges available to other juveniles. Mentally ill youth often interpret this situation as resulting from staff being "unfair," and they may become angry and resentful. Furthermore, if youth are indeterminately sentenced to a facility (which typically entails release only after youth successfully complete a juvenile justice program), mentally ill juveniles can remain under juvenile justice supervision longer than nonmentally ill peers who have similar or less serious committing offenses. This lengthier confinement often has more to do with a lack of ability to complete a program the way it was initially designed (*i.e.*, for young offenders without mental health disorders) versus purposefully choosing not to comply with program requirements.

Differences clearly exist between the mental health and juvenile justice systems. An argument is neither being made that juvenile justice facilities should become "treatment" facilities, nor that mental health facilities should accept all juvenile offenders with mental health disorders. These options are not likely to occur, and they are not necessarily the most appropriate solutions. The population of youth residing in juvenile justice facilities is increasingly similar, if not almost the same, as the population of youth residing within mental health programs.

Therefore, additional mental health resources must be implemented within already-existing justice programs. At a minimum, these resources should include:

- The hiring/contracting of clinical staff
- Individualized need-focused interventions
- Staff training in mental health

Even if juvenile justice facilities had the resources to provide the number and types of services required of many mentally ill juvenile offenders, challenges still exist. One significant hurdle relates to the current philosophy of juvenile justice: changes over the past decade have resulted in the provision of treatment becoming less of a priority.

 Changes in the Juvenile Justice System

Our society's response to juvenile offending behavior has gone through many changes. Historically, youth were viewed as having the same cognitive, emotional, and moral processes as adults. So, youth and adults were treated in a similar fashion if they engaged in law-breaking behavior. Not until the early 19th century did society stop viewing children as miniature adults. They were then seen as individuals who had not yet fully developed all of their abilities. At this time, delinquent juveniles began to be placed in their own facilities, separate from adult offenders. By the beginning of the 20th century, specific courts were developed for juvenile offenders, with a primary goal of protecting them—particularly when their parents were unable to provide appropriate guardianship and care.

In contrast to the criminal justice system for adults, juvenile courts were fairly informal. Youth who engaged in delinquent behavior were recognized as needing treatment and appropriate supervision. Providing intervention and support for troubled youth was the primary mission of the juvenile justice system, versus punishment and discipline. Juvenile court

10

Juvenile Offenders with Mental Health Disorders: Who Are They and What Do We Do With Them?

judges paid specific attention to an individual youth's particular issues and circumstances. It was the juveniles' needs that primarily determined the disposition plan, not the offense the youth committed.

By the 1960's there was concern that the juvenile justice system's mission to rehabilitate juveniles was not as effective as had been hoped. In addition, youth advocates were concerned that the rights of juveniles were being violated. For example, some youth were held in restrictive environments for significant periods of time to receive "treatment." In response to these concerns, juvenile courts became more formal, and youth were given many of the legal rights afforded to adults in the criminal justice system. However, there was also an emphasis on keeping youth who engaged in status offenses (*e.g.*, running away, truancy, uncontrollable behavior) out of the juvenile justice system. But by the 1980's, there was growing concern that crime and violence among young people was increasing and that the juvenile justice system was too lenient. Policy changes were made and several laws were modified, which resulted in the juvenile justice system more closely resembling the adult criminal justice system.

The 1990's were a period of significant toughening on criminal behavior committed by juveniles. It became easier to transfer youth from the juvenile justice system to the adult criminal justice system. Depending on the nature of their crime, some youth were automatically sent to the adult system, bypassing the juvenile system altogether. Presently, the juvenile justice system seems to have a different mission from its initial inception. Rather than primarily focusing on young offenders' circumstances and specific needs for treatment, much of the emphasis in today's juvenile justice system is directed toward:

- Holding youth accountable for their behavior

- Protecting the community

- Deterring future criminal behavior
- Providing restitution to those harmed
- Allocating sanctions consistent with the nature of youths' crime

(Snyder & Sickmund, 1999)

Although some states have moved toward emphasizing the development of youth competencies and skill-building, these objectives are usually secondary to those of accountability and sanctions. The challenge for the juvenile justice system today is to achieve a balance between offender accountability, community protection, appropriate sanctions, and the provision of appropriate evaluation and rehabilitation/ treatment services. This is a tall order—particularly in the face of the significant numbers of youth involved with the system and the often-limited resources.

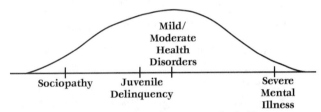

Figure 1. Normal curve of youth in a juvenile facility.

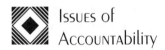 Issues of Accountability

Mental illness is not an excuse for negative behavior within a juvenile justice facility. Juvenile offenders should be held accountable for their behavior, whether or not they suffer from a mental health disorder. However, juvenile offenders with psychiatric disorders should also receive appropriate mental health treatment. Juvenile offenders do not represent a homogeneous group of young people. Each youth has his or her own individual characteristics and circumstances. It can be helpful to view these youth on a normal curve (*see* Figure 1). At one end of the spectrum are the types of youth who would be described as "antisocial" or "sociopathic." They know exactly what they are doing when they commit criminal acts, are aware that these acts are against the law, and do them anyway. They repeatedly violate the rights of others and experience little to no remorse about the damage they inflict upon other people or others' property. They are typically chronic and repeat offenders, and they have every intention of continuing their criminal behavior once released from a juvenile justice facility. Regardless of the type of juvenile justice programming, treatment, or intervention services they receive, these offenders will likely make minimal, if any, long-term positive behavior change. Ironically, these youth can move through juvenile programs fairly quickly because they know what they should say and do to give the impression they are "reforming." As young offenders meeting this description age, they are likely to

---

Youth with Attention-Deficit/ Hyperactivity Disorder are often more impulsive than peers and less skillful in planning ahead.

---

eventually become involved with the adult criminal justice system. Although the media often portray this type of youth as the *typical* juvenile offender, such youth probably do not represent the majority of youth who come into contact with the juvenile justice system.

On the other end of the spectrum are those youth who are very seriously mentally ill. These juveniles may experience extremely psychotic thinking (*i.e.*, losing touch with reality), as well as exhibit unusual and bizarre behaviors. Some may have even been psychotic at the time that they committed their crime. Youth with severe mental health problems may repeatedly engage in dangerous, self-injurious/self-mutilating behavior or make recurrent serious suicide attempts. Or they may have substantial cognitive deficits, resulting in minimal understanding of their crimes, as well as what behaviors are expected of them during incarceration.

Juveniles who are severely mentally ill typically do not belong in the juvenile justice system and require intensive services from the mental health system. These youth may have ended up in the juvenile justice system because their mental illness was not emphasized during court proceedings. Or if it was emphasized, it may have been hoped that juvenile justice would provide the youth with protection and intervention services. This is not unusual if previous mental health services had proven ineffective or unresponsive. Although a number of youth in the juvenile justice system fit this description, these youth are still likely to comprise only a minority of the juvenile offender population.

Between the two categories described above is a category containing youth who engage in various criminal acts and who also suffer from a mild-to-moderate mental health disorder (although their mental health can be severe at times). These youth are sometimes known as "double jeopardy" youth, due to having simultaneous problems related to both delinquency and mental illness. Many youth involved with the juvenile justice system know exactly what they are doing when they commit their crime and engage in the behavior anyway. For example, they are typically aware that stealing a car is wrong, selling drugs is against the law, assaulting someone could get them in trouble, and so forth. Many youth involved with the juvenile justice system, however, also suffer from disorders such as Attention-Deficit/Hyperactivity Disorder, Learning Disabilities, Major Depression and Mental Retardation. This category of youth is likely to be a much larger group than the other two categories of youth described above. Does this imply that young offenders who stole cars, stole the cars because they have Attention Deficit/Hyperactivity Disorder? Or that assaultive behavior is a direct result of youths' depression? Not necessarily. Delinquent behavior stems from a combination of a variety of different factors, including the individual characteristics of juveniles, their family, peers, school, community, and current laws. This does not mean that juvenile offenders' mental health disorders play no role in their criminal behavior. They may or

12

Juvenile Offenders with Mental Health Disorders: Who Are They and What Do We Do With Them?

may not. For example, youth with Attention-Deficit/Hyperactivity Disorder are often more impulsive than peers and less skillful in planning ahead. These youth may not have seriously considered the consequences of their actions, or may not have planned their delinquent behavior well enough to avoid being caught.

In addition, adolescents who suffer from Major Depression are often extremely irritable, which can make it more likely that they will be involved in a physical altercation. Even if mental illness does play a role in their criminal behavior, it usually does not *cause* juveniles to break the law. Therefore, when they commit criminal offenses, juveniles should be held accountable (other than in extreme cases, which are rare). Having a mental health disorder is not an excuse to avoid taking responsibility for engaging in delinquent acts. A mental health disorder is also not a legitimate reason for youth to evade tasks or duties they view as undesirable once under juvenile justice supervision. If mentally ill juveniles engage in negative behaviors, they should receive consequences for their actions. However, in addition to issues of accountability, juvenile offenders with mental health disorders should be evaluated and provided appropriate intervention services. Addressing delinquent and mental health issues simultaneously is critical when supervising juvenile offenders with psychiatric disorders. These youth may require:

- Modifications in juvenile justice programming
- Additional intervention services
- Psychotropic medication

Moreover, substance abuse among juveniles is significantly related to both delinquent behavior and mental illness. Ignoring or dismissing any one of these key areas (delinquency, mental health, substance use) is likely to result in negative outcomes for juvenile offenders with mental health disorders, as well as for the juvenile justice system as a whole.

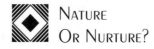

NATURE OR NURTURE?

One of the most common questions asked by juvenile justice professionals relates to whether mental health disorders are associated more with nature or nurture. Is mental illness due to biological factors or environmental influences? New information about mental health disorders continues to be discovered, and the mental health field is constantly evolving. Yet the current consensus in the field indicates that the answer to the above question is "yes." Yes, biological factors play a role in many forms of mental illness and yes, environmental factors play a role in many forms of mental illness. For most juvenile offenders, their mental health disorders are likely related to an interaction between these two influences.

Presently, there is general agreement that many mental health disorders are the result of an interaction between individuals' predisposing vulnerabilities and the stressors they experience in their lives. This *diathesis-stress* model of illness has been applied to various medical disorders (*e.g.*, heart disease, cancer), as well as mental health disorders (*e.g.*, Major Depression, Bipolar Disorder, Schizophrenia). A "diathesis" refers to being vulnerable to, or having a predisposition to, develop a particular disorder. Psychopathology is thought to result when a diathesis interacts with stressful life events, unless there are ample protective factors or resources to offset it (Hakim-Larson & Essau, 1999). If an individual's parents or other close family members have heart disease or cancer, the individual is typically at risk to develop the same illness. Not all individuals with a family history of heart disease or cancer acquire those conditions. But they are more likely to than someone who does not have these medical disorders in their family. The same is true regarding mental health disorders such as the mood disorders and Schizophrenia. Youth whose relatives (*e.g.*, parents, grandparents, siblings, aunts, uncles,

Youth With Mental Health Disorders in the Juvenile Justice System cousins) have Bipolar Disorder or Schizophrenia are at higher risk of developing these disorders themselves in comparison to peers without these disorders in their family history.

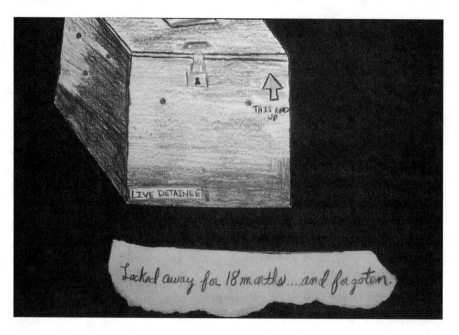

The exact mechanism related to how mental illness is transmitted within families is not yet clear. But research has consistently shown that heredity plays a role in many of the major psychiatric disorders. For example, youth may inherit certain brain chemistry, particular ways of processing or organizing information, or an overly reactive nervous system. A significant number of juvenile offenders have parents and other close relatives who suffer from a variety of mental health disorders. Inheriting a biological predisposition to a psychiatric disorder makes it more *likely*, but it does not *guarantee,* that the youth will develop a similar mental health disorder as well.

Youth differ in their response to stressful life experiences. Some juvenile offenders can tolerate large amounts of stress and not develop a mental health disorder, even when they have inherited a biological vulnerability to do so. Other youth may develop mental health symptoms after exposure to only minor stressful experiences. In fact, juvenile justice professionals are often puzzled by youths' different responses to stress. Some juvenile offenders who have experienced horrific events can function at an adequate level. In contrast, other youth may appear fragile, and emotionally and/or behaviorally decompensate in response to much-less-severe stressors. The actual occurrence of a mental health disorder is likely the result of a combination of juveniles':

- Inherited biological or psychological vulnerabilities
- Environmental stressors
- Environmental supports
- Particular abilities and coping skills

Youth who have significant mental illness in their families, a variety of psychosocial stressors, and poor coping skills are likely at highest risk for mental illness. Many juvenile offenders fit into this category.

A considerable number of juvenile offenders lead lives filled with a variety of environmental stressors. Many are raised in single-parent homes and are from low socio-economic backgrounds. Their parents may have divorced or never married; some young offenders do not know their fathers. Juvenile offenders raised in one-parent or two-parent families have often witnessed domestic violence in their homes. Many juvenile offenders have been raised by a parent who is mentally ill and/or uses drugs and alcohol; this can result in a chaotic home, poor parental monitoring, and a lack of emotional support.

A significant number of these youth have been placed outside of their family homes: some have spent much of their childhood years in foster care, justice facilities, or moving from one relative's residence to another. In addition, many juvenile offenders have experienced physical abuse, sexual abuse and/or caregiver

14

Juvenile Offenders with Mental Health Disorders: Who Are They and What Do We Do With Them?

neglect. Some of these youth have been exposed to a variety of toxins while in utero (*e.g.*, drugs, alcohol), and/or their mothers may not have received adequate prenatal or perinatal care. Many juvenile offenders live in neighborhoods inundated with crime, drugs, and violence. Walking down the streets of their community can be a dangerous endeavor. Moreover, many of these youth have experienced trauma to their heads while growing up (*e.g.*, abuse from adults, accidents, physical altercations with peers), with some to the point of being knocked unconscious. A number of juvenile offenders have also experienced the death of individuals close to them (*e.g.*, parents, siblings, friends, neighbors, relatives), with some of these deaths being violent in nature.

The effects of biological and environmental factors related to mental illness vary among the different mental health disorders, as well as among individuals. Biological influences may play a more significant role in youths' Mental Retardation or Attention-Deficit/Hyperactivity Disorder. Environmental influences may be more significant for youth suffering from Post-traumatic Stress Disorder.

Juvenile offenders are clearly at high risk for developing and manifesting a variety of mental health disorders because:

- Many have a high degree of mental illness among family members
- Many have been exposed to a significant number of environmental stressors

The Stress of Incarceration

The stress of incarceration can have a negative affect on the mental health of youthful offenders'—particularly if they have a biological predisposition to develop a mental health disorder. Some professionals working within juvenile justice facilities question the legitimacy of youths' mental health symptoms. This can be particularly true if these juveniles did not exhibit psychiatric symptoms during previous stays at a facility or if there is no report of the

youth exhibiting mental health symptoms in the community. Juvenile justice professionals often assume that youth are pretending to be mentally ill in order to receive certain benefits (*e.g.*, staff attention, medication, transfer to a psychiatric facility) because the symptoms seemed to have appeared out of nowhere. For example, youth may not exhibit depressive symptoms in the community, but they become suicidal soon after arriving at a justice facility. Youth with no history of self-injury/self-mutilation may begin cutting and carving their skin while incarcerated. Or youth with no history of mental health treatment may report hearing voices. When these behaviors appear without a prior history, juvenile justice professionals often become suspicious.

Incarceration can be an extremely stressful experience for young people—especially for youth arriving at a juvenile justice facility for the first time. Not knowing what to expect and fearing the worst can be frightening, particularly for youth of small stature and minimal criminal offending histories. The following is a sample of the many reasons why incarceration at a juvenile justice facility can be stressful for youth:

- Lack of freedom
- Minimal contact with friends and family
- Being told what to do and when to do it (*e.g.*, eating, showering, using the bathroom)
- Constantly interacting with bigger and tougher youths
- Being observed, supervised and monitored 24 hours a day by authority figures
- High degree of structure in all activities
- Numerous rules and being held accountable when rules are violated
- Having to participate in an academic setting for several hours a day
- Little to no choice regarding anything (*e.g.*, how they spend their time, with whom they spend their time)

- Conflicts with staff members (*e.g.*, different personality styles of staff, inconsistent management styles from shift to shift)
- Minimal access to being outside
- Little to no access to peers of the opposite sex
- Institutional food (*e.g.*, few to no choice in the type or amount of food they eat, unappetizing food, food they do not typically eat)
- Crowding
- Intimidation or threatening by peers
- No privacy (sometimes including having to shower with other youth)
- Being unaware of the legal process and what will next occur (*e.g.*, preliminary court dates, trial, sentencing, transfer to the adult criminal justice system)
- Uncertainty about when they will be released from a facility
- Uncertainty about where they will go after release (some youth are unable to return to their families or do not have families to which to return)
- Placement in isolation or seclusion rooms
- Having to discuss personal, and often painful, issues in front of strangers
- Having to go to bed several hours earlier than what youth is used to
- Having to wake up several hours earlier than youth is used to
- Minimal access to recreational activities or any type of physical activity
- Small sleeping rooms that contain minimal personal items (this can feel claustrophobic to some)
- Large sleeping rooms that are shared with a significant number of other offenders
- Undesirable peers as roommates (*e.g.*, a rival gang member, an aggressive or severely mentally ill youth, a sex offender)

- Confrontation regarding their offending behavior
- Fear of being raped
- Fear of being assaulted

A variety of factors related to incarceration can result in feelings of fear, anxiety, frustration, disappointment, or anger. These feelings are not uncommon among youth involved with the juvenile justice system, regardless of whether or not they are residing in a juvenile justice facility.

When juvenile offenders become distressed in the community, they usually engage in a variety of coping behaviors that are not available after incarceration. For example, when juvenile offenders become stressed or upset "on the outs," they often smoke cigarettes or consume alcohol and other drugs. For some youth, becoming aggressive or engaging in delinquent behavior makes them feel better during difficult times. Others may engage in sexual behavior or run away when experiencing unpleasant emotions. These youth may not have exhibited classic mental health symptoms in the community because they were self-medicating with these behaviors/substances. A number of juvenile offenders deal with negative feelings by making suicide attempts or cutting or carving their skin in acts of self-injury/self-mutilation. Understandably, none of these behaviors is allowable in juvenile justice facilities and if engaged in, typically results in a variety of negative consequences and/or serious sanctions. Even youth who engage in socially appropriate coping behaviors in the community when distressed—talking with close friends or listening to their favorite music—soon find that they have minimal to no access to these behaviors after being locked up.

It can be extremely challenging for youth to experience the significant stressors associated with incarceration without being able to use their typical coping mechanisms. Although these coping strategies usually are not the most prosocial choices, they often helped these juve-

16

Juvenile Offenders with Mental Health Disorders: Who Are They and What Do We Do With Them?

niles manage during significant times of stress, even if only temporarily. Helping young offenders acquire new and more socially appropriate ways of coping with negative emotions is one of the goals of the juvenile justice system. But until these new skills are developed (if they are ever developed), juvenile offenders often experience a variety of negative emotions during their stay in juvenile justice facilities. This does not mean that incarceration should be more pleasant for youths or that juvenile offenders should have access to destructive ways of managing their distress. However, adults working with incarcerated youth should not lose sight of the demanding and challenging conditions in which these youth are often placed. Further, youth with mental health disorders may have an even more difficult time adjusting to a juvenile justice environment than non-mentally ill peers. Youth who have a biological vulnerability to mental illness and/or those who have experienced mild mental health symptoms in the community may manifest significant mental health symptoms after incarceration. The combination of environmental stressors and the loss of typical coping strategies can result in:

- The emergence of mental health symptoms never before observed
- An exacerbation of psychiatric symptoms previously experienced
- Mild symptoms that may dissipate after youth have adjusted to the system

Juvenile justice professionals can lose sight of the stressors associated with residing in a juvenile justice facility—particularly if they have been working in this type of environment for a significant period of time. Both new and veteran staff should keep in mind that when psychiatric symptoms emerge or worsen among incarcerated youth, these symptoms are usually associated with the youth:

- Having difficulty living in a demanding environment
- Lacking the ability to cope versus avoiding responsibility

- Wanting to obtain special treatment/ attention

Not all juvenile offenders find incarceration a stressful experience, however. For some youth, juvenile justice facilities offer a safe and protective environment in comparison to their lives in the community. A number of juvenile offenders feel closer to juvenile justice professionals than members of their own families. This is particularly true among youth who have been repeatedly incarcerated within the same facility. Experiences in a juvenile justice facility (*e.g.*, particular staff members, structured environment, reinforcement of successes, school achievement) often provide these youth with a sense of competency, consistency and security they have never experienced. For this particular group of offenders, *release* from a juvenile justice facility may be the time when psychiatric symptoms begin to emerge or worsen.

The identification and management of juvenile offenders with mental health disorders is challenging due to the:

- Variation among youth in the juvenile justice system
- High numbers of mentally ill youth in the juvenile justice system
- Complexity of mentally ill youth in the juvenile justice system
- High numbers of youth using drugs and alcohol
- Present underlying philosophy of the juvenile justice system
- Limited mental health resources within the juvenile justice system
- Physical environment of most juvenile justice facilities
- Lack of mental health training for juvenile justice staff at all levels
- Effects of incarceration on mental health systems

CHAPTER 2

The Diagnosis of Mental Health Disorders

"Six different doctors have given me six different diagnoses. Guess nobody can figure out what the f_ _k is wrong with me."

Luke, 16

There is often a great deal of confusion within juvenile justice regarding mental health diagnoses. Many juvenile justice professionals have misconceptions about the mental health diagnostic process and the rationale underlying it. Some of these professionals believe certain diagnostic categories are so overapplied among juvenile offenders (*i.e.*, Attention-Deficit/Hyperactivity Disorder, Conduct Disorder, Bipolar Disorder) that these diagnoses have lost their ability to provide helpful information (*see chapters 3-9 for detailed information on common psychiatric disorders among juvenile offenders*). Some juvenile justice professionals oppose the use of all mental health diagnoses because of a concern that youth will be labeled and then stigmatized. In addition, a number of juvenile justice personnel believe that mental health professionals assign psychiatric diagnoses to youth in a fairly arbitrary manner—rendering the information conveyed by a diagnosis meaningless.

Not surprisingly, our thoughts, beliefs, and attitudes about mental illness, the diagnostic process, and specific mental health disorders

are significantly influenced by our own personal experience. Most adults working in the juvenile justice system know someone (*e.g.*, relative, their own child, friend, spouse, coworker) who has received some type of mental health diagnosis. Some have been exposed to portrayals of mental illness in the media. Some may have themselves received a mental health diagnosis for a psychiatric condition. These personal experiences can bias, positively or negatively, juvenile justice professionals' understanding of psychiatric diagnoses, as well as their responses to mentally ill juvenile offenders. This chapter is designed to clarify how and why mental health diagnoses are given to individuals, and specifically address issues related to diagnosing juvenile offenders.

Based on decades of clinical practice and scientific research in the area of mental health, more is known now about psychiatric disorders than ever before. However, there is still a great deal related to this topic that we do not know. Are mental health professionals being too liberal, and assigning psychiatric diagnoses to

18

Juvenile Offenders with Mental Health Disorders: Who Are They and What Do We Do With Them?

youth who do not really have the disorder? Are there certain mental health diagnoses that have lost their meaning because they are given out to such large numbers of youth? Are there certain diagnostic categories that are being overused among juvenile offenders in particular? Unfortunately, at this point, we do not know the answers to these questions. These issues have not been studied enough to say for sure one way or the other. Some mental health professionals are probably providing psychiatric diagnoses to youth who do not have the disorder. It is just as likely, however, that some youth who should be diagnosed with a mental health disorder have never been evaluated. Or when they are evaluated, these youth are not diagnosed with a disorder when they should be.

Some mental health diagnoses (*e.g.*, Attention-Deficit/Hyperactivity Disorder, Conduct Disorder, Bipolar Disorder) are currently being given to juveniles in a fairly liberal manner by certain clinicians. This can result in a loss of value when subsets of youth are described as suffering from a mental health disorder with very specific symptoms. However, when youth are evaluated appropriately and accurately, mental health diagnoses can provide a wealth of information about youths' challenges, and possible directions for effective treatment.

What about juvenile offenders? There is clear evidence that a significant number of youth in the juvenile justice system are suffering from serious emotional and behavioral disorders. Some of these youth have been correctly diagnosed, some have been misdiagnosed, and some have never received a psychiatric diagnosis at all—despite the presence of a serious psychiatric disorder.

This entire publication focuses on the topic of identifying and managing juvenile offenders with mental health disorders. It is designed to help professionals who work with those youth in the juvenile justice system who meet specific criteria for one or more mental health *diagnoses*. Many, if not most, youth in the juvenile justice system have a number of mental health "issues"

and could benefit from some type of mental health intervention. Given the large number of juvenile offenders and the current level of mental health resources, however, providing formal mental health treatment to every youth in the system is an unrealistic expectation.

A subset of juvenile offenders have serious emotional and behavioral difficulties. These difficulties are often serious enough that these youth (as well as their families/caretakers) experience significant distress, and/or the difficulties impair the youths' ability to function in their everyday lives. Many of these juveniles are suffering from mental health "disorders" and require appropriate mental health evaluation and treatment. A mental health disorder refers to a clinically significant psychological or behavioral syndrome or pattern that occurs in an individual and is associated with suffering and disability. Regardless of what caused the disorder, the psychological, behavioral, or biological dysfunction is seen as being within the individual (American Psychiatric Association, 2000). Due to limited mental health resources, the juvenile justice system must be strategic. It must ensure that young offenders most in need of mental health services are indeed those who receive it. Using mental health diagnoses for juveniles who have mental health disorders is one way to identify those youth most in need.

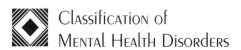 Classification of Mental Health Disorders

Being able to classify mental health disorders (*e.g.*, assign a diagnosis to a certain set of symptoms) has several benefits. First, it facilitates communication between various mental health professionals, including both clinicians and researchers. By grouping specific emotional and behavioral symptoms into certain diagnostic categories, communication is typically clearer and more time-efficient. For example, when referring to youth diagnosed with Bipolar

> **THERE IS CLEAR EVIDENCE THAT A SIGNIFICANT NUMBER OF YOUTH IN THE JUVENILE JUSTICE SYSTEM ARE SUFFERING FROM SERIOUS EMOTIONAL AND BEHAVIORAL DISORDERS.**

Disorder, most mental health professionals have a general knowledge of the symptoms being discussed without having to address them all individually. Second, classifying mental health disorders helps educate mental health professionals about the various abnormal emotional and behavioral syndromes from which individuals may be suffering. Third, when specific mental health symptoms are placed into diagnostic categories, researchers can be more systematic in asking questions and more strategic in selecting data to collect. When specific categories of psychiatric disorders are discovered, research can help guide the types of assessments that best identify individuals who have (or do not have) the particular disorders. Research can also determine which treatment approaches are most effective with particular types of mental health disorders/diagnostic categories. Therefore, having knowledge about youths' psychiatric disorder greatly impacts the type of intervention strategies chosen to alleviate the youths' difficulties. Fourth, third parties (*i.e.,* insurance companies, Social Security, Division of Developmental Disabilities, school districts) often make decisions about reimbursement, financial assistance, or eligibility for specialized services based on the presence or absence of certain mental health disorders. Finally, classifying mental health symptoms into diagnostic categories assists in the collection of prevalence data. Important information can be collected about the percentages of individuals suffering from various mental health symptoms (*e.g.,* in the general population, adolescents versus adults, males versus females).

Each of these benefits is relevant to the classification of youth with mental health

disorders within the juvenile justice system. When mental health diagnoses are used:

- Communication among mental health, health and juvenile justice professionals can be improved
- The formulation of research questions regarding mentally ill juvenile offenders is more systematic
- Assessment and treatment decisions are more strategic

The use of mental health diagnoses facilitates the collection of prevalence data, resulting in a more accurate allocation of both juvenile justice and mental health resources. Formal classification systems (*i.e., Diagnostic and Statistical Manual of Mental Disorders*) reduce the likelihood that clinicians will indiscriminately assign diagnostic labels to juvenile offenders who do not have a mental health disorder. They also help clinicians identify those offenders who truly do have a disorder.

In addition, once juvenile justice professionals become aware that particular youth have been diagnosed with a mental health disorder, many often change their perception of those youth. Juvenile behavior that used to be seen as solely oppositional and purposeful may be interpreted another way and no longer immediately sanctioned. These adults may be more patient with mentally ill youth and/or provide them with additional reminders. Once they are aware that youth have a mental health diagnosis, some juvenile justice professionals develop creative management strategies to help these young offenders better control their behavior and function more successfully.

 ## The Diagnostic and Statistical Manual of Mental Disorders

Medical illnesses are classified into different categories (*e.g.,* Diabetes, Arthritis, Pneumonia), which enables doctors to diagnose patients based on a set of symptoms. Similarly, the field

20

Juvenile Offenders with Mental Health Disorders: Who Are They and What Do We Do With Them?

of mental health also has diagnostic categories that help classify disorders containing a specific set of symptoms (*e.g.*, Mental Retardation, Schizophrenia, Attention-Deficit/Hyperactivity Disorder). One way the field of mental health attempts to keep the classification of mental health disorders as systematic as possible is to use the *Diagnostic and Statistical Manual of Mental Disorders (DSM)*. The *DSM* is a manual that serves as the main resource tool for mental health professionals (*e.g.*, psychologists, psychiatrists, social workers, psychiatric nurses) when providing mental health diagnoses. The main purpose of the *DSM* is to "provide clear descriptions of diagnostic categories in order to enable clinicians and investigators to diagnose, communicate about, study, and treat people with various mental disorders" (APA, 2000).

Mental health experts and clinicians from a variety of backgrounds and theoretical orientations develop each version of the *Diagnostic and Statistical Manual of Mental Disorders*. These individuals use existing research from across the country, as well as all over the world. The *DSM* only includes those mental health disorders where enough scientific data exists to describe the disorders. The manual is widely accepted on an international basis as a means to describe and classify mental health disorders among diverse populations of children, adolescents, and adults. However, the *DSM* does not classify individuals. It classifies the various mental health disorders that individuals may have.

The *Diagnostic and Statistical Manual of Mental Disorders* lists more than 100 mental health disorders and provides descriptive information about each one of them. Each disorder has a specific set of criteria associated with it; disorders are typically based on patterns or clusters of several mental health symptoms. For example, the diagnosis of Major Depression is not provided to youth solely because they are sad or withdrawn. Youth must be experiencing a certain number (five or more) of specific emotional and behavioral symptoms associated with Major Depression for a specified period of time

(two weeks or more). Also, the symptoms must represent a change from the juveniles' typical functioning. In addition to what should be present, there is often a list of characteristics or factors that should *not* be present to qualify for a particular diagnosis. For example, some youths' symptoms of depression are primarily due to the effects of drugs or alcohol, or the direct result of a medical condition. In either case, the diagnosis of Major Depression would not be given because another diagnosis would be more accurate.

The *Diagnostic and Statistical Manual of Mental Disorders* is meant to be descriptive only; it does not provide any information regarding the etiology of the psychiatric disorders. The *DSM* also does not provide any treatment recommendations or report the effectiveness of particular treatment strategies when used with specific mental health disorders.

In addition to providing diagnostic criteria, the *DSM* also provides information about emotional and behavioral characteristics commonly *associated with* each of the mental health disorders. These characteristics are not *required* for an individual to qualify for a specific diagnosis, but they are often observed among individuals who manifest certain psychiatric disorders. Such characteristics can help mental health professionals diagnose youth, as well as facilitate a better understanding of the youths' difficulties. If certain physical or physiological findings are commonly associated with a particular disorder, the *DSM* notes these. Prevalence, familial patterns, and the typical course of each mental health disorder are also listed. The *DSM* also contains information on any known cultural variations in the way individuals present particular mental health symptoms or disorders. For example, individuals from some cultures may manifest a depressed mood in somatic symptoms such as stomachaches or headaches versus sad moods and crying. Additionally, the *DSM* provides information about how to differentiate certain mental health disorders from those that may look somewhat similar. This can

The Diagnosis of Mental Health Disorders

be critical, as many of the mental health disorders contain overlapping symptoms. Discriminating between two possible diagnoses can sometimes be very difficult. The information associated with each of the mental health disorders helps clinicians provide the most accurate diagnosis possible. The more information clinicians have about a specific disorder (based on the latest research and current clinical practice), the better they can distinguish which diagnosis best fits a particular youth's emotional and behavioral symptoms. Although the specific key symptoms related to each of the mental health disorders are critical, the additional information associated with each of the psychiatric disorders is important as well.

There have been several editions of the *Diagnostic and Statistical Manual of Mental Disorders*, and the manual is revised every decade or so. With each new edition, revisions to existing disorders are made, a few disorders are removed, and some new disorders are added. Changes occur when discoveries are made in clinical practice or when additional empirical research data becomes available. *The Diagnostic and Statistical Manual of Mental Disorders—4th edition, Text Revision* (DSM-IV-TR) is the most recent version of the manual. It is the most empirically based *Diagnostic and Statistical Manual* in comparison to editions that have come before it.

The *DSM* is a multiaxial system, and mental health professionals typically assess youth on several axes when making decisions about diagnosis and treatment. By using all five axes contained in the *DSM*, evaluations of youth with mental health disorders are more likely to be thorough and comprehensive. The five axes contained in the *DSM* system of classification include:

Axis I—Clinical Disorders and Other Conditions That May Be A Focus of Clinical Attention

The main mental health disorders included in the *DSM* are listed on this axis (*e.g.*, Major Depression, Posttraumatic Stress Disorder, Attention-Deficit/Hyperactivity Disorder, Conduct Disorder, Methamphetamine Abuse). Personality disorders and Mental Retardation are not included on this axis. If youth have more than one mental health diagnosis on Axis I, all are listed, with the primary disorder listed first.

Axis II—Personality Disorders and Mental Retardation

If juveniles suffer from a personality disorder or Mental Retardation, these disorders are listed on this axis. Mental Retardation can often be overlooked, particularly when youth are also suffering from a diagnosis that is listed on the first Axis. For example, an aggressive youth who hurts others, breaks into neighbors' homes, and runs away from home may easily be identified as having Conduct Disorder. However, this type of behavior may overshadow the fact that this youth is also suffering from Mental Retardation, especially if the Mental Retardation is in the mild range.

Axis III—General Medical Condition

Many juvenile offenders have medical conditions that affect or are related to their mental health diagnosis. For example, when youth are evaluated for possible depression, it is important to note if they are suffering from Hypothyroidism; symptoms of a low thyroid condition can be misinterpreted as depressive symptoms. Juveniles suffering from depressive symptoms may have recently been in a severe car accident, leaving them unable to use their legs. If this medical condition is playing a significant role in the youths' mood disorder, it should be listed on Axis III. In addition, some juvenile offenders may have recently been shot or knocked unconscious in a fight. Thus, they may be suffering from emotional and behavioral symptoms due to the physiological effects of either of these events. Paying attention to medical issues facilitates a more thorough and comprehensive examination. Mental health

22

Juvenile Offenders with Mental Health Disorders: Who Are They and What Do We Do With Them?

professionals should always be aware of youths' medical conditions because they can significantly affect decisions about mental health diagnoses, as well as treatment strategies.

Axis IV—Psychosocial and Environmental Problems

Many youth in the juvenile justice system have a variety of negative events occurring in their lives (*e.g.*, domestic violence, suspension from school, parents refusing to let them return home, death of a parent, death of a sibling/close friend, miscarriage, abortion, rape, physical abuse, arrest, incarceration). Mental health professionals must consider youths' environmental circumstances when making a mental health diagnosis. The context within which juveniles are functioning can trigger or exacerbate their mental health symptoms. Conversely, youths' mental health symptoms may be contributing to their psychosocial or environmental problems. Clinicians typically focus on major problems within the past year. But if an incident prior to the preceding year is clearly related to youths' current mental health disorder, the incident may still be noted (*e.g.*, witnessing a murder as a child may be noted for an adolescent suffering from Posttraumatic Stress Disorder).

Axis V—Global Assessment of Functioning

Clinicians are asked to rate juveniles' current level of functioning on this axis. Most mental health professionals refer to the youths' functioning for the previous week, although longer time frames can be used as well. The *DSM* contains a scale with 10 ranges of functioning to reduce the subjectivity of a clinician's rating. The Children's Global Assessment Scale (CGAS) (Dryborg *et al.*, 2000) is similar to the scale in the *DSM*, but the CGAS is specifically developed for assessing children and adolescents. Therefore, the CGAS can also be used to provide ratings for Axis V. Identifying those areas where youth are currently having the most problems helps determine which specific areas should be

targeted in treatment. In addition, subsequent ratings can be used as a comparison point to assess whether youths' functioning is improving or worsening.

By using all five axes instead of just providing an Axis I diagnosis, clinicians are able to convey a more holistic impression of youths' mental health symptoms; this includes medical issues, youths' current level of functioning, and the context of the youths' lives. This practice can decrease the tendency of clinicians (as well as other professionals) to view youth based purely on a single presenting problem or a few obvious symptoms. Clinicians are not required to use all five axes and may choose to provide only the appropriate diagnoses for Axes I-III. Although this is perfectly acceptable, care should still be taken to explore all relevant factors related to youths' functioning. This way, important information related to a mental health diagnosis is not overlooked or disregarded.

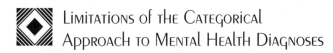

Limitations of the Categorical Approach to Mental Health Diagnoses

Classifying various emotional and behavioral symptoms into discrete categories and providing mental health diagnoses to individuals suffering from these symptoms has many benefits (*e.g.*, facilitates communication, guides research, directs treatment strategies). However, there are some limitations as well. Systems that classify clusters of mental health symptoms (*e.g.*, depressed mood, insomnia, difficulty concentrating) into discrete categories (*e.g.*, Major Depression, Posttraumatic Stress Disorder, Marijuana Abuse) work best when particular disorders are either present or absent within youth; juveniles either have the disorder or do not. This practice can be tricky with some mental health disorders because many emotional and behavioral symptoms are present in a variety of individuals, to a greater or lesser degree. The categorical approach also works best when individuals diagnosed with a specific mental health disorder are very similar to (if not the same as) others who have been diagnosed with the same disorder. Further, these individuals should be very different from others who have been diagnosed with a different mental health disorder, and from individuals without a mental health diagnosis (*e.g.*, the behavior of youth with Schizophrenia should be similar to the behavior of other youth with Schizophrenia. But these youths' behavior should be dissimilar to youth with ADHD and youth with no mental health disorder at all.) Each of these three groups should be distinct from the others, which is not always the case.

Depending on which particular symptoms youth exhibit, the behavior of two juveniles with Attention-Deficit/Hyperactivity Disorder may look very similar or very different— even when both have received an accurate diagnosis.

To meet the diagnostic criteria for a specific mental health disorder, juveniles typically do not need to exhibit all the possible symptoms of a particular disorder. Most disorders require youth to possess three to five of a longer list of symptoms. Depending on which particular symptoms youth exhibit, the behavior of two juveniles with Attention-Deficit/Hyperactivity Disorder may look very similar or very different—even when both have received an accurate diagnosis. Therefore, there is no assumption in the mental health field that two individuals with the same diagnosis will present in the exact same way. Moreover, two youths appropriately diagnosed with Attention-Deficit/Hyperactivity Disorder may not only look similar to each other but also look similar to youth in a manic phase of Bipolar Disorder (*e.g.*, distractible, talkative, increased activity). This situation can occur even though the youth

with ADHD are not suffering from a mood disorder.

There is also no assumption in the mental health field that each of the psychiatric disorders is completely separate from each of the other disorders. An overlap of symptoms from one mental health diagnosis to another is not unusual. Common psychiatric symptoms such as irritability, appetite and sleep disturbances, and difficulty concentrating can be indicative of Major Depression, Bipolar Disorder, Dysthymic Disorder, Alcohol/Drug Intoxication or Alcohol/ Drug Withdrawal. Hallucinations (*i.e.*, hearing voices), or bizarre thinking can be associated with Schizophrenia, Bipolar Disorder, Major Depression, or high levels of drug use. Youth with mental health disorders can often be reliably distinguished from youth without mental health disorders. However, the differentiation of youth who have particular categories of psychiatric disorders is much more difficult (Reeves, Werry, Elkind & Zametkin, 1987). Because of symptom overlap, juveniles can be misdiagnosed if a mental health professional does not conduct a thorough and comprehensive evaluation before assigning a psychiatric diagnosis.

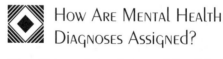 How Are Mental Health Diagnoses Assigned?

The diagnosing of mental health disorders should always be taken seriously due to the significant ramifications associated with being classified as mentally ill. The only individuals who should assign mental health diagnoses are those with the experience and training to do so. Formal training in the screening and assessment of mental health disorders, as well as in the provision of psychiatric diagnoses, is required. The *DSM* offers diagnostic guidelines, but it is not designed to be used in a cookbook fashion by individuals without this type of training (APA, 2000). Clinical psychologists and psychiatrists are the professionals most likely to

24

Juvenile Offenders with Mental Health Disorders: Who Are They and What Do We Do With Them?

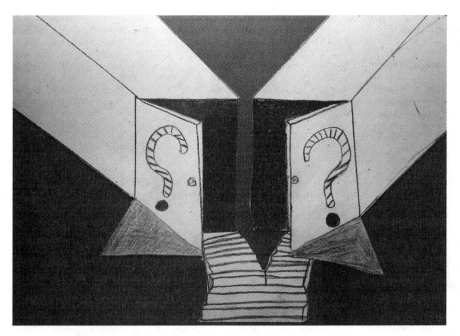

cal trauma to the youths' brain/head, or a chaotic home environment. One or all of these factors might be playing a significant role in youths' clinical presentation.

A systematic and detailed approach is needed when assessing juvenile offenders. Clinicians need to speak at length with youth and with individuals who can provide critical information that juveniles might not report. It is important for clinicians to speak with key individuals who can describe youths' behavior and functioning—both in the present and the past. Depending on the particular juvenile, these individuals could include parents/caretakers, previous caretakers, teachers, juvenile justice facility staff, probation/parole staff, mental health/health treatment, substance abuse treatment providers, and the like. Clinicians do not need to engage in long, in-depth interviews with these individuals but should spend enough time to gather relevant information about the youths' functioning and behavior.

Multiple methods are often used to collect the information needed to make a mental health diagnosis. In addition to interviews, some clinicians use standardized screening and assessment tools. Many psychological instruments and questionnaires must be directly administered to youth by a mental health professional. But some can be given to juveniles for them to complete themselves. Checklists or questionnaires may also be given to parents/caretakers, teachers, or juvenile justice staff to have them describe or rate youths' behavior. Previous records and reports (*e.g.*, mental health, health, juvenile justice) may be used as well *(please see Chapter 13 for more information on screening and assessment of juvenile offenders with mental health disorders)*.

provide youth with diagnoses for mental health disorders. However, depending on their particular training, school psychologists, psychiatric nurses, social workers, and the like, may also assign psychiatric diagnoses to youth. When providing diagnoses to individuals, clinicians use a significant degree of clinical judgment. When working with juvenile offenders in particular, clinicians should have training and experience related to the various mental health disorders, and also related to:

- Normal adolescent development
- Interactive effects of mental illness and substance use
- Effects of trauma
- Common cognitive, emotional, behavioral, and lifestyle characteristics specifically associated with delinquent youth.

Psychiatric diagnoses should be assigned only after a comprehensive and thorough mental health evaluation is conducted. Many juvenile offenders exhibit a multitude of emotional and behavioral symptoms. Some of their difficulties may be related to a mental illness. They could also be due to the effects of drug and alcohol use, significant life stressors, physi-

The Diagnosis of Mental Health Disorders

A clinician should gather a significant amount of information about youth and their circumstances before assigning a psychiatric diagnosis. Examples of the type of information that should be collected include, but are not limited to:

- Current/previous mental health symptoms (*e.g.*, depression, hyperactivity, hallucinations, self-injurious behavior)
- Current/previous suicidal thoughts/ behavior
- Previous mental health evaluations
- Current/previous mental health treatment (*e.g.*, inpatient, outpatient, psychotropic medication)
- Current/previous drug and alcohol use
- Current/previous drug and alcohol abuse treatment (*e.g.*, inpatient, outpatient)
- Relationship between mental health symptoms and substance use
- Cognitive/intellectual limitations
- Recent/previous traumatic event(s)
- Current/previous aggressive or violent thoughts and behavior
- Level of emotional distress or functional impairment
- Home environment/relationships with family and/or caretaker
- Family history of mental health and substance use disorders
- Any incidents of abuse and neglect
- Out-of-home placements
- School/vocational history and status
- Health/medical issues
- Delinquent behavior/juvenile justice involvement
- Recent stressors
- Coping/problem-solving abilities
- Current support system
- Hobbies/interests
- Strengths/resiliencies

- Degree of insight regarding mental health symptoms

When collecting this information, clinicians should always consider the influence of cultural issues (*e.g.*, racial/ethnic background, gender, urban/rural lifestyle, sexual orientation). Clinicians do not look solely for signs and symptoms that indicate a particular mental health disorder. They also look for characteristics and factors that would rule out the possibility of particular disorders. For example, a clinician might suspect that a juvenile has Attention-Deficit/ Hyperactivity Disorder due to his or her overly active behavior, disorganization, and forgetfulness at home. Discovering that the youth is calm, organized, and task-focused in school suggests that the juvenile's difficulties may be associated with something other than that disorder.

Before assigning a psychiatric diagnosis, clinicians should conduct a *mental status examination* of youth. Mental status examinations typically include an observation of youths' appearance and behavior, as well as their affect (emotions) and mood. Clinicians pay particular attention to juveniles' thought processes, including their attention and memory, as well as the rate, tone and volume of their speech.

Even when clinicians carefully conduct detailed evaluations of youth, errors can still occur due to the following factors:

- Youth can be purposefully dishonest about their mood and behavior
- Youth may provide inaccurate information because they did not understand what was being asked of them
- Adults rating, or reporting on, youths' behavior may be biased in their perceptions of the youth

In addition, no mental health assessment tool is 100 percent accurate, even when it is highly structured and standardized. The role of the mental health professional's clinical judgment is critical and fundamental to the entire diagnostic process. However, even well-trained

26

Juvenile Offenders with Mental Health Disorders: Who Are They and What Do We Do With Them?

clinicians are vulnerable to bias (McClellan & Werry, 2000).

 The Challenge of Diagnosing Juvenile Offenders Who Have Mental Health Disorders

As previously discussed, classifying mental health disorders and providing mental health diagnoses has its benefits and limitations. Clinicians face additional challenges when diagnosing juvenile offenders with mental health disorders.

The *DSM* lists specific diagnostic criteria for each of the psychiatric disorders. The *DSM* is most helpful when an individual fulfills the required diagnostic criteria for one particular disorder and does not fulfill criteria for the other disorders. Unfortunately, some youth involved with juvenile justice have a few symptoms from one mental health disorder and a few symptoms from another mental health disorder. But they do not have enough symptoms from either disorder to qualify for a full diagnosis. Juvenile offenders typically do not fit as neatly into the discrete psychiatric categories as their peers in the general population. Their clinical presentations are often complex and confusing, with obvious emotional and behavioral symptoms, as well as subtle ones. For the juvenile offenders who do meet full diagnostic criteria for a mental health disorder, most meet criteria for more than just one. Meeting diagnostic criteria for two, three, four or even five psychiatric disorders at the same time is not unusual among this population of youth. For example, a juvenile offender may be diagnosed with Conduct Disorder, Attention-Deficit Hyperactivity Disorder, a Learning Disorder, Alcohol Abuse, and Marijuana Abuse. In addition, the same youth may also be suffering from Major Depression, Dysthymic Disorder, or Posttraumatic Stress Disorder. Having more than one mental health disorder simultaneously is referred to as *co-morbidity* and is often the norm, rather than

the exception among youth within the juvenile justice system. In addition, many juvenile offenders have experienced trauma to their head and/or brain. Differentiating the effects of mild injuries to youths' head or brain from symptoms of mental illness can be difficult.

Another challenge when diagnosing juvenile offenders with mental health disorders is distinguishing the role of youths' alcohol and drug use on their emotional and behavioral symptoms. Many signs associated with particular mental health disorders can also be directly caused by drug and alcohol intoxication or withdrawal (*e.g.*, irritability, insomnia, difficulty concentrating, depressed mood, elation, restlessness, rapid speech, disorganized behavior). Some youth have both a mental health and a substance use disorder, and each disorder may be influencing and interacting with the other. Juveniles who concurrently meet diagnostic criteria for both a mental health and substance use disorder are referred to as having *co-occurring* disorders. Diagnosing youth with co-occurring disorders can be complex and challenging *(see Chapter 10 for more details on youth with co-occurring disorders)*.

Youths' emotional and behavioral symptoms can be greatly affected by situational factors. Depending on when an evaluation is conducted, a mental health professional may or may not capture juvenile offenders' typical functioning. Youths' emotions and behavior are likely to be different immediately after incarceration versus two years after residing at a juvenile justice facility. Other situational factors that can impact juveniles' functioning including the following:

- Being considered for transfer to the adult criminal justice system

- Being arrested for the first time and feeling fearful

- Being directly admitted from the community with drugs and alcohol still in their system

- Receiving bad news about their friends or family

- Being aware the judge is making placement decisions based on the youths' current behavior

Clinicians should take into account juvenile offenders' context (*e.g.*, legal status, where residing, upcoming transfer to another facility, approaching release date) when providing psychiatric diagnoses because situational factors can dramatically influence the emotions and behaviors exhibited by youth.

In addition to current situational factors, some juvenile offenders display emotional or behavioral symptoms in relation to events that

---

MOST MENTAL HEALTH PROFESSIONALS WORKING WITHIN JUVENILE JUSTICE FACILITIES, OR CONTRACTING WITH JUVENILE JUSTICE AGENCIES, HAVE LARGE CASELOADS WITH NUMEROUS YOUTH TO EVALUATE.

---

have happened to them in the past. Many youth involved with the juvenile justice system have experienced physical and/or sexual abuse. Some have witnessed deaths of friends, siblings, or parents. Even if juveniles are not suffering from Posttraumatic Stress Disorder, they still may exhibit a variety of emotional or behavioral effects from previous traumatic experiences. Being raised in an environment of domestic violence, being neglected by parents/caretakers, or being placed repeatedly in different foster homes can all have a negative affect on youth. Symptoms of anxiety, depression, or irritability can result from any of these experiences. Some juvenile offenders have difficulty regulating their emotions, and/or appear detached and insensitive to others. These youth may be misdiagnosed if clinicians do not take into account the negative life events—and possible traumatic incidents—many of these youth have witnessed or experienced.

Receiving a thorough and comprehensive mental health evaluation can be a challenge for juvenile offenders. Depending on when and where an evaluation is requested, there may not be access to mental health professionals who are adequately trained in providing mental health diagnoses. There may not be enough time to complete the type of detailed mental health assessment required to provide an accurate psychiatric diagnosis. Most mental health professionals working within juvenile justice facilities, or contracting with juvenile justice agencies, have large caseloads with numerous youth to evaluate. Time limitations often prevent these clinicians from assessing juvenile offenders in the same manner as if time were not an issue. In such a case, mental health professionals can give a "provisional" diagnosis. Clinicians note the psychiatric disorder they believe best fits the youths' presentation but convey there is not enough information to be certain. Some clinicians use the term "rule out" to communicate the same idea. Axis I from the *DSM* might have the listing "Rule Out Posttraumatic Stress Disorder." This does not mean that Posttraumatic Stress Disorder has been ruled out. A clinician believes Posttraumatic Stress Disorder is the most likely diagnosis for a particular youth, but due to limited time or information, cannot be sure. This practice is one way to convey to the next clinician evaluating the juvenile that additional information should be gathered. Once this information is obtained, the second clinician can confirm whether the current diagnosis is correct or whether it should be *ruled out*.

Special care should be taken when using mental health diagnoses in court-related matters with juvenile offenders. Terms such as "mental health disorder" or "psychiatric disorder" can be misunderstood or misused. During legal proceedings, youths' mental health may be called into question. Being diagnosed with a mental health disorder—even a serious and debilitating disorder—does not necessarily answer questions regarding juveniles' level of competency (youths' ability to understand the nature of the proceedings against them and ability to assist

Juvenile Offenders with Mental Health Disorders: Who Are They and What Do We Do With Them?

their attorney) or juveniles' degree of criminal responsibility. Additional information must be gathered about a particular youth's functioning and capabilities to help answer these types of legal questions.

 ## Mental Health Diagnoses Within Juvenile Justice Facilities

Many juvenile justice professionals would like to do away with mental health diagnoses altogether. They often report that juvenile offenders "hide behind their mental health diagnosis." Or, they believe these youth use their psychiatric disorder as an excuse for negative behavior or to avoid participating in aversive tasks. Some offenders certainly engage in such behaviors. But most mentally ill youth are embarrassed and ashamed of having a mental health diagnosis; they typically do not want others to know about it. Within the juvenile justice system, strength, toughness, and resiliency are typically valued and respected among peers, while weakness, vulnerability, and limitations are usually looked down upon. Because of these dynamics, most juveniles would prefer to hide that they have been diagnosed with a mental health disorder. Having a psychiatric diagnosis in a juvenile justice facility can reduce youths' status in the eyes of other juveniles—as well as result in verbal teasing and physical victimization.

While attempting to provide youth with appropriate mental health treatment, the juvenile justice system itself can sometimes inadvertently penalize juveniles for having a mental disorder. Many lower-risk offenders who have received diagnoses for psychiatric disorders are ineligible for placement at minimum-security settings—particularly work camps, ranches, etc. Smaller and/or lower security facilities and settings often do not have adequate medical or mental health resources to appropriately monitor youth with significant mental health needs. These youth are typically placed in facilities where there is greater access to both mental health and medical professionals. This situation is particularly true when juveniles have been prescribed psychotropic medication for their illness. Due to limited resources, most health/mental health services are concentrated in the larger and more restrictive facilities. Ironically, if mentally ill youth choose not to take psychotropic medication, their mood and/or behavior is likely to worsen, typically resulting in a more secure placement. A survey of adult correctional agencies found that (in almost all of the states that responded) psychiatric diagnosis not only affects initial facility placement but also subsequent placements as well (Miller & Metzner, 1994).

While some juveniles suffering from mental health disorders cannot adequately be managed at less secure settings, some likely can be. A number of youth who have received a mental health diagnosis have gone years without exhibiting mental health symptoms. These juveniles may have initially been misdiagnosed, their mental illness may be in remission, or their emotions and behavior may have stabilized due to effective intervention strategies. Requiring juveniles to reside at more restrictive settings solely due to having a psychiatric diagnosis is unfortunate—particularly when their criminal behavior would indicate a less restrictive setting. If youth are exhibiting significant mental health symptoms, placement in a secure facility with a greater degree of mental health resources is clearly justifiable. However, if juveniles' emotions and behavior appear to be stable for a significant period of time, these youth should be re-evaluated by a mental health professional. The clinician should determine whether a given psychiatric diagnosis is currently accurate, and whether the youth can be appropriately managed in the least-restrictive setting for which they are eligible. Not all mental health disorders remain consistently active over time.

Problems Associated With Over-Reliance on Mental Health Diagnoses

Youth with mental health disorders are commonly identified in the juvenile justice system by whether they have been assigned an Axis I diagnosis from the *DSM*. Although this practice is an important way to identify youth with psychiatric disorders, it can also be problematic if certain issues are not kept in mind:

Not all juvenile offenders have been evaluated

Although many youth involved with the juvenile justice system have been evaluated by a mental health professional before, during or after arrest/incarceration, many of them have not. In fact, some juvenile offenders with diagnosable mental health disorders have never been evaluated for psychiatric symptoms. This oversight may be due to a variety of factors including, but not limited to:

- Families/caretakers did not know how to obtain an evaluation

- Families/caretakers may have sought out others besides mental health professionals for advice or an opinion (*e.g.*, clergy, extended family, tribal leader)

- Families/caretakers resistance due to stigma of mental illness

- Families/caretakers did not notice anything was wrong because they exhibit the same symptoms as the youth

- Families/caretakers did not want mental health professionals to know personal details about the families (*e.g.*, abuse, neglect, parental substance abuse)

- Families/caregivers and/or teachers had a high tolerance for unusual behavior

- Professionals responded to youth by referring them directly to the juvenile justice system

- Once involved with juvenile justice, youth were not referred for mental health services

- No one may have been aware of the youths' psychiatric difficulties because the youth never disclosed them to anyone (*e.g.*, feelings of depression, suicide attempts, self-injuring behavior, anxiety)

In addition, different families have different tolerance levels related to problematic behavior. Some families might view a youth who stands up at the dinner table twice while everyone is eating as "hyperactive" and in need of a psychological evaluation. Other families may view a youth who cannot sit still, continuously climbs on everything, constantly fidgets, and talks incessantly, as a child "with a lot of energy." They may see no need for an evaluation. Families experiencing significant stressors or in constant disarray may be less attuned to the psychiatric symptoms displayed by their children. Just because juveniles have not been given a psychiatric diagnosis does *not* mean they do not have a mental health disorder.

Not all mental health professionals conduct thorough and comprehensive evaluations

Even if youth are referred for a mental health evaluation, some clinicians do not complete thorough-enough evaluations with juvenile offenders to identify the presence of a mental health disorder. Some clinicians specialize in evaluating youth with a particular mental health disorder (*e.g.*, Attention-Deficit/Hyperactivity Disorder, Bipolar Disorder, Conduct Disorder). Once they see a few signs of the disorder with which they are most familiar, these clinicians may too hastily apply that diagnosis to youth. However, in truth, the youth may actually meet diagnostic criteria for another (or additional) psychiatric disorder. Juvenile justice professionals throughout the country have described working with clinicians who consistently diagnose youth with the exact same disorder, regard-

30

Juvenile Offenders with Mental Health Disorders: Who Are They and What Do We Do With Them?

less of the juveniles' clinical presentation. This practice is not helpful, and it is a waste of valuable resources.

Many parents/caretakers bring their children to family doctors for an evaluation of mental health symptoms. This type of physician is not likely to have an extensive period of time to conduct a comprehensive mental health assessment. Diagnoses of Attention-Deficit/Hyperactivity Disorder, Major Depression and Conduct Disorder have been given after a 30-minute meeting with youth and their parent/caretaker. This short meeting is typically not enough time to thoroughly evaluate juvenile offenders, due to their complex clinical presentation. In addition, mental health professionals who contract with juvenile courts or juvenile justice facilities (as well as those employed by juvenile justice agencies) usually have large caseloads and limited time to conduct comprehensive evaluations. Some clinicians rely purely on an interview with juveniles in order to gather information to make a mental health diagnosis. Although this information is critical, it should not be the sole source of data when determining the presence of mental illness.

Some juvenile offenders have been misdiagnosed

Some juvenile offenders have received a psychiatric diagnosis that does not accurately represent their mental health disorder. Juvenile offenders commonly receive the sole diagnosis of Conduct Disorder. However, many of these youth are suffering from an additional psychiatric disorder as well. This situation occurs because juvenile offenders often present with a variety of behaviors symptomatic of Conduct Disorder. They may have threatened others, initiated fights, run away from home, been truant from school, or stolen things. These behaviors are obvious to observers and upsetting to a variety of individuals in the juveniles' lives. If clinicians focus exclusively on these behaviors and solely assign the diagnosis of Conduct Disorder, they are likely to miss addi-

tional psychiatric disorders that may be present. Some aggressive youth have an underlying mood disorder. Many youth who are truant from school have a learning disorder. Some youth who run away from home have been severely physically or sexually abused and may be suffering from Posttraumatic Stress Disorder. The less thorough a mental health evaluation, the more likely juveniles will be misdiagnosed or additional psychiatric diagnoses will be overlooked.

Due to the often-complex clinical presentation of juvenile offenders, assigning an accurate mental health diagnosis can be challenging. Symptoms of Attention-Deficit/Hyperactivity Disorder and anxiety can look similar to one another. Symptoms of Attention-Deficit/Hyperactivity Disorder and the manic phase of Bipolar Disorder can look similar to one another. Hallucinations and delusions related to Schizophrenia or a mood disorder can appear similar to hallucinations and delusions related to heavy methamphetamine or other substance use. Effects of trauma, being raised in a nonstructured and chaotic environment, living in a violent neighborhood, and multiple incarcerations can significantly impact youths' emotions and behavior—and their ability to manage stressful situations. The timing of a mental health evaluation can influence youths' diagnosis (e.g., prior to a trial, upon admission to a juvenile justice facility, prior to release from a juvenile justice facility). Depending on juveniles' cultural background, age, or level of cognitive functioning, they may not fully understand a clinician's questions during an interview. They may also not understand questions on a psychological test. When English is not the primary language for juvenile offenders and/or their families/caretakers, information collected is likely to be affected. Misdiagnosis can easily occur when clinicians do not conduct detailed evaluations, making sure to take into account the multitude of possible factors influencing youths' functioning.

Some juvenile offenders may no longer be suffering from a mental health disorder

Juvenile offenders may have been adequately assessed and accurately diagnosed in the past, but they may no longer be suffering from a mental health disorder. Although many youth do not outgrow their psychiatric disorder, some do. If youth are not re-evaluated (and many juvenile offenders are not), their original psychiatric diagnosis continues to be placed in file after file and communicated to juvenile justice professionals who work with the youth. Professionals are likely to interact with the juveniles as if they still had the disorder. For example, a female offender may have suffered from Major Depression at the age of 13. At the age of 17, she may have no current symptoms of depression, and she may not have had any within the past four years. However, when staff read this young woman's file, they will likely assume she is still depressed. A 16-year-old young man may have been accurately diagnosed with Attention-Deficit/Hyperactivity Disorder at the age of seven and placed on psychostimulant medication with positive effects. This juvenile may have stopped taking medication at the age of 10 and shown few to no symptoms of hyperactivity, impulsivity or inattention since the early teens. If this offender is never re-evaluated, juvenile justice personnel will assume he continues to suffer from Attention-Deficit/Hyperactivity Disorder (which may or may not be correct) if that is what is written in his file. Along the same lines, a juvenile diagnosed with Posttraumatic Stress Disorder after a rape may no longer meet diagnostic criteria for the disorder after participating in therapy.

 ## Cultural Issues and the Diagnosis of Mental Health Disorders

Challenges can arise when clinicians are asked to evaluate youth from cultures or ethnic backgrounds different from their own. Lack of familiarity with youths' culture can result in the over-diagnosis or under-diagnosis of psychopathology within a particular youth. The *DSM* is used to classify mental health disorders among diverse populations of individuals from a variety of cultures around the world. To decrease the likelihood of bias when assigning mental health diagnoses, the *DSM* includes cultural information to help clinicians diagnose individuals from different backgrounds. Cultural variations in the way particular mental health disorders are expressed are noted, as are possible cultural explanations for individuals' behavior.

Previous studies have found that race and ethnicity influence psychiatric diagnoses. African-American and Asian-American adults were more frequently diagnosed with organic/psychotic disorders (including Schizophrenia) in comparison to Caucasians and Latinos. Caucasian adolescents were more frequently diagnosed with mood disorders, anxiety disorders and substance abuse disorders in comparison to African-American adolescents (Flaskerud & Hu, 1992; Kilgus, Pumariega, & Cuffe, 1995). These diagnoses may reflect the true occurrence of these psychiatric disorders in youth of different races. Or, the difference in mental health diagnoses may be related to other factors. For example, African-American youth have been found to have more face and head injuries versus Caucasian youth, which may account for the greater number of organic (medical) diagnoses (Lewis, Shanok, Cohen, Kligfeld, & Frisone, 1980). However, African-Americans do not seek mental health services as often as their Caucasian counterparts. Perhaps African-American families have more tolerance for mental health symptoms, so only the most seriously disturbed African-American youth receive psychiatric diagnoses. African-Americans are under-represented in the mental health system and over-represented in the juvenile justice system. Therefore, some African-American youth with mental health disorders likely are sent directly to the juvenile justice system, instead of receiving mental health evaluations and treatment for their behaviors.

32

Juvenile Offenders with Mental Health Disorders: Who Are They and What Do We Do With Them?

Another factor that may be playing a role is possible bias in the mental health assessment tools being used. Clinicians often use psychological testing results when formulating mental health diagnoses. Many psychological measures have been developed for middle-class Caucasian males. When youth of other races, backgrounds or gender are assessed with these tools, the results may or may not be valid. Just because youths' answers are *different* from the correct answer, it is not necessarily indicative of psychopathology. Similarly, it is also possible that clinicians are misinterpreting youths' interview responses as manifestations of mental illness primarily because they are unfamiliar with the juveniles' background (*e.g.*, culture, race, gender, sexual orientation). For example, in some cultures, having visions of deceased relatives during periods of grieving is an accepted experience and not viewed as hallucinatory. In addition, juvenile offenders' reality-based reactions (*e.g.*, paranoia, fear, extreme religiosity) may be perceived as symptoms of mental illness.

Clinicians must be careful not to attribute psychopathology where none exists. Likewise, clinicians must not overlook or automatically dismiss psychiatric symptoms among youth from different backgrounds due to an automatic assumption that the symptoms are culturally sanctioned phenomena. When mental health professionals rely on stereotypes related to individuals different from themselves (*e.g.*, youth from various ethnic/racial backgrounds, females, juvenile offenders, homosexual youth), they may miss significant signs of disturbance, assuming, "That's just the way they are." This type of bias has been reported in relation to African-American youth in the juvenile justice system. Professionals were failing to notice, or were rationalizing, youths' psychopathology as part of the African-American culture—even when the behavior was considered inappropriate or deviant by the youths' families/caretakers. In comparison to Caucasian youth, African-American youth needed to display extremely obvious and excessive mental health symptoms to secure an appropriate mental health evaluation and treatment. And even those conditions were no guarantee (Lewis, Balla, & Shanok, 1979).

 MENTAL HEALTH DISORDERS VERSUS NORMAL ADOLESCENT BEHAVIOR

One source of confusion associated with mental health disorders is related to what distinguishes psychopathology from normal adolescent behavior. Some juvenile justice professionals have stated that "adolescence itself seems like a mental health disorder!" This statement is not the least bit surprising, based on their experience working with large numbers of adolescents, many of whom are experiencing psychiatric symptoms. Part of the confusion on this issue arises from society's lack of understanding about what constitutes healthy adolescent development. It is important for adults working within juvenile justice to understand "normal," healthy adolescent development (including *expected* behavior during this time of life). Once normal adolescent behavior is clear, it is easier to notice when youths' behavior is pathological.

Normal Adolescent Behavior

Adolescence is a period of significant physical, emotional, intellectual, and social, development. For some youth, the changes are dramatic; for others, the changes are more slow and gradual. During this phase of life, children are transitioning into adulthood. They are discovering who they are, what they like and do not like, with whom they want to spend their time, and how they want to spend their future. Compared to when they were younger, adolescents spend more time with their friends and less time with their families. They may experiment with various styles of clothes, music, and even hair color. Their bodies grow larger and hormones are produced. As their brains continue to develop, adolescents are able to think abstractly, opening up new realms of possibilities regarding things to try and places to go. Adolescence is often an exciting time, full of discovery and opportunities.

For many years, experts believed that adolescence was a period of tremendous "storm and stress" and that all youth experience tumultuous emotions and relationships during this developmental stage. It is now clear that this is not so for all youth. Many young people pass through the teen years with little upheaval or upset. Although this stage of life is not as traumatic as once was thought, the adolescent years can be more difficult than other periods of life—difficult for juveniles, as well as for those around them (Arnett, 1999). For example, adolescents experience their emotions in an extreme fashion, particularly negative feelings. Physical changes occurring in their bodies, transitions within the educational arena, and initial experiences with dating may play a role in mood changes during adolescence. Teenagers report more anxiety, loneliness, embarrassment and self-consciousness in comparison to their parents. Negative moods are more likely if youth are not doing well in school, are not popular with peers, or if there are problems within the family unit. Although negative emotions are more common during adolescence, most youth do not experience them to the degree that would qualify as a mental health disorder.

There is also an increase in conflict between parents and their children during the adolescent years. This heightened level of conflict typically occurs in early adolescence and eventually decreases during late adolescence. Most disagreements are related to everyday issues such as chores, curfew, and homework. Despite this increase in conflict, most parents and their adolescent children report having a positive and close relationship in which they share common values.

It is also during the teenage years that risk-taking behavior begins to increase. Delinquent behavior, alcohol and drug use, and risky sexual behavior are most prevalent among adolescents and young adults (Arnett, 1999). Although not every youth engages in high-risk behavior, most adolescents will at one point take part in some type of risky activity.

Each juvenile's experience during the adolescent years is individualized and influenced by his or her family/caretakers, culture, and community. The combination of increased risk-taking behavior, conflict with parents, and extreme emotional experiences can make the developmental stage of adolescence more difficult for youth (as well as those closest to them) in comparison to either childhood or adulthood. However, despite these challenges, the majority of teenagers:

- Feel positive about their lives
- Get along with their parents
- Have friends to whom they feel connected
- Have a positive view of their future

Pathological Adolescent Behavior

A critical task for mental health professionals is to determine whether adolescents' behavior is normative for their developmental stage or pathological and in need of intervention. About 20 percent of adolescents suffer from a true mental health *disorder* (Weiner, 1990). Many adolescents display extreme emotions, engage in risk-related behavior, and experience increased conflict with parents. But this behavior does not interfere with most young people's ability to accomplish everyday tasks. Activities such as delinquent behavior or drug and alcohol use are not necessarily pathological. In fact, most adolescents have experimented with or occasionally used drugs and alcohol. In addition, a large number of adolescents have engaged in delinquent behavior for which they could be arrested. In and of themselves, these behaviors do not indicate psychopathology. These behaviors are actually the norm during the teenage years. However, there is a subset of youth for whom emotions and/or behaviors deviate significantly (quantitatively or qualitatively) from most youth in the general population, and for whom intervention is warranted.

There are no hard-and-fast rules in determining which youth are engaging in normal adolescent behavior and which youth are displaying symptoms of a psychiatric "disorder." Often, it is a matter of degree or frequency. Experimenting with drugs and alcohol a few times is not the same as engaging in this behavior on a daily basis. Becoming irritable and getting into frequent disagreements with one's parents is different from throwing things at or physically assaulting one's parents. Psychiatric symptoms are often similar to normal adolescent behaviors but more extreme. Emotions and behaviors become pathological—and worrisome—when they cause youth (and/or others in their lives) significant distress and/or interfere with juveniles' ability to function in activities related to daily life (*e.g.*, family relationships, school, job, friendships).

Particular features of adolescent development are related to future emotional and behavioral difficulties. The following behaviors can be an indication that something has gone awry:

- Social isolation
- Lack of friends
- Strange or unusual thoughts or behaviors
- Odd usage of language
- Extreme emotional instability
- Declining academic performance
- Extreme and continuous rebellion
- Loathing or hate of one's parents
- Repetitive and serious criminal behavior
- Frequent drug or alcohol use

The above behaviors are not typical of healthy adolescent development and should not be ignored (Weiner, 1990). Youth exhibiting these behaviors should be evaluated to determine whether a mental health disorder is present or is in the early stages of development. When professionals attribute pathological behaviors to "typical adolescence," juveniles in serious need of treatment do not receive appropriate mental health services. For many youth, mental health symptoms and functional impairments during the adolescent years persist into adulthood, reinforcing the importance of early identification and intervention (Ferdinand & Verhulst, 1995).

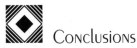 Conclusions

Although the current state of classifying and diagnosing mental health disorders is far from perfect, it is more advanced than ever before. Discrete mental health categories are based on decades of clinical practice and empirical research. When used appropriately, the *Diagnostic and Statistical Manual of Mental Disorders* decreases the subjectivity involved in providing psychiatric diagnoses and improves communication, research and education related to psychopathology. The accurate diagnosis of mental health disorders among juvenile offenders can be challenging; it requires clinicians with training and experience in mental health, normal adolescent development, substance use, and characteristics specific to juvenile offenders. An awareness of the way youths' culture, gender, and age affects the manifestation of mental health symptoms is also critical.

Psychiatric diagnoses should be based on a comprehensive evaluation of juveniles, with information gathered from a variety of methods and a variety of sources. Knowing the limitations of the current diagnostic system and using it appropriately can result in accurate mental health diagnoses that guide effective intervention strategies. The current diagnostic system, the *DSM*, is based on present knowledge within the field of mental health. As new information is discovered, it is likely that revisions to existing disorders will be made, a few mental health disorders removed, and new categories added.

CHAPTER 3

Oppositional Defiant Disorder and Conduct Disorder

"I thought the only difference between a kid with Conduct Disorder and a 'mental health' kid was that the youth with Conduct Disorder needed punishment, and the mentally ill youth needed treatment."

Detention Youth Specialist

Craig, 14, has been refusing to go to school. He continues to get into fights with his older sister, and recently he pulled a knife on her. He steals money out of his mother's purse and has been caught stealing a pair of shoes from a department store. Lately, he has been starting fires in the basement when no one is home. His parents think he may be using drugs and do not know what to do about him.

Shawna, 15, continues to talk back to her mother. She stays out past her curfew every weekend and when her mother restricts her from the telephone as a punishment, Shawna makes phone calls anyway. Shawna is constantly taunting her younger brother and seems to be annoyed at everything her mother says. Her stubborn behavior and irritable attitude have made the whole household a tense and unpleasant place to live for the entire family.

Oppositional Defiant Disorder and Conduct Disorder are often referred to as "disruptive disorders." Youth who suffer from these mental health syndromes display behavior that is typically annoying, *disruptive*, and often danger-ous to those around them—adults and peers alike. Youth with Oppositional Defiant Disorder and Conduct Disorder are often seen as juve-niles who just need "to be taught a good lesson" or just need more "structure" or "punishment." But these disorders are much more complicated than that. Such beliefs are based on the assump-tion that the behaviors are volitional and pur-poseful, or stem from an underlying disease process or psychopathology solely *within* the youth. These beliefs do a disservice to juveniles and dismiss the complexity of these disorders. Environmental factors play some role in most of the mental health disorders from which juvenile offenders suffer. However, the role of environ-mental factors is particularly critical for these two disorders, especially Conduct Disorder.

Environmental factors play a significant part in both the development and the management of juvenile offenders with Oppositional Defiant Disorder and Conduct Disorder. In addition, although youth with these disorders can victimize other individuals, many suffer a great deal themselves.

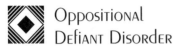

Oppositional Defiant Disorder

Youth who have been diagnosed with Oppositional Defiant Disorder display a pattern of behavior that is angry, disruptive, and disobedient to adults, primarily authority figures (APA, 2000). These juveniles are typically stubborn and spiteful, and may purposefully engage in behaviors that they know will annoy or irritate others. They rarely take responsibility for their negative behavior and instead blame others or external circumstances. They are often irritable and easily annoyed. Juveniles with Oppositional Defiant Disorder do not like to be told what to do and often blatantly ignore rules or requests. Most youth, particularly adolescents, may engage in this type of negative behavior at various times. But youth with Oppositional Defiant Disorder behave this way significantly more than their same-age peers. These youths' behavior is so frequent and intense that it interferes with their ability to function adequately at home, school, or work. These behaviors are not caused by another psychiatric disorder (*e.g.*, Major Depression, Dysthymia, Psychosis).

Oppositional Defiant Disorder can be difficult to diagnose because it is not exactly clear how youth with this disorder differ from youth without Oppositional Defiant Disorder. Many "normal" youth display similar types of behaviors throughout their development. There is much less known about youth who have Oppositional Defiant Disorder in comparison to Conduct Disorder. Approximately 2-16 percent of youth in the general population suffer from Oppositional Defiant Disorder, and this rate is significantly higher among juvenile offenders. Many juveniles who display symptoms of Oppositional Defiant Disorder will outgrow these negative behaviors by mid-to-late adolescence without any untoward effects. However, there is a subset of youth that will go on to develop the more severe behavioral disorder, Conduct Disorder. Oppositional Defiant Disorder is typically a disorder of noncompliance toward authority figures. In contrast, Conduct Disorder is typically a disorder in which there is a violation of the rights of others and the rules of society (*e.g.*, breaking laws, fighting, displaying cruelty to animals). Viewing these two mental health disorders as two points on a continuum versus two separate mental health disorders can be helpful. Most youth with Conduct Disorder begin with Oppositional Defiant Disorder-like behaviors (Kazdin, 1989). Therefore, early intervention with oppositionally defiant youth may help prevent the development of more serious negative behavior. The *exact* relationship between Oppositional Defiant Disorder and Conduct Disorder is not yet known. Although many youth with Oppositional Defiant Disorder go on to develop Conduct Disorder, some do not.

This chapter is primarily focused on juvenile offenders with Conduct Disorder. The reason for this is two-fold: much more is known about the etiology of Conduct Disorder, the developmental course of Conduct Disorder, and the ways to manage youth with Conduct Disorder (in comparison to what is known about Oppositional Defiant Disorder); and most juvenile offenders exhibiting *oppositional* behaviors have already progressed to the more serious and dangerous behaviors of Conduct Disorder.

Conduct Disorder

Conduct Disorder is one of the most complex and challenging psychiatric disorders among juveniles. Youth with this mental health diagnosis can present with very different behaviors.

Some juveniles with Conduct Disorder begin engaging in delinquent behavior as teenagers, but they outgrow it by early adulthood. Other youth have long histories of aggressive and antisocial behavior and have spent years in juvenile justice facilities. Conduct Disorder is one of the most common psychiatric disorders among youth referred to mental health facilities, inpatient and outpatient.

Conduct Disorder is often not taken as seriously as some of the other psychiatric diagnoses that can be applied to youth, particularly in the realm of juvenile justice. However, most antisocial youth experience tremendous challenges during their youth, as well as in adulthood. As children and adolescents, youth with Conduct Disorder tend to have more difficulty in the areas of:

- Academic achievement (*e.g.*, having poor grades, dropping out)

- Interpersonal relationships (*e.g.*, rejection by same-age peers, conflict with both peers and adults)

- Drug and alcohol use

As adults, they are more likely to have marital difficulties, suffer from both physical and other psychiatric illness, get into accidents, use welfare services, and experience long periods of unemployment (Patterson, DeBaryshe, & Ramsey, 1989).

In addition to the impairment youth with Conduct Disorder experience, the youths' antisocial behavior results in negative consequences for others as well. For example, many antisocial acts are committed against other people. Antisocial youth have committed acts of assault, theft, rape, and/or property damage against their own families and friends, as well as strangers, neighbors, and business owners. Given the nature of conduct-disordered juveniles' behavior, many parents and siblings are too frightened to allow their antisocial child back into the family home. They may fear the youth will steal money or family possessions, or become angry and aggressive toward them.

Antisocial acts also have significant monetary consequences. In the United States, almost one-half billion dollars is spent repairing school vandalism (Feldman, Caplinger, & Wodarski, 1981). And more than one billion dollars per year is spent to maintain the juvenile justice system (Patterson, *et al*, 1989). Youth with Conduct Disorder are also one of the most frequent users of special services within social service agencies, including mental health, foster care, and special education services.

Anyone working with juvenile offenders has interacted with youth diagnosed with Conduct Disorder. These youth have often been arrested more than once and some have spent time in juvenile detention facilities on three, four or even 14 different occasions.

Juvenile justice professionals are often bewildered by some youths' lack of remorse or guilt for the damage caused to a random stranger, a neighbor or even a loved one. This can make it more difficult for staff to emotionally relate and connect with these youth—as well as see hope for positive change.

These youth often challenge the authority of juvenile justice personnel and continue to break rules, even when residing in a juvenile justice facility. They have little to no respect for authority, and the treatment programs that are effective for many juvenile offenders may have little impact on these youth. Some juveniles with Conduct Disorder have been involved with the juvenile justice system since they were very young. They are familiar with how the "system" works and often know exactly what to do and what not to do to be a "model resident." They may only receive a few sanctions while incarcerated, and some may even receive extra privileges or an early release date due to good behavior. Once these juveniles are released back in the community, however, their antisocial behavior returns; they are often aggressive, deceitful and cruel. Conversely, some juveniles with Conduct Disorder may continue to display aggressive and antisocial behavior throughout their incarceration. Such behavior typically

Juvenile Offenders with Mental Health Disorders: Who Are They and What Do We Do With Them?

results in increased sanctions, often including a loss of privileges and/or room confinement or seclusion.

Conduct Disorder is by far the most common psychiatric diagnosis given to youth who are involved with the juvenile justice system. Rates as high as 81-91 percent (Student & Myhill, 1986; Halikas, Meller, Morse, & Lyttle, 1990; Davis, Bean, Schumacher, & Stringer, 1991) of incarcerated youth have been identified as meeting diagnostic criteria for Conduct Disorder, compared to 3-9 percent (Anderson, et al., 1987; Kashani, et al., 1987) of youth in the general population. However, incarceration does not automatically imply that youth have Conduct Disorder. Youth who engage in behavior that breaks the law (i.e., commit a crime) and are arrested and processed through the juvenile court system are labeled "juvenile delinquents" or "juvenile offenders." These are legal terms. Conduct Disorder is a psychiatric term. It refers to youth who exhibit certain types of behaviors including, but not limited to, those that are against the law. Many juvenile delinquents/ juvenile offenders suffer from Conduct Disorder, particularly those with the most frequent and severe antisocial behaviors (West & Farrington, 1977). However, not all youth involved with juvenile justice are conduct-disordered.

Almost all youth engage in some behavior that is against the rules or the law. For example, lying, stealing and non-compliance are common at various points of childhood. Sixty percent of teenagers report that they have committed more than one antisocial act (e.g., vandalism, arson, drug abuse, aggression); 45 percent say they have destroyed someone's property; 50 percent have stolen something; and 35 percent have assaulted someone (Kazdin, 1994). However, most adolescents will reduce or completely stop this behavior as they age. A subset of these youth will be referred for mental health evaluation and/or treatment. Most children and adolescents do not suffer any major negative consequences as a result of briefly engaging in these antisocial behaviors. In addition, these

behaviors typically do not interfere with their ability to function within their families, school, or social environment.

Diagnostic Criteria for Conduct Disorder

According to the DSM-IV-TR (APA, 2000), youth who have Conduct Disorder have a repetitive and persistent pattern of violating the rights of others and/or violating the norms of society (antisocial behavior). These youth are often aggressive. They bully, threaten, and intimidate others in order to get what they want (e.g., money, sex, drugs). These youth often engage in physical fights with others, with and without weapons, and may be physically cruel to animals as well. Juveniles with Conduct Disorder often destroy the property or belongings of others. They may steal from stores, family members, friends, or strangers, and many have broken into schools, cars, and houses. A significant number of youth with Conduct Disorder manipulate and lie in order to get what they want, including tricking and conning others. Staying out all night, not going to school, and running away from home are common, even before the adolescent years.

Although non-conduct-disordered youth may engage in some of the above activities, the pattern of their behavior is very different. Rule-breaking behavior is often a response to specific stressors in the lives of non-conduct-disordered youth (e.g., change or problems at home or in school). Or it may be related to a desire to fit in with peers. The lawbreaking behavior of non-conduct-disordered youth typically occurs as one or a few isolated incidents. Once the stressors are resolved or peers move on to new activities, the antisocial behavior tends to diminish. In addition, youth without Conduct Disorder typically engage in only one or two types of antisocial behavior (e.g., stealing, being aggressive, setting fires, manipulating, being truant). Youth with Conduct Disorder, however, engage in antisocial behaviors repeatedly, sometimes for several years or more. Their incidents of theft and aggression are often

Oppositional Defiant Disorder and Conduct Disorder

serious and cause great suffering to those around them. They typically engage in a *variety* of antisocial behaviors in a *variety* of settings and against a *variety* of individuals. The antisocial behavior of youth with Conduct Disorder significantly interferes with their ability to function at home, school, work, and/or interpersonally. Their behavior is often serious enough that they are referred to the mental health system and/or the juvenile justice system.

Juveniles can suffer from *mild, moderate,* or *severe* forms of Conduct Disorder. This distinction is based on the number of conduct problems the youth have and how much harm other people have suffered as a result of those problems. Keeping in mind the social and economic context in which youths' behavior occurs is important. Some juveniles may engage in intimidating behavior, or take things that do not belong to them, as a means of survival in their community, neighborhood, or social environment. For these youth, antisocial behavior may actually have been adaptive in one social context, but the behavior is problematic in others. Juveniles who meet diagnostic criteria for Conduct Disorder have a *persistent pattern of antisocial behavior* that *significantly interferes* with their ability to function in their daily life.

Associated Features of Conduct Disorder

Aggression and antisocial behavior are the most common features seen among youth with Conduct Disorder. In addition, many of these youth are impulsive and restless. Learning disorders are common among youth with Conduct Disorder, with many having a difficult time reading, writing and doing mathematical calculations. These youth are often placed in special educational classes due to learning and behavioral problems. Because of their academic difficulties, school can become a frustrating place for youth with Conduct Disorder. Many experience a great deal of failure and shame. One common response to this frustration and

embarrassment is for youth to become increasingly disruptive, oppositional, and sometimes aggressive in the classroom. Another common response is to avoid the negative feelings associated with school by missing certain classes or skipping full days of school.

Because of the juveniles' often angry and oppositional behavior, teachers may not be as motivated to provide extra assistance to these juveniles. Teachers may initially try to provide aid to the youth, but after several negative interactions, these efforts are likely to decrease. Both truancy and disruptive behavior in the classroom often result in these youth being sent home from school for the day—or suspended for several days, or even weeks. Because of their academic difficulties, juveniles with Conduct Disorder often fall behind in classroom assignments, as well as homework. Being sent home from school and/or suspended typically results in these youth falling further behind academically. They may feel even more lost, confused and frustrated when they return to the classroom. This may partially explain why many youth with Conduct Disorder do not return to school and drop out of junior high or high school before graduation.

Juveniles with Conduct Disorder tend to have few to no *meaningful* relationships with youth their own age or with family members. Many of these youth never developed appropriate social skills, so they rely on intimidation, coercion, and manipulation in their interpersonal relationships. They find it hard to trust others (including juvenile justice staff and teachers), so most of their relationships are superficial.

Some youth with Conduct Disorder do have individuals whom they consider to be "friends" (usually other youth with Conduct Disorder). However, deep levels of empathy and trust are still typically limited. Many youth with Conduct Disorder are focused on getting their own needs met and have little concern for what others may want or feel. Some youth with Conduct Disorder have learned to outwardly express guilt or

Juvenile Offenders with Mental Health Disorders: Who Are They and What Do We Do With Them?

shame for their antisocial behaviors in order to avoid negative sanctions or punishment. Differentiating between when these juveniles are expressing genuine, heartfelt remorse for their behavior versus superficial, detached emotional expressions to avoid negative consequences can be difficult.

One of the reasons juveniles with Conduct Disorder have difficulties with interpersonal relationships is that they often misperceive social interactions. These youth are more likely to misperceive the intentions of peers and adults as *more* hostile and threatening than are actually true—especially in situations that are uncertain or ambiguous (Dodge, 1985). As a result, youth with Conduct Disorder often respond with aggression and feel completely justified in their behavioral response. Additionally, juveniles with Conduct Disorder are more likely to perceive their own behavior as *less* hostile and threatening than is really the case. Thus, many juveniles with Conduct Disorder continually perceive themselves as "victims" even when they have been observed aggressing against someone else.

JUVENILES WITH CONDUCT DISORDER TEND TO HAVE FEW TO NO *MEANINGFUL* RELATIONSHIPS WITH YOUTH THEIR OWN AGE OR WITH FAMILY MEMBERS.

For example, a youth with Conduct Disorder may be walking down a crowded hallway with peers when another youth accidentally bumps into him or her. The juvenile with Conduct Disorder is likely to think the other youth intentionally ran into him or her as a means of disrespect and/or intimidation. As a result, the youth with Conduct Disorder may respond with verbal aggression, and possibly physical aggression. This youth is likely to perceive his or her actions as completely reasonable given the context of the situation. Unfortunately, the recipient of the aggression is often puzzled and

caught off guard, unable to comprehend why the youth with Conduct Disorder over-reacted. Sometimes the recipient of a verbal or physical assault also has Conduct Disorder or has a tendency toward aggression. When this situation occurs, there is likely to be a physical fight, with both individuals at risk for injury. Not surprisingly, this situation is not unusual in juvenile justice facilities, due to the high numbers of youth with Conduct Disorder involved in the juvenile justice system.

Youth with Conduct Disorder are less likely to defer to, and behave politely with authority figures such as parents, teachers, police officers, and juvenile justice professionals. They can be rude and oppositional, and most individuals (adults and same-aged peers) do not seek them out to spend time with them. The youths' negative behavior can result in the youth being socially isolated and without models for healthy behavior. Juveniles with Conduct Disorder often brag about themselves and may be vulgar or sarcastic to those around them. It is not unusual for these youth to be socially rejected by non-conduct-disordered peers in their school or community. This rejection may partially explain why juveniles with Conduct Disorder tend to "hang out" together, regardless of the social context. Many youth with Conduct Disorder have never learned how to interact appropriately with others. They have difficulty understanding how those around them feel, and they are often unaware of how their aggressive or oppositional behavior affects the people in their lives. These youth also have a limited repertoire of behaviors to use in interpersonal situations. When faced with problems in social relationships, juveniles with Conduct Disorder typically over-rely on what they know best: manipulation, lying, intimidating, and coercing. Alternative ways of dealing with situations may not even come to mind.

It is common for juvenile offenders with Conduct Disorder to misperceive the intent of others. For example, when juvenile justice staff provide a standard directive or command to

Oppositional Defiant Disorder and Conduct Disorder

juveniles with Conduct Disorder, the youth may perceive it as a direct personal attack. These youth often view juvenile justice professionals as having hostile and threatening motives, and perceive much of staff behavior in that context. Juvenile justice professionals are often perplexed by what appears to be an inappropriate and angry response from youth after fairly neutral requests are made of them.

Juveniles with Conduct Disorder also tend to have difficulty regulating their anger. They are often irritable and easily agitated. Due to their low frustration tolerance (insistence on having their needs met immediately), these youth may engage in temper tantrums and/or explosive angry outbursts. Sometimes these angry outbursts are in response to something that appears minor or trivial to, observers . Oftentimes, it is the juveniles' responses to not getting what they want at the time they want it.

Although they appear to be strong and tough in the way they present themselves to the outside world, many youth with Conduct Disorder experience feelings of low self-esteem. In addition, some of these youth have feelings of fear and anxiety that they are trying to contain. They may be confident about their behaviors related to delinquent activities, their ability to intimidate others, and other antisocial behavior. However, youth with Conduct Disorder often experience feelings of low self-worth in relation to more prosocial activities and behaviors related to school, work, family, and interpersonal relationships.

There are some gender differences among juveniles with Conduct Disorder. This disorder is more common in males than females, particularly in childhood versus adolescence. Males with Conduct Disorder tend to be more confrontational and outwardly aggressive toward others. Males are also more likely to participate in physical fights, steal from individuals or businesses, display disruptive behavior in school, and vandalize property. On the other hand, females are more likely to engage in antisocial behaviors that are less confrontational. They

may run away from home, skip school, engage in drug use, and participate in prostitution.

Alcohol and drug use are common among youth with Conduct Disorder. For some of these youth, substance use precedes their antisocial behavior, while others initiate drug and alcohol use subsequent to their antisocial behavior. Substance use can lower juveniles' inhibitions, which can increase the likelihood they will engage in a variety of negative behaviors.

Because many youth with Conduct Disorder are impulsive, they frequently engage in high-risk behavior. Unprotected sex is common among these youth. Males with Conduct Disorder are often unselective regarding sexual partners and may use manipulation and/or coercion in order to engage in sexual activities. Females with Conduct Disorder are often sexually promiscuous, and they may engage in prostitution. The behavior of both genders is likely to result in the juveniles obtaining sexually transmitted diseases and experiencing unplanned pregnancies. The risk-taking behavior of juveniles with Conduct Disorder can also result in significant physical injury from automobile or other types of accidents, as well as physical fights.

Developmental Course of Conduct Disorder

Although the developmental course of Conduct Disorder is variable, almost all youth begin to exhibit the disorder before the age of 16. Some youth may display oppositional and aggressive behaviors as early as preschool or kindergarten. But most youth with Conduct Disorder begin exhibiting conduct problems during late childhood or early adolescence. The frequency and severity of behaviors associated with Conduct Disorder typically increases throughout the teenage years. This increase is probably due to the expanded opportunities afforded to adolescents, as well as the cognitive and physical changes that occur during this period of development. However, there is a subset of youth with Conduct Disorder—typically those with

Juvenile Offenders with Mental Health Disorders: Who Are They and What Do We Do With Them?

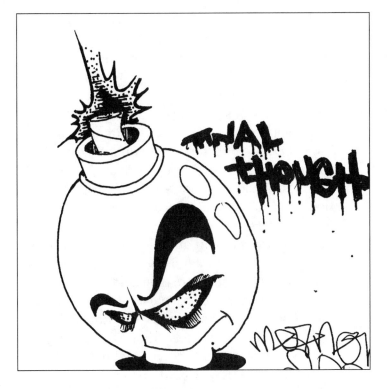

severe symptoms—who engage in very dangerous and aggressive behaviors even at a very young age. Some youth with Conduct Disorder will lead productive lives and show few, if any, antisocial behaviors during adulthood. But, a significant portion will continue engaging in behaviors that violate the rights of others and/or are in conflict with the norms of society. Once they reach 18 years of age, youth belonging to this group will likely meet diagnostic criteria for Antisocial Personality Disorder. These adults are manipulative, deceitful, and often cause significant harm to others due to their disregard for, and violation of, the rights of other people.

Juveniles whose Conduct Disorder began at the age of 10 years or younger tend to have significantly more difficulties in life than youth who develop the disorder during adolescence. These youth are typically male, more aggressive, have more interpersonal problems, and are more likely to manifest an Antisocial Personality Disorder as they age. Youth with an *early onset* of Conduct Disorder also tend to be more impulsive and have more problems with school.

Compared to youth whose Conduct Disorder began after the age of 10, as these juveniles get older, they are more likely to have continued problems in their relationships with others, difficulties with work, and greater use of alcohol and other drugs. Juveniles whose Conduct Disorder became evident during the adolescent years are more likely to engage in *delinquent* activities versus *aggressive* behaviors. Their antisocial behavior is typically not as serious or frequent as those with an earlier onset, and treatment interventions are more likely to be effective (Alexander & Barton, 1995; Kazdin, Siegel, & Bass, 1992).

Conduct Disorder tends to be stable over time (Loeber, 1991), particularly if youth have an early onset and engage in a variety of antisocial behaviors. This behavior is not only likely to endure throughout the juveniles' entire lives but also likely to affect their own children. Youth diagnosed with Conduct Disorder in childhood have a higher chance of raising children who display similar behavior. Even grandchildren are at a higher risk of displaying antisocial behavior if their grandparents did (Glueck & Glueck, 1968). Youth with severe Conduct Disorder typically experience a variety of problems and difficulties in many areas of their adult lives. As adults, they are more likely to physically abuse their spouses and/or children and drive under the influence of alcohol (Kazdin, 1989). All juveniles with Conduct Disorder are at increased risk for developing other mental health disorders as well. Aggression is one of the most stable personality traits (remains constant throughout individuals' lives), and antisocial behavior often continues into adulthood (Olweus, 1979). Therefore, viewing severe cases of Conduct Disorder as *chronic* conditions that will require long-term treatment services can be helpful.

Co-Existing Mental Health Disorders

Many youth in the juvenile justice system with

Oppositional Defiant Disorder and Conduct Disorder

Conduct Disorder meet diagnostic criteria for another psychiatric disorder(s) as well. Attention-Deficit/Hyperactivity Disorder (ADHD) is very common among youth with Conduct Disorder, and juveniles who have both ADHD and Conduct Disorder have significant adjustment problems. These youth have more academic difficulties, lower intelligence, and more problems within their families than youth who have only one of these mental health disorders (Moffitt, 1990). In addition, many juvenile offenders with Conduct Disorder also suffer from Major Depression, Dysthymic Disorder, Posttraumatic Stress Disorder, learning disorders, and/or substance abuse disorders. A number of youth diagnosed with Conduct Disorder suffer from hallucinations, delusions, and/or neurological problems, although these symptoms may be overlooked or misidentified (Lewis, Lewis, Unger & Goldman, 1984). And assaultive youth are at higher risk of suicide than nonassaultive youth (Cairns, Peterson, & Neckerman, 1988). Too often, medical, mental health, juvenile court, and juvenile justice facility personnel narrowly focus on youths' aggressive and delinquent behavior. This focus typically results in continuous referrals made to the juvenile justice system and these youth not receiving appropriate—and much needed—mental health assessment and treatment services.

What Causes Conduct Disorder?

Conduct Disorder is a very heterogeneous disorder, and youth with this diagnosis can behave very differently. Some youth with Conduct Disorder may have written graffiti on private property and been truant at school, while others may have raped and murdered. Just as there is no "typical" youth with Conduct Disorder, there is no single *cause* of this very complex disorder. However, a variety of risk factors are typically associated with Conduct Disorder. When a number of these risk factors occur together, the likely result is a juvenile who repeatedly breaks rules and laws, and who

violates the rights of others around him or her. Most of what is known about Conduct Disorder is associated with male juveniles with the disorder; much less is known about females with Conduct Disorder.

A variety of social/environmental factors are also associated with Conduct Disorder. One of the strongest predictors of Conduct Disorder is a parent who is abusive and physically harmful to his or her child. Conflict within a marital relationship and parental substance abuse and/or mental illness are also significantly related to juvenile development of Conduct Disorder. The same is true of parental neglect and multiple placements in foster care (Alexander & Pugh, 1996). Some juveniles have been left alone with few to no rules and as a result, continually have engaged in unsupervised activities. Spending time with peers who engage in delinquent activities is strongly related to youth development of Conduct Disorder. When youth are not supervised, there is no one to direct them away from deviant and antisocial peers. Youth who have intellectual difficulties and/or speech and language problems are also at risk for Conduct Disorder, as are youth with chronic physical illnesses. For juveniles who already have some of the above risk and social/environmental factors for Conduct Disorder, unsupervised viewing of violence (real-life or televised) can also result in violent behavior (Murray, 1980).

Conduct Disorder appears to have at least some biological component. Heredity likely plays a role, but exactly how and what is inherited is not yet clear. If biological parents display aggressive and antisocial behavior, there is an increased likelihood their children will display aggressive and antisocial behavior as well. This situation is also true if adoptive parents are antisocial, but the effects are lessened (Kazdin, 1989). This finding implies that there is at least some genetic component to the disorder but that environmental effects of parental modeling are also important. Juveniles are also at higher risk for Conduct Disorder if they have a sibling who has Conduct Disorder. Biological abnor-

44

Juvenile Offenders with Mental Health Disorders: Who Are They and What Do We Do With Them?

malities (*e.g.*, in the brain and central nervous system) have been found in some youth that have Conduct Disorder. These abnormalities may be due to exposure to toxins (*e.g.*, lead) in early childhood. Or, because the majority of juveniles with Conduct Disorder have experienced verbal, emotional, and/or physical abuse as children, the biological differences may be a result of emotional trauma. More violent juvenile offenders tend to have had higher rates of birth complications (*e.g.*, premature birth, lack of oxygen to the brain) and abusive trauma to the head and face (Lewis, Shanok, & Balla, 1979).

It is probably the combination of environmental factors and genetic influences that results in the juvenile development of patterns of behavior consistent with Conduct Disorder. The disorder is not necessarily due to "bad" parenting and blaming parents is not helpful. Some parents are unable to provide what their children need for a variety of reasons including, but not limited to:

- Parental mental illness
- Parental substance abuse
- Significant social stressors (*e.g.*, poverty, unemployment, lack of stable residence)
- Never learning how to parent effectively

In addition, some juveniles with Conduct Disorder were moody and irritable from the day they were born, as well as throughout their infancy. Many of these youth do not feel easily soothed by their parents. In fact, some infants even dislike being touched or held by anyone, including their mother. The interaction between parent and child typically flows two ways, with each party influencing the behavior of the other.

Youth with Conduct Disorder can *learn* to use aggression and antisocial behavior in a variety of ways. If they receive inconsistent or harsh discipline from parents, these juveniles are more likely to develop maladaptive ways of interacting within their own families. Some families unwittingly reward aggressive behavior by paying attention to youth or giving youth

what they want when they become angry or loud. These families may not pay much attention to youth when they are behaving quietly or asking for things politely. In some families, intimidation and coercion are the typical way family members interact with each other.

Many youth diagnosed with Conduct Disorder have lived in various out-of-home placements (*e.g.*, foster care, group homes) during their formative years, sometimes with loving adults, sometimes with abusive ones. Some juveniles have run away or been thrown out of their family home and forced to live on the streets at a young age. These youth may have learned to use antisocial behaviors as a means to survive on their own. Running away from home is not always an act of defiance; some juveniles are attempting to escape an intolerable situation, such as physical and/or sexual abuse (Boesky, Toro, Wright, & Wolfe, 1997).

If they learn that aggression is an effective way to get their needs met within their families, juveniles may never learn prosocial ways of interacting with others. Using the same aggressive strategies in a classroom or with non-aggressive peers is likely to result in negative consequences. Rejection by nonaggressive peers is common among juveniles with Conduct Disorder because most youth do not want to spend time with peers who are intimidating, aggressive or manipulative. Youth with Conduct Disorder are likely to seek out peers who behave similarly to themselves (*e.g.*, delinquent, aggressive). As these antisocial youth continue to interact with each other in negative ways, their behavior becomes further ingrained.

Conduct Disorder can develop in a variety of ways; it is a very heterogeneous disorder with several different causes. The circumstances of youth with Conduct Disorder differ due to the variability in youths' biological make-up and the social context in which they were raised. Environmental factors play a large role in the development and maintenance of this disorder. Therefore, viewing Conduct Disorder as an underlying mental illness intrinsic to individual

Oppositional Defiant Disorder and Conduct Disorder

youth is misleading. Such a view typically results in intervention services provided solely to juveniles for *their* problem. Risk factors for Conduct Disorder are related to family interaction patterns, academic achievement, peer relationships, and the like. Thus, family members, school personnel, peers, and individuals from any other relevant systems should be involved in intervention strategies with juveniles diagnosed with Conduct Disorder.

Management of Juvenile Offenders with Conduct Disorder

Because Conduct Disorder is a complex and challenging disorder, it requires long-term treatment interventions. There are no short-term "cures" for juvenile offenders with Conduct Disorder. Many programs and therapeutic modalities that have attempted to intervene with youth suffering from Conduct Disorder have been unsuccessful. This is particularly true for conduct-disordered youth once they reach their adolescent years and/or those suffering from severe Conduct Disorder. Some mental health and juvenile justice professionals have reached the conclusion that youth with Conduct Disorder are *untreatable.* However, in recent years, new intervention strategies and programs have been developed that have shown some success with this very difficult to treat population of youth (Henggeler, Melton, & Smith, 1992; Henggeler, Schoenwald, Rowland, Borduin, & Cunningham, 1998).

Because conduct-disordered youth typically exhibit multiple behavior problems in different settings and with a variety of individuals, effective treatment strategies must intervene in each of these areas. Recently developed treatment strategies for these youth take into account the multi-determined nature of this syndrome. Interventions focus on the primary areas within the youths' life, including family, school, peers, and community, and target factors associated with the development of Conduct Disorder. Treatment plans are individualized for youth and their families.

Intervention strategies emphasize empowering parents and helping them develop more effective child-rearing strategies with their children. All of the systems and agencies with which a juvenile is involved (*e.g.*, mental health, juvenile justice, education, child welfare) coordinate and collaborate with each other in order to provide integrated treatment services. The good news is that most of these interventions can be delivered on an outpatient basis in the youths' community, and often in the youths' home. These programs have been used with juvenile offenders with Conduct Disorder. They are cost-efficient and show positive outcomes related to:

- Decreased criminal activity
- Decreased aggression
- Decreased substance abuse
- Increased feelings of family closeness

The bad news is that most of these interventions are difficult to deliver within a juvenile justice facility given the current level of resources of most juvenile justice agencies. In addition, some youth are unable to benefit from these interventions in the community due to an unwilling parent or adult surrogate. Many of these new treatment programs for youth with Conduct Disorder are time-intensive, staff-intensive, and require specialized training of staff.

Youth with Conduct Disorder typically experience difficulties related to aggression, family relations, school, and interpersonal relationships with peers. Therefore, a comprehensive intervention strategy is needed to have a significant impact on these youths' behavior. Given the large numbers of youth in the juvenile justice system diagnosed with Conduct Disorder—as well as current funding levels of the system—this type of comprehensive intervention has not been undertaken on a widespread basis. However, some states, counties, and cities have begun to implement all or some of the components of these multisystemic interventions for a subset of their juvenile

Juvenile Offenders with Mental Health Disorders: Who Are They and What Do We Do With Them?

offenders. This has occurred more often for youth on probation or parole.

Sometimes the experience of being detained in a juvenile justice facility, and the fear associated with it, can decrease future antisocial behavior. This response, however, is most common among youth with a very mild case of Conduct Disorder. Juvenile offenders with mild, moderate, and severe Conduct Disorder can take advantage of the "rehabilitation" services offered at many juvenile justice facilities throughout the country. Although most juvenile justice facilities do not offer extensive treatment programs, many offer rehabilitation groups such as anger management, conflict resolution and victim empathy. Attempts are made to teach juvenile offenders new ways to think about their antisocial behavior, as well as develop new skills to help them participate in prosocial activities

Most juvenile justice facilities do not have the resources to provide comprehensive *treatment* services to all youth with Conduct Disorder residing in their facilities. However, there are still many strategies available to effectively *manage* juvenile offenders with Conduct Disorder while they are under juvenile justice supervision. These strategies should not be viewed as an attempt to "cure" or eradicate all of youths' antisocial attitudes or delinquent behavior.

Instead, the strategies can serve as a first step toward positive behavior change and the development of more adaptive and prosocial skills. This step can significantly influence youths' future behavior and how they view themselves and others. The step can also prepare the youth to participate in community-based interventions. Within juvenile justice facilities, such management strategies can help staff maintain a safer living unit, as well as a more enjoyable working environment.

Increasing juveniles' success in daily activities, as well as reducing aggression and antisocial behavior, are primary goals of managing juvenile offenders with Conduct Disorder. Although these strategies may help youth

decrease their delinquent behavior once they return to the community, there is no guarantee that this will occur. Eradicating delinquent behavior requires an intensive and comprehensive set of interventions. Juvenile justice professionals should keep this point in mind when they work with juveniles with Conduct Disorder. This will help to minimize frustration among youth, as well as the staff.

The following strategies are important for staff to consider when they are working with juveniles who have Conduct Disorder.

ASKING THE QUESTION: WHAT ELSE IS GOING ON?

Given the complex clinical pictures commonly observed among juvenile offenders, the question *What else is going on?* should always be asked if youth are solely assigned the diagnosis of Conduct Disorder. Many youth diagnosed with Conduct Disorder also suffer from Attention-Deficit/Hyperactivity Disorder, Major Depression, Posttraumatic Stress Disorder, learning disorders, substance abuse disorders, as well as other mental health disorders. With regard to juvenile offenders in particular, having another mental health disorder co-exist with Conduct Disorder is often the rule rather than the exception.

Attributing offenders' aggression and disruptive behavior solely to Conduct Disorder without considering the co-existence of additional mental health disorders can be a disservice to youth. Such a limited diagnosis can prevent them from obtaining mental health services they need. Youth displaying *significant* aggressive and/or oppositional behavior should be referred to mental health/health professionals. Providing comprehensive evaluations in order to rule out all possible psychiatric illnesses that may account for these youths' negative behavior is critical. Due to the often disruptive and dangerous behaviors of youth with Conduct Disorder, serious symptoms of other mental health disorders are frequently overlooked. When these juveniles are accurately diagnosed, appropriate treatment services can be provided, decreasing the likelihood of aggression and antisocial behavior.

SUPERVISING PEER ACTIVITIES

Research has shown that association with deviant and antisocial peers increases antisocial behavior, especially in the early adolescent years (Lipsey & Derzon, 1998). Juveniles with Conduct Disorder tend to socialize with other juveniles with Conduct Disorder. Antisocial attitudes and behaviors can become further embedded as they are accepted and reinforced by young offenders' social group. Research has shown that peer-group intervention with adolescents can actually *increase* youths' delinquency, substance use and violence. This type of "deviancy training" is particularly true for juveniles who have poor interpersonal relationships and who have already engaged in at least moderate levels of delinquent behavior (Dishion, McCord and Poulin, 1999).

Juvenile justice professionals should assign activities or tasks that can be done in pairs or groups, while placing conduct-disordered youth with peers with whom they do not typically "hang out." This way, youth with Conduct Disorder can be exposed to alternative (and more prosocial) ways of thinking and behaving. The goal is to provide these juveniles with opportunities to interact with less aggressive individuals whose lifestyles are less delinquent and more adaptive.

One of the unfortunate effects of incarceration is that youth with mild Conduct Disorder typically reside with youth who have more serious and dangerous antisocial attitudes and behaviors. Youth who do not have significant behavioral problems may adopt some of the antisocial behavior and attitudes of youth who are seriously conduct-disordered. To the extent possible, juvenile justice professionals should closely supervise juvenile offenders as they interact with each other, to decrease the number of discussions about criminal activities or maladaptive behaviors.

In addition, youth who already have risk factors for Conduct Disorder are more likely to display aggressive behavior after viewing violence, whether in real life or televised (Murray, 1980; Offord, 1989). Most juvenile offenders have several risk factors for Conduct Disorder or already suffer from the disorder. Therefore, juvenile justice professionals should carefully select, and then monitor, the television programs and video rentals the juveniles are viewing.

REMOVING FROM SOCIAL ENVIRONMENT

Some juvenile offenders with Conduct Disorder engage in behavior that is so dangerous, they cannot be in close proximity to peers, teachers, or juvenile justice professionals. These youth may be so aggressive that they continually destroy property or assault others in the living unit or in the classroom. If juveniles are unable to control their aggressive behavior, they may need to be removed from the social environment for a *temporary* period of time. This action protects the rest of the group from being injured, and can be done in a variety of ways. A teacher may request that juveniles leave the school area and return to their living unit. Youth may be removed from a group activity in the living unit or a recreational activity in the gymnasium and placed in their room. Or youth may be physically escorted to a locked room with little to nothing in it in a living unit or in another location (*e.g.*, isolation room, seclusion room, quiet room).

Placing youth in a room that is away from social reinforcement for a short period of time can serve a variety of purposes. This practice allows youth a quiet space with no one around so that they can calm themselves down. Some juveniles with Conduct Disorder have difficulty regulating their anger. They may need several minutes or hours before they are calm enough to return to a living unit or classroom to interact with others. Removing youth from their social environment can also provide juvenile justice professionals, teachers or peers a period of time

Juvenile Offenders with Mental Health Disorders: Who Are They and What Do We Do With Them?

to calm themselves down as well. This break period may be especially necessary if the incident preceding the "time-out" response was severe. Most incidents of seclusion involve a small subset of juveniles with serious behavior problems. Youth suffering from the co-existing disorders of Conduct Disorder and ADHD often have the highest rates of time-out or seclusion (Atkins & Ricciuti, 1992).

Placing youth in time-out or seclusion (whether in their own room or a room designed

---

SOME JUVENILE OffENDERS WITH CONDUCT DISORDER ENGAGE IN bEHAVIOR THAT IS SO dANGEROUS, THEY CANNOT bE IN CLOSE PROXIMITY TO PEERS, TEACHERS, OR JUVENILE JUSTICE PROFESSIONALS.

---

particularly for the purpose of behavioral control) is not intended to cause *suffering* for the youth. This strategy is designed to help juveniles regain control of their emotions, particularly their anger, and their behavior. As soon as youth appear calm, staff should talk with them about the incident and discuss what the youth would do differently the next time they are in a similar situation. Youth then should be removed from the room and allowed to return to the group. Juveniles should never be isolated and/or secluded for prolonged periods of time.

Various mental and behavioral disturbances can be created if juvenile offenders are isolated for a significant period of time (*e.g.*, aggression, impulsivity, paranoia, mood disturbances; Mitchell & Varley, 1990). Juvenile justice professionals should make repeated attempts to assess whether youth have met the criteria for returning to the group. In addition, peers and staff members should not be allowed to distract or provoke youth during this "time-out" period. Staff should speak to these juveniles in a "matter of fact" tone, repeatedly assessing whether the youth are able to move to a less restrictive environment.

In rare instances, isolating an out-of-control youth with Conduct Disorder may not be enough to contain their behavior. Some juvenile justice facilities use mechanical restraints/ therapeutic restraints to further calm youth or prevent injury to them or those around them. Juveniles should never be placed in restraints for the purpose of discipline/punishment, and restraints should only be used when less restrictive interventions have proved ineffective. It is recommended that restraints be made of fleece-lined leather, canvas or rubber. Because serious injuries can occur with the improper use of restraints, juvenile justice professionals should be thoroughly trained in how to use them. Placing youth in restraints should require approval from administration (*i.e.*, superintendent/director or designee) and a qualified health care authority. Due to the potential negative physical and psychological effects of restraints, health and mental health professionals should assess restrained juveniles' physical and psychological condition. Medical and mental health authorities should also advise whether restrained youth should be transferred to a medical/mental health facility for emergency treatment. If restrained youth remain in a juvenile justice facility, they should be under continuous visual observation by appropriately trained juvenile justice staff. Specific and individualized plans should be developed for each youth in relation to releasing them from restraints as soon as possible. Many juvenile justice facilities are able to manage juvenile offenders in their facilities effectively without using restraints, or using them in very limited ways. Therefore, this type of management strategy is not recommended (Mitchell & Varley, 1990). (Please see Chapter 16 for additional information on seclusion and restraint.)

COMMUNICATING WITH SCHOOL/ VOCATIONAL PERSONNEL

Because low academic achievement is significantly related to antisocial behavior, educational involvement should be emphasized with juve-

Oppositional Defiant Disorder and Conduct Disorder

niles who have Conduct Disorder. Many juvenile offenders with Conduct Disorder suffer from learning disorders in reading, writing and/or mathematics. These youth have often had very negative academic experiences and many have dropped out of school. Oppositional and disruptive behavior in the classroom can keep the focus off youths' learning problems and instead place it on their behavioral difficulties. Because of this, many conduct-disordered youth with learning disorders have never received any type of tutoring or academic remediation. Those who have been placed in Special Education classes often were placed there because of unmanageable behavior versus learning difficulties. While incarcerated, juveniles with Conduct Disorder may have no motivation to attend the available school services. Receiving a high school diploma or a GED may be of no interest to them. Unfortunately, academic underachievement can have long-term consequences, making it much more difficult for youth to find quality employment when they return to the community.

To help them develop prosocial skills, juvenile offenders with Conduct Disorder should be encouraged to attend academic classes or some type of vocational training. Tutoring may be needed in one or several subject areas. Attempts should be made to discover what topics are of most interest to youth, and identified topics should be incorporated into classroom and homework assignments. A primary educational goal is to motivate juveniles to participate in academic studies. Doing so can help youth develop important skills for functioning in the community. If juveniles neither work nor attend educational classes upon release, they will be left with an excessive amount of free time on their hands. This idleness often leads to feelings of boredom and a search for adventure and excitement. Such youth are likely to occupy their time engaging in delinquent and antisocial activities.

Incarceration can provide one of the best opportunities for youth with Conduct Disorder

to become reacquainted with education. Smaller classrooms, more individualized instruction, and a drug-free environment often helps motivate these youth to learn. This is particularly true for youth who have already dropped out of school in the community. Many youth with Conduct Disorder have significantly raised their academic skills while residing in long-term juvenile justice facilities. A considerable number of these youth receive high school diplomas or GEDs each year. These accomplishments are important factors for increasing youths' chances for positive adjustment once they are released back into the community.

Juvenile justice professionals should be in communication with school teachers/vocational training supervisors regarding the behavior of juveniles with Conduct Disorder. All professionals working with these youth should communicate with each other regarding effective and ineffective management strategies—what is and is not working with particular youth.

When supervising juveniles with Conduct Disorder who are aggressive, juvenile justice professionals and teachers/vocational supervisors should agree upon a consistent way of responding when youth become hostile or disruptive. It is best when selected responses are agreed upon *before* youths engage in negative behavior so that consequences are swift and clear. In addition, all adults working with conduct-disordered youth should emphasize the juveniles' strengths and communicate with each other when youth demonstrate appropriate and constructive behavior (versus only problematic behavior). Managing youth with severe Conduct Disorder can be extremely frustrating, and juvenile justice professionals may find it helpful to talk with others who have worked with the same youth. These individuals can often empathize and offer suggestions about possible management strategies that have been effective in the past. Many teachers within juvenile justice facilities have been specifically trained to work with youth who exhibit behavior problems and learning disabilities. Rather than reinvent-

50

Juvenile Offenders with Mental Health Disorders: Who Are They and What Do We Do With Them?

ing the wheel, juvenile justice professionals and teachers should work together to creatively manage this often difficult-to-supervise population of youth

PROVIDING PSYCHOTROPIC MEDICATION
Medication is not typically prescribed for the treatment of Conduct Disorder because there has not been one class of medication shown to be particularly beneficial. If youth with Conduct Disorder are prescribed psychotropic medication, it is typically prescribed for the symptoms of a co-existing disorder. Psychostimulants (*e.g.*, Ritalin®, Dexedrine®, Adderall®) can be prescribed for concurrent problems with impulsivity and hyperactivity. An antidepressant (*e.g.*, Prozac®, Zoloft®, Tofranil®, Wellbutrin®) or mood stabilizer (*e.g.*, Depakote®, Lithium®, Tegretol®) may be prescribed if youth with Conduct Disorder are also experiencing feelings of depression or an extremely agitated, irritable mood. Mood stabilizers may also be prescribed if these juveniles' behavior is out of control and/or very aggressive. Medication can help youth with a co-existing mental health disorder, making it more likely they will be able to participate and benefit from the intervention strategies specifically designed to address conduct problems.

A small subset of youth with severe Conduct Disorder may be so out of control and dangerous that they are prescribed antipsychotic medication (*e.g.*, Risperidal®, Zyprexa®, Haldol®, Thorazine®). These medications can have a strong sedating effect, which may be necessary in short-term/acute situations. Sometimes, this type of medication is prescribed for longer periods of time if youth with Conduct Disorder are chronically agitated. For example, long-term medication may be prescribed when youths' seriously aggressive behavior cannot be completely managed by behavioral strategies. Antipsychotic medication may also be prescribed for youth with Conduct Disorder if they are experiencing strange or bizarre thoughts and/or exhibiting strange or bizarre behavior. Caution should always be used with antipsy-

chotic medication, especially in a juvenile population. This type of medication can have profound and serious side effects.

Several variables should be present before medication is prescribed to youth with Conduct Disorder, if the primary goal is to treat symptoms of that particular disorder:

- Youths' aggressive behavior should be severe and occur over a significant period of time
- A highly structured environment and behavior management strategies have not been effective in decreasing the youths' aggression
- Youths' aggressive behavior has serious negative implications for either the juveniles or those who come into contact with them
- Youth are willing to take the medication consistently as prescribed

Many juvenile offenders with Conduct Disorder are resistant to taking psychotropic medication due to the negative stigma often associated with it. They do not want to be perceived as "crazy" or "mental." Because of the high rate of substance abuse among youth with Conduct Disorder, caution should be taken when psychotropic medication (*e.g.*, Ritalin®, sleep medication) is prescribed for them. These youth may abuse the medication themselves or sell/trade the medication to peers.

DEVELOPING SKILLS

Anger Management/Interpersonal Problem-Solving Training
Because many juveniles with Conduct Disorder have difficulty controlling their anger, they often become aggressive toward others. *Anger management* programs can help youth develop or increase their anger management skills. A variety of programs have been designed for this purpose (Cullen and Wright, 1996; Goldstein & Glick, 1994; Weisinger, 1985), and some have shown positive effects when delivered in a juvenile justice setting (Goldstein, Glick, Reiner,

Zimmerman, & Coultry, 1986). Anger management programs can be provided in an individual or group format.

Most programs of this type spend some time educating young offenders about the biological factors underlying their anger. Such knowledge helps juveniles identify the bodily cues that can alert them when they are beginning to get angry. Regaining control of their anger at the trigger point is easier than when they are already "worked up." Some programs use relaxation and visualization exercises as well.

The way juvenile offenders perceive a situation is often more important than the situation itself. Because youth with Conduct Disorder often interpret neutral or ambiguous situations as hostile (Dodge, 1985), they tend to behave aggressively in order to protect themselves. In addition, when these youth find themselves in problematic and/or conflicted social situations, they are often limited in the number of solutions they generate. They often rely on aggression, coercion, and manipulation to deal with conflict. A primary focus of anger management training is to teach youth adaptive problem-solving skills to use in interpersonal situations—instead of relying on the antisocial tactics they have always used. Youth are taught to identify situations in which they typically become verbally and/or physically assaultive and instructed on how to use prosocial skills when coping with those situations.

Youths' beliefs about anger affect how they react towards others, so identifying what types of things juveniles say to themselves when they become angry or aggressive is important. For example, many juveniles with Conduct Disorder believe engaging in antisocial behavior (*e.g.*, lying, stealing, using aggression) is the only way to get their needs met.

Because of their attributional bias (*i.e.*, perceiving others intentions as more hostile than they really are), many of these youth say to themselves: "He is trying to disrespect me," "I cannot show weakness, no matter what," or "They are a threat to me and I need to protect

A PRIMARY FOCUS OF ANGER MANAGEMENT TRAINING IS TO TEACH YOUTH ADAPTIVE PROBLEM-SOLVING SKILLS TO USE IN INTERPERSONAL SITUATIONS—INSTEAD OF . . . ANTISOCIAL TACTICS . . . .

myself, no matter what the cost." In anger management training, young offenders are taught that when they are being provoked or feeling angry, they should pay attention to their thoughts. Teaching juveniles with Conduct Disorder to use new self-statements such as "Hitting him isn't worth losing all my free time," "That punk isn't worth my time and energy," "Even if it feels like I am going to explode—I won't," can be helpful. Youth with Conduct Disorder are also taught to use behaviors other than verbal and physical aggression when they are angry: walking away from a situation, ignoring a provoking peer, taking deep breaths while counting to ten, and so forth.

Anger management programs are only effective if juveniles learn specific, practical skills to use in situations where they are likely to become angry. Program leaders (*e.g.*, juvenile justice professionals, mental health/health professionals) should not only *talk* about new skills but also *model* appropriate responses, as well as participate in role-playing with youth. During role-playing, adults and peers typically provide feedback regarding what youth are doing well and where they need improvement. Role-playing provides an opportunity for juveniles to portray themselves and practice newly learned anger management skills in a non-threatening environment. In addition, when peers or adults play the role of juveniles with Conduct Disorder, the youth experience first-hand how their anger affects those around them.

Many anger management programs have been criticized for being unrealistic and contrived, especially when working with juveniles who have severe conduct and anger control

52

Juvenile Offenders with Mental Health Disorders: Who Are They and What Do We Do With Them?

problems. Making the training applicable to the social context in which youth interact is critical. "Walking away" from an enemy may be viewed as weak and unworthy of respect for some youth involved in gang activity. This action can lead to the youths' enemies "jumping" the youth at a later time. Juveniles with Conduct Disorder may not be able to "ignore" peers' provocative behavior if peers hit them or have a weapon. Therefore, providing realistic scenarios from juveniles' own lives, as well as problematic situations they are anticipating in the future is essential.

For many juveniles with Conduct Disorder, anger is a large part of their self-identity—of how they view themselves. Many of these youth grew up in environments where they felt powerless and out of control. Their anger provides them with a sense of strength, authority, and power. As a result, these juveniles are often *attached* to their anger and not motivated to give it up. Many of them cannot remember an age that they were *not* angry. Their anger may even have been adaptive in the past given the youths' families, neighborhoods, schools, or communities. Juveniles with Conduct Disorder often fear that they would be weak and vulnerable if they were to give up their anger. Leaders of anger management programs should discuss these issues explicitly with youth who have Conduct Disorder at the beginning of the intervention—otherwise, motivation to participate in the program is likely to be low.

Even when all of the above issues are taken into account, instilling long-term positive change related to youths' anger and aggression is still difficult when working with youth who have Conduct Disorder. This is particularly true for those with moderate to severe difficulties. Many juveniles are able to learn new anger management skills and demonstrate them while under juvenile justice supervision. However, retaining these new ways of thinking and behaving upon returning to the community (and interacting with their families and peers again) is more difficult. Old habits die hard.

Basic Social Skills Training

Juveniles with Conduct Disorder often threaten, force or manipulate others in order to get what they need. This behavior tends to be their primary mode of interaction with family members, peers, and teachers. Many youth with Conduct Disorder are deficient in positive and prosocial ways of interacting with others. Some of these juveniles may never have learned how to achieve goals in an adaptive and legitimate manner because they were raised by parents who also have Conduct Disorder. Social skills training attempts to teach youth, in a concrete and practical manner, the interpersonal skills needed for everyday living. Depending on how they were raised, some youth will experience this type of training as a re-education process, while others will be learning the skills for the first time.

Social skills training can encompass a wide range of skills needed to interact effectively with others, and it can be provided in an individual or group format. Some youth with Conduct Disorder need to begin with very basic skills, such as social participation skills (*e.g.*, how to initiate a conversation, how to enter a group of peers). Many juveniles with Conduct Disorder are limited regarding what topics they discuss, and conversations with peers usually revolve around delinquent activity or drug use. Boasting and bragging are common. These youth need practice talking about other areas of their lives and other interests. Skills related to conflict resolution, effective negotiation, and compromise are often lacking and can be addressed by this type of training. Youth with Conduct Disorder often need to be taught:

- How to accurately read other people's body language

- How to listen to others

- How to communicate in a "give and take" manner, instead of monopolizing conversations

Social skills training should include a variety of techniques (Sarason & Ganzer, 1969). Program leaders (juvenile justice professionals, mental health/health professionals) should always model the appropriate way of behaving for youth. Role-playing is effective in having juveniles try out new social behaviors that may initially feel foreign and uncomfortable. During role-playing, adults (or peers, if applicable) should provide specific feedback to youth with Conduct Disorder regarding areas in which improvement is needed. Feedback also should be provided when youth are able to demonstrate appropriate new skills. Youth should be encouraged to practice their newly learned social skills with peers and juvenile justice professionals in between formal training sessions. It is not enough for staff to formally role-play appropriate social behavior with conduct-disordered youth. Staff should always model prosocial skills during their day-to-day interactions with these youth.

For this type of training to be successful, the skills being taught must take into account juveniles' social environment. Describing their current interpersonal relationships and providing examples of "typical" social interactions is important for the youth. If role-playing is not reflective of the types of social situations youth encounter, the training will not have long-term benefits. Statements by juveniles with Conduct Disorders such as, "I would appreciate it if you would not talk to me in that way," would be met with laughter and endless teasing by peers in most inner-city neighborhoods. New skills should take into account the community in which youth will be interacting, as well as individual youths' personal style.

EFFECTIVE BEHAVIOR MANAGEMENT
One of the most beneficial interventions for managing youth with Conduct Disorder is providing effective behavior management. The following are important issues that should be kept in mind when using behavior management strategies with juvenile offenders with Conduct Disorder:

Clear Expectations
Knowing exactly what is expected of them is critical for youth with Conduct Disorder. The rules and expectations of a juvenile justice facility should be simple and clear. In addition, they should be explained verbally to youth and clarified if there is any confusion. Rules and expectations should also be visually displayed. Youth with Conduct Disorder should be told what behaviors staff would like them to engage in, rather than focusing solely on what behaviors the youth should stop doing. Youth with Conduct Disorder often *increase* their negative behavior as soon as they are told to *stop* doing it. For example, telling juveniles, "Only items belonging to you are allowed in your room," is more helpful than saying, "No borrowing" or "No stealing." If youth are told to "Speak at a conversational level," there is no need to say, "Stop yelling."

By teaching and reminding juveniles with Conduct Disorder what they are *supposed* to be doing, their behavior can be corrected. And they also have an opportunity to learn something new. When they are told only what to stop doing, some of these juveniles may truly not know what alternative behavior to use in its place. Directing them to what they should be doing can also help to reduce some of the power struggles with these youth. New, alternative behaviors do not usually come naturally. These replacement behaviors must be modeled, and youth must practice them.

Consistency
Many youth with Conduct Disorder were raised in environments where inconsistent discipline was the norm. At times, punishment may have been harsh and even abusive. At other times, there may have been little to no limit set on their behavior. Being consistent when responding to a conduct-disordered youths' behavior, therefore, is critical. When youth with Conduct Disorder break a rule, they should receive a negative consequence that is commensurate with their misbehavior (*e.g.*, loss of points from the level system, removal from an activity, time in their room, placement in a seclusion room). This consequence should occur immediately after the infraction, every single time youth

54

Juvenile Offenders with Mental Health Disorders: Who Are They and What Do We Do With Them?

break that rule. In addition, all adults interacting with youth (*e.g.*, juvenile justice professionals, mental health/health professionals, teachers, mentors, volunteers, recreational staff) should reward the same behaviors and discipline the same behaviors. This is why expectations and rules need to be clear and easy to understand—so both the youth and the staff understand them.

Although consistency is essential, achieving it can be a major challenge in juvenile justice facilities, due to the nature of shift work and the various personality styles of staff. Communication between all adults working with conduct-disordered youth is key—to make sure that everyone is managing the juveniles in a similar manner. Sometimes staff are unable to communicate with each other verbally about particular youth, due to scheduling conflicts. Communicating through supervisors or providing written communication in a log book is typically sufficient.

> Although disciplining youth for disruptive behavior might result in better behavior the following day, a more effective strategy for long-term results is to help juveniles experience success in the classroom.

Reinforcement of Success

Strict discipline is not enough to modify antisocial youths' behavior. Interventions that primarily rely on coercion and control of youth will not be effective if the intent is to modify the juveniles' behavior long-term. The goal is not for juveniles with Conduct Disorder to become "good residents." *The goal is to help them develop the skills that will help them function effectively while residing in a juvenile justice facility, and ultimately, the community.* Providing positive consequences when youth behave in a prosocial and adaptive manner is just as important as

disciplining antisocial or aggressive behavior. Every time youth fulfill an expectation or complete an assignment, they should receive a positive consequence (*e.g.*, points on level system, verbal praise from staff, eligibility for a specific privilege). This reward should happen immediately (or as soon as possible) after completion of the behavior.

Because Conduct Disorder is usually a chronic condition, every success, no matter how small, should be acknowledged and rewarded. When these youth begin to experience success, they are more willing to expand their behavioral repertoire beyond the antisocial behaviors to which they are accustomed. When they are frequently punished and receive no praise, they become demoralized, discouraged, and even more committed to their antisocial ways. Youth with Conduct Disorder who have repeated failure experiences in school may try to be removed from that environment by becoming increasingly disruptive in the classroom. Although disciplining youth for disruptive behavior might result in better behavior the following day, a more effective strategy for long-term results is to help juveniles experience success in the classroom. For example, teachers can allow youth to write a report on a topic of their choosing. Or teachers can provide youth with extra assistance on a generic assignment so that they can actually complete it. These successes can result in juveniles beginning to feel more positively about school and their performance in the academic arena. If youth no longer feel inadequate about education and become interested in a particular subject area, their need to be disruptive tends to diminish. In addition, these juveniles learn valuable academic skills and are more likely to try additional assignments or subject areas in the future.

One of the most effective ways of decreasing youths' disruptive and aggressive behavior is to help them feel successful in an area that is of interest to them. Many juvenile offenders continue to engage in delinquent activity because it is something in which they are skilled.

Or, at least, they *think* they are skilled at it. Many of these youth know about drugs: they know how to buy drugs, they know how to take drugs, they know how to sell drugs, and some even know how to grow or make drugs. Some juvenile offenders know all about cars: how to break into a car, how to hot-wire a car, and so forth. A significant number of juvenile offenders (many of whom have been diagnosed with Conduct Disorder) acquire their sense of self-worth and pride from their behavior in the arena of delinquency.

Therefore, a primary goal with these juveniles is to help them develop feelings of self-worth and pride in relation to prosocial activities instead of antisocial activities. A first step toward achieving this goal is to reward these youth when they do something positive and prosocial, no matter how trivial it may appear.

Continuing to discipline youth, over and over, with no teaching of skills or reinforcement of positive behavior, results in youth feeling dejected and hopeless. This process often reconfirms in the juveniles' own mind that the only thing they will ever be good at is antisocial activity. This can result in them becoming even more resistant to discontinuing negative behaviors. This process also sets up a dynamic where youth begin to fear or hate juvenile justice professionals or teachers who repeatedly punish them. The youth may then be motivated to become verbally or physically aggressive with those particular adults as an attempt to regain some control or "save face," even if the youths' behavior results in additional restrictions and sanctions. Not surprisingly, when they are upset or in need of support or advice, these juveniles are also less likely to turn to those adults. A possible life-changing relationship for both individuals is never given the opportunity to develop.

Token Economy

Many juvenile justice facilities use a *token economy* (*i.e.*, point system, level system) where youth receive a certain number of points for accomplishing pre-determined chores, tasks, and assignments. As they attain a greater number of points, juveniles are typically eligible for certain privileges (*e.g.*, later bedtime, extra snack, increased personal items in room, less restrictive supervision). Points also can be taken away if youth engage in behavior that violates the rules of the facility.

The most effective token economy programs are those in which expected behaviors are *objectively* defined. When expected behaviors are specifically described and observable, staff and youth will both be clear on whether or not youth engage in particular behaviors (positive or negative). Objective behavioral expectations can significantly reduce conflict between juvenile justice professionals and youth with Conduct Disorder. Rewards and "punishments" are not given out on a personal basis but solely based on youths' *behaviors*. Objectively defined behavioral expectations also reduce conflict between various juvenile justice professionals who may not agree on whether or not youth "deserve" certain privileges or sanctions. Decisions regarding privileges and sanctions should not be based on staff members' subjective opinions but instead based directly based on youths' behavior.

To have the maximum effect on behavior change, token economies should emphasize reinforcement of juvenile offenders' strengths. The focus should be on earning points for accomplishing tasks, demonstrating prosocial skills, and participating in activities versus removing points for noncompliance. This focus develops an atmosphere that is more conducive to learning new, more adaptive behaviors. Discipline should be provided when necessary. However, it should be paired with reinforcement for any and all adaptive behaviors exhibited by youth.

Some juveniles with Conduct Disorder have difficulty earning points or progressing to the next level of a token economy system. When this situation occurs, staff should re-evaluate whether expectations for a particular youth are too high. Behavioral expectations for individual offenders may need to be lowered slightly so there is a chance to reinforce the juveniles' positive behavior. Once youth begin to experience success, there is a greater chance they will continue to behave in a positive manner. Juveniles who remain on the lowest level of a token economy system (with few to no privileges) for a significant period of time will typically begin to feel hopeless and demoralized. At this point, the juveniles may feel they have "nothing to lose." This often results in youth continuing to display negative behaviors and abandoning any attempts to engage in prosocial behaviors. When this dynamic occurs, it is a negative and downward cycle that is difficult to break by either the youth or the juvenile justice professionals managing them.

Some juveniles seem unable to display any appropriate behaviors, no matter how minimal. When this situation occurs, it is likely that juvenile justice professionals have not yet identified (or sufficiently provided) meaningful reinforcement for those particular youth (Moss, 1994). The behavior of some juvenile offenders with Conduct Disorder may seem so out of control and aggressive that adults believe "nothing works." In these cases, juvenile justice professionals, as well as the other adults involved with the youths' treatment, should continue searching for what specifically motivates the youths' behavior (*e.g.*, eliciting attention, being placed in seclusion, tension release). Once they identify what particular juveniles find reinforcing, staff should make every effort to provide this reinforcement when the youth are *not* engaged in negative behaviors. For example, most youth with Conduct Disorder realize that being disruptive and aggressive results in a great deal of staff attention. Providing attention to these youth when they are not being disruptive and aggressive may decrease their motivation to engage in these behaviors, because their need is being met.

Along the same lines, there is a small but troublesome subset of conduct-disordered youth that find time spent in a seclusion room very reinforcing. Seclusion allows these youth time away from:

- Annoying peers
- All adults
- Tasks they need to complete
- Schoolwork
- Expectations in the living unit

Some juveniles with Conduct Disorder engage in specific negative behaviors they know will result in them being placed in seclusion—which is exactly what they want to occur. Offering time in a seclusion room as *reinforcement* for positive behavior may seem contradictory since isolation from others is typically viewed as a disciplinary action. But for youth who enjoy it, seclusion should be treated as a privilege. Using seclusion as a "reward" can be effective in getting these youth to engage in behaviors staff would like the youth to do. Juveniles end up getting their needs met, and staff do not have to contend with the youths' negative behavior. The entire unit is likely to run more smoothly and safely.

There will be some youth for whom no type of reinforcement appears to work. Staff should look more closely at what appears to motivate these youths' negative behavior to discover what it is the juveniles are truly after. Once they know what drives a particular juvenile's behavior, staff can be more strategic in their management strategies with the youth. Juvenile justice professionals often need to be incredibly creative in order to manage the most disruptive and out-of-control youth with Conduct Disorder.

The goal of an effective behavior management program is not for youth to just comply with rules in order to reach the top of the "level system"—which results in increased rewards. The goal is for youth to develop and demonstrate prosocial behaviors (including individually driven treatment goals) that will help them successfully function within a facility and the community at large. Behavior management programs (*e.g.*, token economy programs) appear straightforward and based on common sense. However, unless these programs are designed and implemented competently, they can be

Oppositional Defiant Disorder and Conduct Disorder

useless at best. At their worst, these programs can actually increase and reinforce the negative behaviors staff are trying to change. Juvenile justice facilities should consult with professionals trained in behavior management principles when developing or modifying these programs.

In addition, effective behavior management should not stop when youth with Conduct Disorder are released from juvenile justice facilities. Conduct Disorder among juvenile offenders is typically a chronic condition. Therefore, these youth also need clear-cut behavioral expectations and consistent responses to positive and negative behaviors from individuals supervising them in the community (*e.g.*, probation officers, parole officers). They also need this type of behavior management in their family homes, group homes, or foster care placements. Anyone supervising youth with Conduct Disorder should be:

- Aware of the principles of effective behavior management
- Able to identify what consequences are rewarding to specific youth
- Able to identify what consequences are punishing to specific youth

Remaining consistent and swift when providing consequences to juveniles' behavior, whether the behavior is prosocial or antisocial, is critical. (*Please see Chapters 5 and 14 for additional information on effective behavior management.*)

RESPECTING YOUTH
Treating youth with Conduct Disorder in a respectful manner can help to decrease their antisocial behavior. Youth provide respect to juvenile justice professionals who display respect for the youth. Providing respect for youth does not reduce juveniles' accountability for negative behavior or decrease resulting sanctions. Staff can hold youth accountable for their behavior and continue to be respectful.

Some youth with Conduct Disorder in the juvenile justice system have little to no empathy for others. These juveniles display little to no remorse for their crimes and/or for the victims to whom they have caused suffering. These youth may be aggressive, assaultive and cruel. They may verbally and/or physically assault peers or juvenile justice staff. Juvenile justice professionals may have a strong negative reaction to this type of youth and want to "teach them a lesson." Sometimes, this type of youth "brings out" the anger within particular staff— especially when the youth focus on personal aspects of staff and/or staff members' lives.

Many of these juveniles were raised in punitive and harsh environments; using conflict and anger is often the way they are most comfortable interacting with others. Juvenile justice professionals must avoid engaging in power struggles with these youth and/or becoming overly punitive, even though it may be difficult. Staff should continue to focus on the youths' *behavior*, hold the youth accountable for their *behavior*, and not let it get personal. No matter how offensive or intolerable their *behavior* is, youth need to be treated with respect. Staff should make it clear to these juveniles that they are not offensive and intolerable, their *behavior* is.

DISPROVING NEGATIVE EXPECTATIONS
Interpersonal relationships are a two-way interaction, with juveniles affecting staff behavior and staff affecting juveniles' behavior. Due to the thinking errors mentioned above, many youth with severe Conduct Disorder *expect* juvenile justice professionals to be controlling and punitive. Ironically, these youth often act in ways that are antisocial and aggressive. This behavior forces juvenile justice professionals to take control of situations and to discipline youths' potentially harmful behavior to maintain a safe and secure environment. Staff's response tends to reinforce juveniles' expectations about how staff will behave. Because of this dynamic, it is important that juvenile justice professionals respond to youths' rule violations and aggressive behavior in a "matter of fact" manner—as objectively as possible—

making sure to keep their own emotions in check. Being objective can be difficult when juveniles are offensive and making direct personal attacks, but it is critical to effectively manage youth behavior.

In addition, juveniles with Conduct Disorder often think that no one cares about them. Most believe that adults cannot be trusted and that the world is a dangerous place, full of people who are out to hurt them (Moretti, *et al.*, 1997). When juvenile justice professionals engage in behavior that is contrary to these beliefs, the youths' worldview begins to change. This is why being consistent and keeping their word or promises with youth who have Conduct Disorder is critical for staff to do. What may appear to be a minor matter to juvenile justice professionals (*e.g.*, meeting with youth for a few minutes at 3:00 p.m. to hear about a recent visit with family members, giving youth a can of soda that was promised) can have a great influence on youth if a commitment is not kept. The goal is to challenge the negative beliefs that youth with Conduct Disorder hold instead of reinforcing the beliefs. Trust is earned over a long period of time with these youth; it slowly develops as juvenile justice professionals stay true to their word on a variety of minor matters. One of the most important factors in helping juveniles with Conduct Disorder stay out of trouble is having a positive relationship with an adult figure (*e.g.*, parent, teacher, coach, neighbor, uncle, grandmother). Juvenile justice professionals are in an ideal position to play this role in young offenders' lives.

INVOLVING THE FAMILY
Because of the large role that family members play in the development and maintenance of antisocial behavior, family members ("family" as defined by the youth) should be involved in youths' rehabilitation plan. Family members should be taught how to provide effective behavior management with youth: reinforcing positive and prosocial behaviors and punishing, or not reinforcing negative and antisocial behav-

iors. Family members should receive weekly updates related to the status of their children's behavior, and family visits should be encouraged. Although scheduling issues can be a challenge, juvenile justice professionals should meet with youths' families during visits whenever possible. Staff can discuss behavior management strategies that have been effective with the youth, as well as address issues related to where the youth will live upon release to the community. Depending on their level of training and/or experience, juvenile justice professionals can also help youth talk about difficult topics with family members and provide support during family conflicts.

 Conclusion

In conclusion, effective and strategic management of juveniles with Conduct Disorder is critical. For many youth with mild Conduct Disorder, the use of effective management strategies can have a powerful and positive effect on their antisocial behavior. For juveniles with moderate and severe Conduct Disorder, effective management strategies can help youth begin taking positive and prosocial steps with regard to their behavior—although these strategies are unlikely to "cure" the youth of their delinquent/antisocial lifestyle. Effectively managing youth with Conduct Disorder can be challenging and time-consuming, and long-term behavior change is often difficult to achieve. The key to effectively managing youth with Conduct Disorder is to provide early prevention and intervention programs that address the family and environmental issues known to play a role in the development and maintenance of this disorder.

Case Example
Anthony, 16, was arrested on a theft charge and brought to juvenile detention. The judge found Anthony guilty of the crime, and he was committed to one of the state

training schools located two hours from his home. He would remain at the detention center over the weekend and would be transferred to the state institution early Monday morning. Juvenile detention staff knew they would need to watch Anthony closely for the next few days. He had been incarcerated at the local detention center a total of eight times for a variety of charges (*i.e.*, possession of marijuana, trespassing, assault, theft, attempted rape), and the staff knew him well. He was known for being an "instigator" and often started trouble in the living unit or in the school. Although he was no more than 5' 10", many of the other youth were afraid of him. Anthony walked around as if he owned the facility, as if nothing and no one could touch him. He often took the other youths' belongings without asking, even taking food off of their plates during meals. If any of the other juveniles stood up to him, Anthony became intimidating and threatening. He was known to slam peers against the wall, hit them on the back of the head, or kick them from behind when staff members were not watching. He was unusually calm, had an air of "coolness" about him, and rarely raised his voice. When he did become angry, his aggression would reveal itself without warning. This behavior made him even more intimidating to peers and more of a management problem for juvenile justice staff.

Anthony takes little to no responsibility for his behavior. When confronted about his aggression toward peers in the living unit, Anthony denies he has any part in the interaction. He repeatedly accuses others of "trying to frame me." He has never admitted to trying to rape his 13-year-old cousin, even though there were four witnesses in the same room when it occurred. He has always maintained that the sexual incident was consensual and that "she wanted me bad and begged me for it" —even though his younger cousin was crying, screaming for him to let her go, and had bruises throughout her pelvic area.

Anthony began harming others when he was 10. He used to beat up his younger brothers when they were in elementary school and used to break the legs of the dogs and cats in the neighborhood. He said he thought it was funny to see the injured animals limp.

There were few rules in the residence where Anthony and his three brothers were raised. They lived with their mother who was addicted to alcohol and cocaine. Anthony's mother often prostituted herself to pay for her drugs, as well as for food for Anthony and his brothers. The boys were typically unsupervised and allowed to wander the neighborhood at all hours of the night. They did not go to school on a regular basis and "hung out" on the streets with older youth.

Various men would stay with the family for weeks at a time, but none of them took an interest in the boys. Anthony remembers several times when he and his brothers were punished for playing too loudly or wrestling in the living room. Some of these men commonly smacked the boys, hit them with their belts, or even locked them in the closet. Anthony's mother would get upset and cry, but she never stopped the men. Anthony began selling marijuana for some of the older boys in the neighborhood when he was 14. He used the money he made to buy nice clothes for himself and spent the rest on beer and marijuana, which he used on a daily basis. Anthony's father is in prison, and the two have never met. Anthony never completed the sixth grade and when asked about his life goals, he replied, "To turn 18."

Juvenile Offenders with Mental Health Disorders: Who Are They and What Do We Do With Them?

CHAPTER 4

Mood Disorders: Major Depression, Dysthymic Disorder and Bipolar Disorder

"When I am depressed, everyone around me gets depressed—I get really mad, and everything gets on my nerves. I think I am Bipolar."

Karin, 15

Devon, 17, has recently begun sleeping 16 hours a day. When he is awake, he mostly stays in his room, listening to music. He will occasionally spend time with his friends, but they have noticed that he has become quiet and guarded. He used to love basketball, was always in a good mood, and seemed to enjoy school. Now Devon's parents are concerned that he will not graduate from high school. His grades have been slipping because of missed classes, he has become increasingly irritable at home, and he has not played basketball in weeks.

Susan, 15, seems overly happy one week and then completely depressed the next. Her friends do not understand why she has become so moody, and her boyfriend is complaining that she is constantly over-reacting to minor events. Susan's family noticed the change in her moods about a month ago when she began staying up all night. When asked about this behavior, she gave several explanations that made little sense to her parents. When Susan is in one of her "low" moods, friends and family try to make her feel better. But she blames them for all of her problems and says "everyone is against her." She has begun picking on her younger brother, acting rudely to her mother, and sporadically complaining that she would be "better off dead."

Adolescence is a time of frequent mood changes and greater extremes of mood (positive and negative) in comparison to preadolescence and adulthood (Arnett, 1999). However, every adolescent should not be diagnosed with a

mood disorder. The term *mood disorder* encompasses a group of diagnostic categories that describe a range of emotional disturbances. *Mood* refers to the feeling or emotional state experienced by an individual (*e.g.*, happy, sad, angry, irritable). Most people experience a wide range of feelings and are able to control them in a socially appropriate manner. For example, when individuals receive good news at the doctor's office, they are likely to refrain from jumping up and down and shouting hallelujah—even if that is how they are feeling inside. Most individuals are aware of their social context and are able to curtail their emotional expressions until an opportune moment. Juveniles with a mood disorder are less able, and sometimes completely unable, to control their emotions. Their moods may be significantly depressed or elevated, which can lead to problems in several areas of their lives. Their intense moods often interfere with daily activities, including their ability to interact with others, attend school or hold a job. They often have physical complaints and may withdraw from friends and family.

Because emotions during adolescence are intense, determining when juvenile offenders have a mood disorder and when they are acting like a typical adolescent can be difficult. Adults usually assume that youths' emotional intensity and mood swings are part of being a teenager and that they will "outgrow it." Unfortunately, this attitude results in many juvenile offenders with serious mood disorders not getting the treatment they need. Without help, they may go on to have more serious, and potentially long-term, psychiatric problems.

Mood disorders are both under-identified and under-diagnosed among the adolescent population (Reynolds, 1994), particularly among youth involved in the juvenile justice system. Adolescent offenders have significantly high rates of mood disorders. Studies have found up to 32-88 percent of incarcerated juveniles met diagnostic criteria for a mood disorder (Davis, Bean, Schumacher, & Stringer, 1991; Timmons-Mitchell, *et al.*, 1997). The three most common mood disorders among youth in the juvenile justice system are Major Depressive Disorder (Major Depression), Dysthymic Disorder (Dysthymia), and Bipolar Disorder.

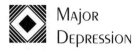 MAJOR DEPRESSION

Identifying which youth are suffering from a major psychiatric disorder and which youth are having a normal reaction to a stressful situation can often be difficult while juveniles are incarcerated. This situation is especially true if:

- youth are residing at a juvenile justice facility for only a short period of time, and/or

- there is not much information on the youths' mood and behavior before they arrived at the facility

A significant number of youth involved with juvenile justice have a great deal to be depressed about. They may have just been arrested, brought to a juvenile detention facility, and separated from friends and family. Many juveniles have to face a judge in a courtroom, and some may be looking at serving a considerable amount of time in a long-term juvenile justice facility. Some juvenile offenders have already been found guilty of a crime and may be serving their sentence at a state training school, work camp, or boot camp. Some youth have been transferred to an adult jail or prison. Is it reasonable to expect these youth to be depressed?

Imagine how it would feel to be in their situation: sleeping in a very small room with minimal personal belongings, authority figures telling you when and where and what to eat, losing most of your freedom, having minimal contact with friends and family, and so forth. While incarcerated, many youth are provoked by bigger and tougher peers, some of whom may be gang-affiliated. Fear, sadness, and anger are common emotions given these circumstances. When some juveniles are initially incarcerated, they may appear depressed—unable to eat, withdrawn, crying. For most of these youth, however, these symptoms discontinue after several days. These juveniles may still be upset about their circumstances, but most are able adjust to a facility's program (*e.g.*, eating at

62

Juvenile Offenders with Mental Health Disorders: Who Are They and What Do We Do With Them?

mealtimes, completing chores, attending school, participating in recreational activities) within 48-72 hours. The vast majority of juveniles adjust within a week. One of the challenges for juvenile justice professionals is to know the point at which they should be concerned about youths' depressive-type behaviors—so that they can make a referral to a supervisor or mental health/medical professional.

Mental health professionals rely on the *Diagnostic and Statistical Manual of Mental Disorders* (*DSM*) in order to diagnose Major Depression among youth. In the current edition of this classification system, the *DSM-IV-TR*, the diagnostic criteria for Major Depression among youth are the same criteria used to diagnose Major Depression among adults (American Psychiatric Association, 2000). Although some symptoms may be more or less common at particular developmental stages, the core symptoms of Major Depression are the same for both adolescents and adults.

Diagnostic Criteria for Major Depression

To receive a diagnosis of Major Depression, youth must experience several specific symptoms. At least one of these symptoms must be "a depressed or irritable mood" or "diminished interest or pleasure in activities." The symptoms of depression must be present most of the day, nearly every day, for at least a two-week period (APA, 2000). *And* the symptoms must cause significant distress or impairment in the youths' functioning (*e.g.*, interfere with school, work, relationships). Major depression can be mild, moderate or severe. Symptoms of depression should represent a *change* from the way juveniles typically feel and behave. The symptoms must be new or significantly worse than what the youth typically experience. This change may be difficult for juvenile justice professionals to observe in some youth if the youth are chronically depressed (*i.e.*, depressed every time they enter a juvenile facility). Because they interact with juveniles for several hours

each day, staff have many opportunities to observe youth behavior. Juvenile justice professionals' observation of youth is critical. When juvenile offenders suffering from Major Depression are directly asked if they are depressed, the majority will say "no." These youth are typically not lying; most are unaware.

All juvenile justice professionals interacting with youth should be alert to the following symptoms and behaviors among the juveniles:

- Depressed or irritable mood
- Loss of interest or pleasure
- Appetite disturbances
- Sleep disturbances
- Restlessness/slowed body movements
- Fatigue
- Feelings of worthlessness
- Difficulty concentrating
- Suicidal thoughts/behavior

DEPRESSED/IRRITABLE MOOD

Although many depressed individuals exhibit a sad mood or describe themselves as feeling "blue" or "down in the dumps," a significant number of adolescents (particularly those involved in the juvenile justice system) manifest their depression in an irritable or agitated mood. They often describe feeling like they have a "short fuse" and are ready to "blow" at any minute. Juvenile offenders suffering from Major Depression tend to get annoyed by others very easily. Even small comments and statements from other people can result in angry outbursts. These irritable/depressed youth might go out of their way to provoke juvenile justice professionals but become upset if negative consequences result.

Some depressed youth are able to control their irritable mood and behavior for short periods of time. For example, juveniles' behavior may improve while they are in court, while they are at school, or while they are talking to a mental health counselor. Depressed youth commonly exhibit their most disruptive

Mood Disorders: Major Depression, Dysthymic Disorder and Bipolar Disorder

behavior when they are at home or in a home-like situation (such as in a living unit or cottage in a juvenile justice facility), or when residing at a group home.

Some depressed youth constantly feel like victims, repeatedly claiming that they are not being treated fairly. No matter what activity is occurring, these juveniles often complain that they did not get as much (e.g., food, time on the phone, time in the shower, shampoo, points for doing chores) as their peers. They may feel that staff are purposely depriving them of their fair share. Some depressed youth will respond to this feeling by becoming increasingly sad and withdrawn. The more irritable depressed youth will become angry, often throwing a "temper tantrum"—regardless of their age.

Because most adults assume that the key symptoms of depression include sadness, crying and social withdrawal, many juvenile offenders suffering from Major Depression are misdiagnosed, undiagnosed, and/or untreated. This fact is particularly true among the more *aggressively* depressed juveniles who are typically diagnosed with Conduct Disorder and provided with little to no mental health treatment. Depressed youth who exhibit extreme irritability and anger tend to receive a significant number of sanctions during incarceration. Consequently, they often spend a considerable amount of time confined to their own rooms or in special seclusion rooms. These youth are typically viewed as "bad" and are rarely referred to mental health professionals for an evaluation.

Major Depression, isolation, and aggression are all significant risk factors for suicide. Therefore, aggressively depressed juvenile offenders are at extremely high risk for a suicide attempt. Because they often do not view these youth as having a mental health disorder, juvenile justice professionals are often less sensitive to these youths' high-risk suicide status (in comparison to youth who express their depression through sadness and tears). Any type of suicidal threat or statement from this type of youth should be taken extremely seriously, regardless of what

juvenile justice professionals believe is the youths' underlying motivation. This type of juvenile can be impulsive and overly concerned with "saving face" in front of authority figures. These youth may make an impulsive suicide attempt when angry at staff members, especially after receiving sanctions for negative behavior. Even if aggressively depressed youth are only trying to scare staff and not really intending to kill themselves, poor planning can result in a completed suicide attempt.

Youth who repeatedly display extreme irritability or aggression may be suffering from Major Depression. They should be referred for a mental health assessment to determine whether additional symptoms of depression are present. Juveniles who are constantly angry tend to be more severely depressed than youth whose anger is connected to particular events. Proper treatment, often including antidepressant medication, can significantly reduce youths' irritable and angry moods. However, just because youth are aggressive does not automatically imply that they are depressed. Several of the other diagnostic criteria for depression must be present as well. Without the youth having a comprehensive mental health evaluation, the likelihood of an aggressively depressed youth receiving appropriate treatment is low—while the likelihood of continued negative and dangerous behavior is high.

SIGNIFICANTLY DIMINISHED INTEREST OR PLEASURE IN ALL OR ALMOST ALL ACTIVITIES

Juveniles suffering from Major Depression often experience *anhedonia*, which refers to youth losing interest in the activities they used to find enjoyable. Some of these juveniles appear bored and uninterested in things that used to interest them. When asked why they are reluctant to participate in activities, youth may say, "It's stupid" or "Only losers do that," even though they used to enjoy the same activities only a short time before. To avoid having to participate in certain activities, youth may:

64

Juvenile Offenders with Mental Health Disorders: Who Are They and What Do We Do With Them?

- Pretend they are ill
- Say they are too tired
- Purposely engage in rule-breaking behavior so that they will be removed from the activity

Recognizing when there is a change in youths' behavior is important for juvenile justice professionals. For example: depressed juveniles who are usually very social often start to isolate themselves and no longer want to be around peers or staff; depressed youth who used to enjoy playing basketball would rather stay back in their room than go the gymnasium to shoot hoops; depressed females who used to enjoy gossiping with the other girls in a unit or styling the other girls' hair may begin choosing to spend time by themselves. Instead of enjoying interaction with peers, depressed youth often find the other juveniles in a living unit annoying and intrusive. Youth displaying a lack of interest in their usual activities for several days in a row should be followed up on—to identify whether feelings of depression may be playing a role.

SIGNIFICANT WEIGHT LOSS/
WEIGHT GAIN OR INCREASE/
DECREASE IN APPETITE
Appetite disturbance and changes in weight are common symptoms of Major Depression. When depressed, some youth may overeat in an attempt to comfort themselves and/or fill up their feelings of emptiness. Some depressed youth, however, lose their appetite and eat very little.

Appetite and weight-related symptoms are often difficult to assess among juvenile offenders in residential facilities. Incarcerated youth may eat more or less than usual for a variety of reasons that are completely unrelated to depression. For example, some juveniles do not like the food in juvenile justice facilities because it is different from what they are used to or because it does not taste good. As a result, they may choose to eat as little of the food as possible. In contrast, some juveniles have been living on the street or in youth shelters before incarceration, so they are extremely hungry when they enter a facility. These youth may be insatiable and eat a great deal more than their peers. When youth are initially withdrawing from drugs and alcohol, they may feel nauseated and unable to eat. A few days later, they may be ravenous and eat everything in sight. When juvenile justice professionals notice that youths' eating behavior is different from other juveniles'—or a change from how the youth typically eat—they should ask the youth about it. A change in eating behavior and/or weight may be a symptom of Major Depression or it may be related to the menu selection of the week.

DIFFICULTY SLEEPING OR
EXCESSIVE SLEEPING
Disturbance of the sleep-wake cycle is common among both youth and adults who suffer from Major Depression. Some youth will want to sleep too much (all day and night), and trying to get them out of bed in the morning can be difficult, if not impossible. Other depressed youth may complain that they cannot sleep at all. Depressed juveniles:

- May not be able to fall asleep at bedtime
- May wake up numerous times during the middle of the night
- May wake up very early in the morning and not be able to fall asleep again
- May have disturbing or frightening dreams when they are able to fall asleep

Similar to appetite disturbances, sleep disturbances are often hard to assess among adolescents residing in a juvenile justice facility. Juvenile offenders may suffer from sleep disturbances for a variety of reasons that have nothing to do with symptoms of depression. Some juvenile justice facilities keep youth constantly involved in activities, whereas in other facilities, youth spend a significant time in their rooms. Depending on the scheduled programming in a facility, juveniles may have the opportunity to

Mood Disorders: Major Depression, Dysthymic Disorder and Bipolar Disorder

sleep several hours during the day. Many youth describe this as an effective strategy for making the time they are incarcerated pass more quickly. Unfortunately, the more youth sleep during they day, the greater the likelihood they will have difficulty sleeping in the evening. The following can also play a role in juveniles' sleeping problems:

- Excessive noise
- Rooms that are lighted all night
- Fear of roommates
- Anxiety
- Side effects from psychotropic medication
- Uncomfortable beds

If they hear youth complain about sleep difficulties and/or notice that youth are not sleeping, staff should ask the juveniles about their typical sleep patterns. Many youth involved in the juvenile justice system stay out very late at night (*e.g.*, 1:00 a.m., 3:00 a.m.) when residing in the community. They often sleep in until late morning or early afternoon. Adjusting to a new routine of going to bed at 9:00 p.m. or 10:00 p.m. and being awakened early in the morning (*e.g.*, 6:00 a.m., 7:00 a.m.) while in a facility can be difficult for them. Sleep difficulties may be related to depression, but they may also be the result of juveniles' sleep cycles being thrown off.

In addition, many incarcerated youth are accustomed to using drugs or alcohol before going to bed. Some juveniles typically have a few beers, or smoke some marijuana, before going to sleep every night. Therefore, these youth might have difficulty falling asleep while they are incarcerated because they are not intoxicated or high. This pattern of needing chemical substances to sleep can be indicative of depression and should be further explored.

Some juvenile offenders, particularly those who have a drug abuse disorder, may complain of sleep difficulties in order to obtain sleep medication. Whenever youth report sleeping problems, staff should pay attention to more than just the youths' subjective complaints. "Sleep logs" can provide important information about youths' sleeping behavior. Staff working the overnight shift are typically required to do routine checks on all youth as they sleep (*e.g.*, every 15, every 20 minutes, every 30 minutes). During regular room checks, staff can use a simple form to document whether or not particular juveniles are sleeping throughout the night. Youth may subjectively feel that they are not sleeping, but when staff regularly check on them, the youth may indeed be asleep. Or staff may discover that these youth are lying awake much of the night.

Staff should inquire about youths' typical sleep/wake patterns if youth are complaining of sleep problems. Some incarcerated juveniles have difficulty awakening in the morning and are slow to get going. Other youth lie in bed for hours before falling asleep. However, these behavior patterns do not necessarily imply that these juveniles are suffering from Major Depression. These patterns of behavior are *signs* for further exploration. Staff should ask these youth whether current sleep difficulties are a change from how the youth normally sleep, and observe the youth for other signs/symptoms of depression.

SIGNIFICANT RESTLESSNESS OR SLOWED SPEECH/BODY MOVEMENT

Youth suffering from Major Depression frequently experience changes in their psychomotor functioning. The pace at which they move and speak may be significantly revved up or slowed down. Some depressed juveniles appear jumpy and nervous. They may fidget with their clothes and other objects, or pace around the room. The restlessness seen in youth suffering from Major Depression can appear similar to the hyperactivity seen in Attention-Deficit/Hyperactivity Disorder (ADHD). Depressed youth may be misdiagnosed with ADHD if a comprehensive evaluation is not conducted. *(Please see Chapter 5 for additional information on ADHD.)*

In contrast, some depressed youth experience a significant slowing of behavior. They may talk very slowly and wait a lengthy period of time before responding to questions. They may move very slowly and are unable to hasten their behavior even when directed to do so. These juveniles are often the ones who lag behind in line; they often move at a much slower pace than their peers when walking from one area of a facility to another.

FATIGUE OR LOSS OF ENERGY

Youth with Major Depression often appear worn-out and exhausted. They lack energy and complain of chronic feelings of fatigue. Small requests may feel burdensome to them, and they may want to do nothing but lie around. Some depressed juveniles will complain of overall feelings of boredom or having the "blahs." Most juvenile offenders cannot wait to go outside and engage in recreational activities. They commonly enjoy roughhousing or horse-play. Youth with Major Depression, however, are often too tired or feel too drained to involve themselves in activities that require physical exertion. Even when fun activities or special events occur, depressed youth often have difficulty summoning the energy to attend the activities or events. If their attendance is mandatory, these youth are not likely to fully participate.

FEELINGS OF WORTHLESSNESS/ EXCESSIVE GUILT

Youth with Major Depression often experience low self-esteem and are preoccupied with past failures and mistakes. These juveniles are often highly critical of themselves, and even small mistakes can cause them tremendous distress. They may take on an appearance of bravado and act as if they do not care what others think about them. But most depressed adolescents are very sensitive to criticism. They perceive any negative feedback as confirmation that they are losers and not as good as everyone else. Juvenile justice professionals may be unaware of

negative remarks made in passing to adolescents with Major Depression. However, these youth can obsess about these negative comments for hours or days. Small failures at games, tasks, or activities can significantly impact depressed juveniles, resulting in intense feelings of sadness or anger.

Depressed youth may exaggerate small mistakes or failures from their past and often believe they should be severely punished for what they have done. But excessive and inappropriate guilt can be difficult to assess among juvenile offenders. Many youth involved with the juvenile justice system have engaged in behaviors and acts for which feeling guilty would be appropriate. For example, youth may feel guilty if they have caused damage to another's property or have physically assaulted someone; feeling poorly about committing these actions is usually appropriate and even adaptive. However, this reaction differs from youth who have been brought in on less serious charges (*e.g.*, making too much noise in a movie theatre, trespassing) who feel a tremendous amount of guilt and shame about "ruining their lives." Juveniles who are depressed experience *excessive* or *inappropriate* guilt. Their guilty feelings can be so strong that they may even feel responsible for causing things that have nothing to do with them.

DIFFICULTY CONCENTRATING/ INDECISIVENESS

Similar to the slowing of speech and body movements among youth with Major Depression, their thinking may also be slowed down. Not surprisingly, this behavior can negatively affect juvenile offenders' schoolwork, their ability to make important decisions, and their capacity to participate in activities in a living unit. Depressed youth may look to juvenile justice professionals to help them with every decision, even those that seem small or trivial. They may also find it difficult to pay attention and concentrate, which can interfere with their ability to follow directions. Depressed youth can

Mood Disorders: Major Depression, Dysthymic Disorder and Bipolar Disorder

appear oppositional and as if they are purposefully not following clearly specified rules. However, their behavior is often a result of difficulty in thinking, remembering, and paying attention. These symptoms are similar to those seen in youth with Attention-Deficit/Hyperactivity Disorder (ADHD), and a comprehensive assessment is needed in order to discriminate between the two disorders.

> SuffERiNg fRom MajoR DepRessioN is a significANt Risk fActoR foR mAkiNg a suicide attempt, ANd the Risk becomes EVEN highER if youth ARE abusiNg dRugs ANd/oR alcohol.

RECURRENT THOUGHTS OF DEATH/ SUICIDAL BEHAVIOR

A significant number of depressed youth in the juvenile justice system have thought about killing themselves. These types of thoughts typically vary in their intensity and specificity. Some youth have brief moments when they wonder what it would be like to be dead. Others may be preoccupied with killing themselves and have a detailed plan as to how and when they will make a suicide attempt.

Juveniles with Major Depression are often attracted to music, books and poetry containing themes of death and destruction. These youth may begin to ask questions about what happens when people die or begin reading books about the afterlife or reincarnation. Suffering from Major Depression is a significant risk factor for making a suicide attempt, and the risk becomes even higher if youth are abusing drugs and/or alcohol. Although many juvenile offenders have had thoughts about killing themselves—particularly during moments of extreme stress—they typically do not design a specific suicide plan or engage in suicidal behavior. Any time youth communicate thoughts about death, wanting to die, or killing themselves, juvenile justice

professionals should take these warnings very seriously. Further evaluation is necessary. *(Please see Chapter 11 for additional information about suicidal behavior among juvenile offenders.)*

Many juvenile offenders will experience the above symptoms of depression at various times and to various degrees. For most youth, however, these symptoms will not occur at a level that interferes with their daily functioning. Major Depression is different from the few hours or days of sadness or irritability seen in youth who are having difficulty adjusting to being arrested and/or incarcerated. To qualify for a diagnosis of Major Depression, youth must have symptoms for at least two weeks. These symptoms must cause the youth *significant distress* or *interfere* with their ability to function in everyday activities (*e.g.*, school, home, juvenile justice facility). The symptoms cannot be caused solely by drug and/or alcohol intoxication or withdrawal. They also cannot primarily be a response to the recent death of someone close to the youth.

Juvenile justice professionals should be aware that youth from various cultures and ethnic groups may present depressive symptoms differently from the symptoms listed above. For example, Hispanic individuals who are depressed may complain of headaches and "nerves". Individuals from Asian cultures may describe feelings of depression as weakness or tiredness (APA, 2000). Whether youths' depression manifests itself in sadness, oppositional behavior, or physical complaints is often related to the norm in their particular culture.

Associated Features of Major Depression

Individuals suffering from Major Depression often experience a variety of additional signs and symptoms. For example, somatic (bodily) complaints such as headaches, stomachaches, and vague arm/leg pains are common among depressed juveniles. These youth may constantly complain of not feeling well and may be worried that they have some type of serious physical ailment, disease or medical disorder. Not surprisingly, depressed juvenile offenders often make repeated requests to see a doctor or nurse.

Youth suffering from severe cases of Major Depression can also experience psychotic symptoms. These youth can actually lose touch with reality and experience *hallucinations*— hearing things that other people do not hear or seeing things that other people do not see. The voices youth hear or the visions they see are typically mood congruent. Because their mood is depressed, they are likely to see and hear things that are negative, pessimistic, and destructive. For example, depressed juveniles may hear voices telling them that they are no good, they are stupid, they will never amount to anything, and that they should kill themselves. *Delusions* also can be present if depressed youths are psychotic. A delusion is a fixed belief that is highly unlikely but which someone holds onto despite logic or contrary evidence. Severely depressed juveniles might believe that parts of their body are rotting away or that they are dying of cancer, despite a thorough medical evaluation and normal medical tests.

Course of Major Depression

Most youth develop the symptoms of Major Depression over a period of several days or weeks. However, they may experience feelings of anxiety and mild depressive symptoms before actually experiencing a full-blown episode of Major Depression. If left untreated, an adolescent can remain depressed for months. Some adolescents can remain significantly depressed for up to two years. Some youth have only one episode of Major Depression during their lives. But, recurrence of episodes is common, and once adolescents experience one major depressive episode, they are likely to experience another one within the following years and into adulthood (Kandel & Davies, 1986; McCauley, *et al.*, 1993).

In addition to their problems with school and academic functioning, depressed youths'

interpersonal relationships are also impaired. Conflict with family members and peers is common. Juveniles with Major Depression may be so irritable and overly sensitive that friends and family find it difficult to spend time with them. Because of isolation and withdrawal, depressed youth can lose the few friends the juveniles had left. This pattern often results in the youth feeling worse about themselves and helps to perpetuate the cycle of depression. Even after the depression lifts, many of these juveniles continue to suffer educational and interpersonal difficulties compared to youth who have never been depressed (Puig-Antich, *et al.*, 1985).

Co-existing Disorders

It is unusual to find a youth diagnosed solely with Major Depression, particularly in the juvenile justice system. Anxiety disorders, Conduct Disorder, eating disorders, learning disorders, Attention-Deficit/Hyperactivity Disorder and substance abuse disorders commonly co-occur with Major Depression. Fifty to 80 percent of depressed youth have one or more psychiatric diagnoses in addition to Major Depression, and most exhibit increased impairment with each additional disorder (Compas, Ey, & Grant, 1993; Kovacs, *et al.*, 1984). Depressed youth who are aggressive and engage in delinquent behavior tend to be more impaired and have higher levels of psychopathology than depressed youth without these additional behaviors. Because they often suffer from Major Depression, Conduct Disorder and one or more substance abuse disorders, youth in juvenile justice are at significant risk for:

- long-term psychiatric problems, and
- impairment affecting several areas of their lives (*e.g.*, family, interpersonal relationships, school, work).

The juvenile justice, mental health and substance abuse systems need to work collaboratively when providing services to depressed juvenile offenders. This increases the

Mood Disorders: Major Depression, Dysthymic Disorder and Bipolar Disorder

likelihood that all aspects of the youths' psycho-pathology are appropriately addressed and treated.

The relationship between Major Depression and substance abuse is not yet clearly under-stood. Youth who are depressed have high rates of drug and alcohol abuse, but whether the substance abuse occurred before or after the depressed mood is not clear. Kandel (1988) suggests that suffering from depression in adolescence increases youths' risk for initiation into drugs. However, others have found that the use of drugs and alcohol precedes the onset of Major Depression (Brook, Cohen, & Brook, 1998; Hovens, Cantwell, & Kiriakos, 1994).

Co-existing psychiatric disorders can occur before, during, and after an episode of Major Depression. Depressed youth should always receive a comprehensive mental health evalua-tion to identify whether they are suffering from another psychiatric disorder in addition to their mood disturbance. If each one of youths' mental health disorders is not identified and appropri-ately treated, sustained positive outcomes are unlikely.

What causes depression?

There is not one unique factor that *causes* Major Depression. The disorder is likely a result of the interaction between juveniles' biological make-up and their environmental circumstances. Factors contributing to the development of Major Depression can be separated into two main categories: biological models and psycho-social models.

BIOLOGICAL MODELS

Major depression appears to have a strong *heritable* component. If one of their parents has Major Depression, youth have a 25 percent chance of developing the disorder themselves. If both parents have depression, the risk can be as high as 75 percent (Gershon, *et al.*, 1982). Similar results are found even when their own biological parents do not raise the youth. Addi-tionally, if one identical twin has Major Depres-sion, the other twin is also likely to have the disorder. Relatives with Major Depression can often be found throughout several generations of depressed youths' families.

Youths' *brain chemistry* may also play a role in the development of depression. Several neurotransmitters, especially norepinephrine and serotonin, have been implicated in the development of Major Depression. After con-ducting many studies, researchers believe that depression may result, at least in part, from an insufficient amount of one or more neurotrans-mitters or an imbalance of these neurotransmit-ters. Researchers have found that serotonin is involved in the systems that regulate appetite, sleep, aggression and motor activity—all of which can be impaired during an episode of Major Depression. In addition, many depressed individuals report a significant decrease in their depressive symptoms while taking medications that increase the availability of serotonin in their brain.

PSYCHOSOCIAL MODELS

Family dysfunction also has been linked to Major Depression among youth. Family conflict, distant and controlling parents, high levels of physical punishment, and minimal time spent in family-oriented activities have all been linked to adolescent depression. Whether adolescents become depressed from having this type of family, or whether the family is behaving this way as a reaction to the depressed youth's behavior is not clear. Parents may spend less time with youth who are irritable and angry. They also may need to assert more controls and punishments in response to depressed youths' negative behavior. Family interaction always flows in two directions, with parental behavior affecting adolescents and adolescents' behavior having an effect on their parent(s). Family interactions with depressed youth can easily become a vicious cycle.

Youth who are depressed report a greater number of *stressful events* in their lives, particu-larly in the year prior to the onset of Major

Juvenile Offenders with Mental Health Disorders: Who Are They and What Do We Do With Them?

Depression. Many juvenile offenders who suffer from depression have experienced significant stresses throughout their childhood, as well as during their adolescent years. Youth involved with the juvenile justice system commonly experience:

- Divorce
- Death of a parent and others close to them
- Family violence
- Physical abuse
- Sexual abuse
- Parental neglect
- Romantic relationship difficulties
- Significant academic difficulties

Sometimes minor events can have a significant negative impact on youth. Incarcerated juvenile offenders have made suicide attempts following incidents such as:

- Being removed from a classroom
- Being removed from a treatment group
- Receiving "room confinement" in response to their negative behavior
- Not having a visitor when one was expected
- Having their date of release from a juvenile justice facility pushed back two weeks

Many youth briefly become upset after these types of incidents but then return to their normal mood. Juvenile offenders with Major Depression, however, can become very depressed after these types of incidents occur. Usually, these minor life events are the "last straw" after a long list of disappointments or altercations (Ingersoll & Goldstein, 1995).

Individuals who are depressed often engage in *distorted thinking*. They tend to hold negative views of themselves, the world, and their future. Depressed juvenile offenders are often very

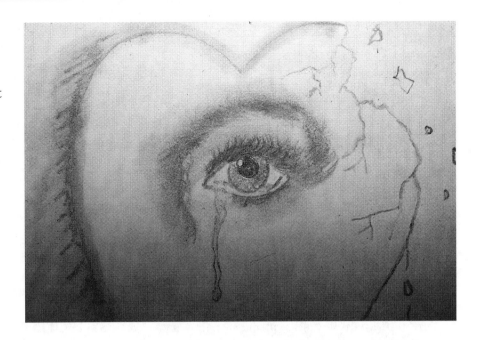

critical of themselves and believe they are worthless and defective. In addition, when these youth look at the world around them, they tend to interpret things in the worst possible light. They often misinterpret the actions of others as a personal slight against them. When depressed youth look at their future, they typically feel hopeless and have a difficult time believing that their circumstances will improve.

How to identify youth with Major Depression

Observing juveniles' behavior is one of the best ways for juvenile justice professionals to identify youth with Major Depression. For example, some depressed juveniles are quiet, socially withdrawn, and want to sleep much of the time. Staff tend to pay the least amount of attention to these youth because they usually make few requests and do not cause much disruption in a facility. Safety and security is of utmost importance in a juvenile justice facility. Most facilities house large numbers of youth, and resources are often limited. Therefore, much of staff time is typically spent with those offenders who are the most disruptive and difficult to manage. The quietly depressed youth may never be identified. Further exploration is warranted if juvenile justice professionals notice youth

Mood Disorders: Major Depression, Dysthymic Disorder and Bipolar Disorder

looking despondent, slowly responding to directions, or spending an excessive amount of time sleeping.

The above description is only one type of adolescent suffering from Major Depression. Another type of depressed youth is irritable, angry, or rebellious and is often the more commonly seen type of depressed youth within the juvenile justice system. Depressed juveniles of this nature may purposely provoke and insult adults and peers. These youth can appear as if they enjoy upsetting those around them. They do not like to follow directions or routines, and they tend to disagree with anything and everything that an authority figure asks them to do. These *aggressively* depressed youth come to the attention of juvenile justice professionals very quickly. However, these offenders are often misidentified as "troublemakers" and in need of swift and strong negative consequences. Youth fitting this description should receive negative consequences for their rule-breaking behavior. But juvenile justice professionals should also refer these youth to a supervisor and/or a mental health/medical professional. An evaluation is necessary to identify whether depression is playing a role in the juveniles' behavior, and if so, to what degree.

Managing Juvenile Offenders with Major Depression

One of the most critical issues in managing juvenile offenders with Major Depression is the identification of these youth. The quiet and withdrawn depressed offenders often slip through the cracks of the system. The irritably depressed youth are typically viewed as solely having "behavior problems." As a result, these irritable youth tend to spend much, if not all, of their time in juvenile justice facilities locked in their rooms because of their disruptive behavior. The first thing juvenile justice professionals need to be aware of is that there may be a mood disorder underlying young offenders' extreme irritability and anger.

The following are important management

strategies to use with juveniles with Major Depression, whether they are sad and withdrawn or angry and irritable.

REFERRAL

If juvenile justice professionals suspect that youth may be suffering from Major Depression, they should refer the juveniles to a mental health/medical professional for further evaluation. If youth meet diagnostic criteria for Major Depression, the following management strategies can be effective in helping the juveniles continue to participate in facility programming—without major disruption to other offenders in a living unit or major conflict with staff.

PSYCHOTROPIC MEDICATION

Antidepressants are the most commonly prescribed medications for Major Depression. One particular class of antidepressant medications, *selective serotonin reuptake inhibitors (SSRIs),* has become increasingly popular over the past few years for the treatment of Major Depression among adolescents. Examples of SSRIs include Prozac®, Zoloft®, and Paxil®. This type of antidepressant medication tends to produce fewer negative side effects and is less toxic than some of the other classes of antidepressant medications. In addition, the SSRIs often target the co-existing symptom of anxiety, which commonly occurs among juvenile offenders suffering from depression. Reducing youths' anxiety can decrease their irritability and help to "take the edge off."

Tricyclic antidepressants (TCAs), such as Tofranil®, Pamelor®, and Elavil®, are also used to treat Major Depression among juveniles. However, cardiac monitoring is necessary if youth are taking this type of antidepressant, as this class of medication can have serious cardiovascular side effects. In addition, the TCAs are highly lethal when taken in large doses. Juvenile justice professionals should be aware of the overdose potential of this type of medication. TCAs might be prescribed to depressed adolescents who are suicidal. Therefore, medical personnel should be immediately alerted if there is even a slight suspicion that youth are not taking their tricyclic antidepressant as prescribed. Further, caution should be exercised if depressed juvenile offenders are provided with a supply of TCA medication when they are released back into the community.

Other medications used to treat depression that do not fit neatly into either of the above categories include Wellbutrin®, Effexor®, and Desyrel® (Trazodone).

Antidepressants typically require youth to be on a therapeutic dose for 10–14 days for the medication to begin working; the full effects of the medication may not be evident for up to six weeks. Sleep and appetite disturbances, however, may improve in a week or less.

DAILY ACTIVITIES
Juvenile justice professionals should encourage depressed youth to participate in daily activities, on and off a living unit, unless it is not safe for the youth to do so. Depressed youth may want to sleep all day. They often want to avoid attending school and may say they are too tired to engage in expected behaviors —such as maintaining their hygiene, completing chores in a living unit, or participating in recreational activities. Irritably depressed youth may become oppositional and angry when they are encouraged to participate in these activities. Depressed youth should awaken according to a unit's schedule, shower, and go to school/vocational activities, if required. Even if depressed juveniles complain of not being hungry, they should be expected to attend meals with the rest of the group. Eating a small amount of food or just picking at what they like is fine. Any food is better than no food, and not eating can increase these youths' crankiness and fatigue. Requiring, in a supportive manner, that juveniles go to school, attend recreational activities (even if they sit on the bench), be present in treatment groups, and the like, is beneficial. These activities help distract the youth from all of the things depressing them

and help them avoid becoming isolated from others.

INTERACTION WITH OTHERS
Helping depressed youth to be socially successful can have a significant impact on the youths' mood. Depressed juveniles commonly want to withdraw and spend time alone. Because of their negative view of themselves and others, depressed offenders often find spending time with others a truly aversive experience. Both the quiet, withdrawn depressed youth and the irritable, explosive depressed youth, typically experience interpersonal difficulties. Peers frequently reject them and do not include them in activities. In addition, both types of depressed youth tend to drive their peers away, which results in the juveniles feeling even more pessimistic and alone. This dynamic can become a vicious cycle, with depressed youth avoiding peers to avoid feeling rejected; the isolation can further decrease their already-low feelings of self-esteem.

Juvenile justice professionals should encourage depressed youth to interact with peers, as well as take the time to engage with the youth themselves. When depressed juveniles spend too much time alone, they typically ruminate about all of the bad things that are happening in their lives. Depressed youth also spend a great deal of time thinking about aspects of themselves that they do not like. The more juvenile justice professionals can keep these youth interacting with others, the less time depressed offenders have to focus on themselves and their problems. Preventing isolation and withdrawal is an important goal.

Interacting with a group of other offenders may overwhelm some depressed juveniles. Or, depressed youth may be so irritable and disruptive that engaging in group activities is too chaotic and dangerous. Pairing a depressed youth with one other peer in a living unit who is mature and/or responsible can be less intimidating than participating with a group. Staff can encourage the two juveniles to engage in an

Mood Disorders: Major Depression, Dysthymic Disorder and Bipolar Disorder

activity together (*e.g.*, fold the laundry, play a board game, serve a meal, clean up the unit, shoot basketball hoops). The activity itself is not as important as providing depressed youth with an opportunity to be socially successful.

Juvenile justice professionals must be strategic when placing depressed juveniles in a group with other offenders. If depressed youth are miserable and withdrawn, they will likely feel uncomfortable around others and will sit silently without participating. When they are feeling low, irritably depressed youth do not get along well with others, are easily annoyed by peers, and may get into fights—verbal and physical. This type of depressed offender often harasses others or purposely annoys/provokes peers, reducing the offender's chances of social success in a group situation. Therefore, putting these youth into a group situation and "hoping for the best" or making them a group leader (which puts a great deal of pressure on the youth) is usually not a good idea. Having them initially interact with one peer in a structured activity is a better option. Typically, it only takes one other juvenile with whom the youth can engage to positively impact the depressed youths' mood. This peer does not have to be a friend, just someone with whom the juveniles feel they can "hang out" or talk.

COMMUNICATION

One of the most important things juvenile justice professionals can do for depressed youth is to *listen to them*—really listen to them. This is much easier said than done. Juvenile justice professionals may not have much time for one-to-one interactions with youth. Even when they have the time, staff may not want to listen to depressed offenders who have been disruptive in a living unit, who have cursed at them, or who have been refusing to listen to their requests or directions. Adolescents with Major Depression typically do not explicitly state, "Hey, I'm upset, and I need to talk to you." In today's society, young men talking about their feelings, especially their fears, is typically not

viewed as masculine. This belief is particularly common among young male offenders who want to project a tough and macho image. Females are somewhat more comfortable talking about their feelings and fears, partly because society deems it more acceptable. However, many of the females involved with the juvenile justice system also have a tough image they want to maintain—for adults, peers, and themselves.

When they are upset, most juvenile offenders do not initially want to go to juvenile justice professionals for support. These youth often believe they do not need help from anyone, especially authority figures. After a period of time, however, they are usually willing to talk to staff about personal issues and problems. Many youth with Major Depression throw out verbal "tidbits" related to their problems to see how staff will respond. If juvenile justice professionals interrupt youth mid-sentence or convey the message (through their words and/or behavior) that they do not have time for the youth, depressed juveniles are likely to:

- Feel badly about the interaction
- Feel personally rejected
- Not reach out for support from those individuals again

Unfortunately, some incarcerated youth report that they purposely act out aggressively so that staff will physically restrain them. These youth state that this behavior guarantees that adults will give them attention, will physically touch them, and will debrief with them at length after an incident. Many depressed juvenile offenders do not know how to ask for help in a socially appropriate manner.

Juvenile justice professionals should approach depressed offenders and engage them, instead of waiting for the youth to seek them out. Staff should express concern for juveniles upon noticing a change in the youths' behavior, such as becoming increasingly irritable or withdrawn. Such action can open up a line of communication with depressed youth. Juvenile

Juvenile Offenders with Mental Health Disorders: Who Are They and What Do We Do With Them?

justice professionals may have to approach offenders with Major Depression several times before the youth feel comfortable talking. The staff members' concern can be reassuring to youth, especially when they are told that staff will be available in the future should the youth need support. Taking time to talk individually with depressed juveniles can be difficult when staff have several other youth to manage. However, a few minutes invested when staff initially notice indicators of depression can potentially save a large amount of staff time, energy, and frustration in the end.

If they listen closely to depressed youth as they rant and rave, juvenile justice professionals can typically hear cues as to what particular issues are contributing to the youths' depressed mood.

Listening to depressed juveniles who are irritable and agitated can be difficult. When juvenile justice professionals ask them what is wrong, these youth may exclaim, "None of your f*****g business! Leave me alone!" Most staff would be more than happy to do that. However, that is typically what aggressively depressed youth want—to push people away so that they can be alone. Approaching and listening to sad and tearful youth talk about what is bothering them is much easier than listening to angry youth. Staff should continue to approach irritable youth during times the youth appear calm. Irritably depressed youth often communicate what is truly bothering them while they are yelling and making demands about something trivial. If they listen closely to depressed youth as they rant and rave, juvenile justice professionals can typically hear cues as to what particular issues are contributing to the youths' depressed mood. Statements are usually made about how staff disrespected the youth, treated

them unfairly, gave other youth extra privileges, and so forth. Or, juveniles may make statements about how they are never going to be released from a facility, how nobody comes to visit them, or how no one cares about them. Youth with Major Depression can get very upset about these types of issues, and the issues are usually only briefly revealed when the juveniles are screaming about something else. Once youth calm down, staff can go back and calmly discuss the juveniles' concerns, clarifying any miscommunication or misperceptions on the part of the youth.

Juvenile offenders with Major Depression often need a great deal of time to develop trust, so repeated attempts at communication are usually the norm rather than the exception. Additionally, depressed juvenile offenders are often extra-attuned to juvenile justice professionals' behavior and will pick up on the little things that staff do to build trust—even when staff are unaware of their own behavior. The following actions can often go a long way when developing trust with depressed juvenile offenders:

- Acknowledging youth when staff first come on shift

- Checking in with youth about a goal they are working on

- Letting youth know that staff take their sleep concerns seriously

- Inquiring about juveniles' visitors or lack thereof

- Following through on promises/ agreements, no matter how small or trivial

Active Listening
When talking to depressed juveniles, juvenile justice professionals should convey that they truly understand what youth are trying to say. Giving their full attention to youth and maintaining eye contact is important. Using sayings such as, "Got it," "Mm-hmm," and "Yeah" can let youth know that staff are paying attention. Active listening seems easy, but it actually takes

a great deal of practice to do comfortably and with skill. The goal is for depressed youth to feel that staff understand and accept youths' thoughts and feelings about a situation, particularly if they are angry or upset.

The following are some communication strategies that adults use when working with depressed youth (Faber & Mazlish ,1980). They are not very effective and can often alienate the juveniles:

- Give advice ("Call your cousin and tell him you aren't going to do that," or "You should go back to live with your mother")

- Be philosophical ("Life isn't fair," or "We don't always get what we want, we get what we need")

- Deny what youth are feeling ("I saw you laughing earlier; I bet you aren't as sad as you think," or "You don't look that mad to me")

- Disagree with them ("That's not what she was trying to do," or "A staff member would never say that")

- Tell youth they are blowing a situation out of proportion ("C'mon, it's not that big of a deal" or "I am sure it is not as bad as you think it is")

- Reassure youth without evidence ("I'm sure everything will turn out fine," or "I am sure that is not what he meant when he said that")

Although adults engage in these strategies to be helpful, and their intentions are usually good, such strategies often invalidate youths' thoughts and feelings. Giving advice to depressed offenders can convey that they are not smart enough to handle the situation and that someone needs to tell them what they should do. Having youth think of solutions on their own is much more effective. Juveniles may need some help with this, but they need to be an active part of the process. Hearing that their experience is not a "big deal" can be demeaning for youth.

When depressed juveniles are emotionally upset, they want someone to listen to them and understand their point of view; they want to feel validated. Statements such as, "I can see why that made you mad," "Yeah, that is scary," and "That *is* a stressful situation" are examples of how juvenile justice professionals can show that they understand what the youth are going through. These statements also help create trust and rapport. Staff do not necessarily need to take the side of juveniles or agree with the youths' assessment of a situation. In fact, staff may think depressed youth are overreacting or being overly sensitive. Just being non-judgmental and listening can go a long way to help depressed youth with their problems.

Relationships with adults are extremely important to youth, particularly those involved with juvenile justice. These juveniles may have had only a few positive relationships with adults in their entire lives. Many juvenile offenders were raised in households full of conflict and strain; many have had negative experiences with teachers and law enforcement. Building a relationship with staff is an opportunity for depressed youth to develop a positive and trusting relationship with adult authority figures.

Not every juvenile justice professional is going to work well with all youth. Each individual staff member has his or her own personal style and will work more effectively with some youth versus others. For example, some juvenile justice personnel view oppositional, disruptive youth as a challenge and enjoy working with these types of youth. Other staff find this type of behavior intolerable. Regardless, being available to listen when youth, especially depressed youth, are ready to talk is important for all juvenile justice professionals.

Unfortunately, juvenile justice professionals often are required to supervise a large number of youth at once, as well as simultaneously complete other required job responsibilities. Therefore, staff may find it difficult to be available to youth the exact moment juveniles need to talk. Juvenile justice professionals can communicate that they are interested in what youth have to say but cannot provide their full attention at that time. Giving a *specific* time when staff will be available to talk with youth individually, even if only for a few minutes, will usually pacify depressed juveniles. However, staff must make sure to follow up on any promises and agreements made. Typically, it is not the duration of time juvenile justice professionals spend with depressed offenders that has the greatest impact. Staffs' undivided attention and genuine attempt to understand the youth is what seems to make the biggest difference.

EFFECTIVE BEHAVIOR MANAGEMENT

Depressed youth, particularly those who are irritable and angry, often engage in behavior that is disruptive to a living unit. This behavior must be attended to and appropriately sanctioned. When most individuals think of behavior management, they usually think of punishing youth to stop unwanted behavior. However, reinforcing desired behaviors is just as important. Staff should make sure to support positive behaviors youth should continue. Reinforcement should be given whenever depressed offenders do something positive: appropriately engaging with other peers, assisting with unit responsibilities, following directions without difficulty, and so forth. Examples of effective reinforcement include:

- A few moments of personal time with staff
- A few extra minutes on a telephone call
- Permission to leave their room for a drink of water before going to sleep

Elaborate reinforcers are not necessary. Smiling, winking, or exclaiming, "Good job!" on the part of juvenile justice professionals can go a long way with depressed youth. Reinforcement can be both easy and efficient, and it typically has a positive affect on staff as well.

Negative consequences for misbehavior are also important. Maintaining security and control within juvenile justice facilities is critical. If depressed youth are engaging in unacceptable behavior, they should be sanctioned. However, harsh and painful consequences are not likely to improve youths' behavior; they also can hurt and humiliate them. Juvenile offenders with Major Depression are particularly sensitive to negative feedback, especially criticism and aversive consequences. Removing offenders from a group and using their room for a "time-out" period can be effective. Rather than being seen as a *punishment*, however, time-out periods should be an opportunity to problem-solve. Youth should be able to identify what triggered their behavior (*e.g.*, thoughts, feelings, behaviors) and how they would handle a similar situation more appropriately in the future. Having youth take a time-out in their room can also be helpful for staff, who may also need a chance to cool off. Depressed offenders can be difficult to work with, and some of these youth repeatedly provoke fights and arguments with authority figures. *(Please see Chapters 3 and 14 for additional information on effective behavior management.)*

HOPE

Many juvenile offenders with Major Depression feel hopeless. They often feel negatively about their current circumstances, as well as what lies ahead for them in the future. Some of these young offenders feel as if they are never going to return to the community. Unfortunately, the reality for some juveniles is that they will be incarcerated for years. Therefore, helping depressed youth focus on positive events (no matter how small) in the future is important. Such events may include a pizza party or movie night at the end of the week, a visit with a favorite relative at the end of the month, or a high school diploma at the end of the year. Giving depressed youth something to look forward to provides them with a sense that things can get better. And it helps keep them motivated to participate in facility programming and treatment. Hopelessness is strongly related to suicidal behavior. Helping youth build hope

Mood Disorders: Major Depression, Dysthymic Disorder and Bipolar Disorder

through small incidents of empowerment and success can help improve their mood, as well as help protect them from suicidal thoughts and behavior.

COMMUNICATION WITH SCHOOL PERSONNEL

School is difficult for many of youth involved in the juvenile justice system, especially those who suffer from Major Depression. Most depressed juveniles have difficulty concentrating and paying attention to their school assignments. Many of these youth also have learning disorders and do not feel they can do anything right in the classroom. They frequently perceive themselves as failures and often have given up trying to achieve in the academic arena.

Offenders who are frustrated in the classroom, and who do not want to be there, often behave in a disruptive manner. This behavior gets them removed from a classroom and sent back to their living unit. Once removed, depressed juveniles miss what is being taught and fall further behind in their academic work. This dynamic typically exacerbates offenders' depressed mood, feelings of hopelessness, and low opinion of themselves. Therefore, juvenile justice juvenile justice professionals must communicate and work collaboratively with educational staff so that depressed youth can remain in the classroom for as much time as possible. Additionally, educational staff may need to provide depressed juveniles with extra time for assignments or remedial assistance, so that the youth can achieve some success in the classroom.

AVOIDING ISOLATION

Some juvenile offenders with Major Depression engage in extreme negative behavior to avoid interacting with others and participating in daily activities. Irritably depressed juvenile offenders are quick to realize which negative behaviors result in room confinement or placement in a seclusion room. These youth may purposefully engage in aggressive behavior with the goal of seclusion in mind. Once confined to their own room or a seclusion room, these youth no longer have to deal with peers, school/vocational responsibilities, or staff. Secluded depressed juveniles are similar to depressed adults who want to pull the bed covers over their head. Once confined in a room, they can sleep all day long. One of the best ways for depressed youth to withdraw socially from others is to be secluded for disciplinary reasons.

When these juveniles are about to be released from seclusion back into the general population, they often engage in behavior that guarantees them additional time in isolation. Isolation from others is not helpful and can be potentially harmful to depressed youth. Depressed youth tend to spend their time thinking about all of the things they are depressed about when alone in a room with minimal stimuli and nothing to do but sleep. This situation is likely to exacerbate these juveniles' feelings of sorrow and loneliness. When the above dynamic becomes apparent with depressed youth, staff should discuss alternative ways of managing the youths' negative behavior. Staff should make sure not to inadvertently reward negative behavior with an opportunity for social withdrawal.

MANAGEMENT OF STAFF EMOTIONS

Working with depressed offenders who are irritable, cranky and explosive can be taxing. These youth often defy authority and refuse to do what is asked of them. Juvenile justice staff may become angry and frustrated with youth who continually blow up, defy them or engage in personal insults. Although these feelings are understandable, they are not helpful to the situation or the youths' behavior. Staffs' ability to help youth engage in alternative and more positive behaviors is significantly compromised when staff themselves are upset. For example, when juvenile justice professionals are angry, they may have difficulty reinforcing depressed juveniles' small successes because all of the youths' behavior seems negative. Moving beyond depressed offenders' annoying and often

78

Juvenile Offenders with Mental Health Disorders: Who Are They and What Do We Do With Them?

provocative behavior can be difficult. But it must be done if a change in youth behavior is the desired outcome.

Juvenile justice professionals must remember that the aggressively depressed offenders are suffering from a mental health disorder. It may be genetic, it may be a result of early childhood losses or abuses, or it may be a combination of all of these. Regardless of the underlying cause, youth with Major Depression did not *choose* to be afflicted with the disorder. Although they may seem to purposely and volitionally provoke staff, this may or may not be the case. Depressed youth may have little control over their irritability and explosive behavior. Although their behavior can feel personal to staff, a closer look typically reveals that depressed offenders behave that way with many individuals. It is true that some juvenile offenders have both Major Depression AND enjoy deliberately irritating and annoying staff. The important thing is not to *assume* that their negative behavior is purposeful until there is clear evidence this is the case.

Taking care of themselves is critical for juvenile justice professionals. Working with depressed offenders can be a difficult and exhausting task. Chronic fatigue, irritability, somatic complaints, insomnia, hopelessness, and lack of motivation can also be signs of depression in adults. The repeated experience of receiving personal insults from depressed juveniles, as well as the level of intensity often needed to manage aggressive and irritable youth, can result in burnout. Staff should be aware of the signs and symptoms of Major Depression and seek treatment for themselves if they begin showing signs of the disorder.

MENTAL HEALTH SERVICES UPON RELEASE

An appointment for mental health services in the community should be scheduled for youth with Major Depression if they are scheduled for release from a facility prior to being seen by a mental health professional. Depressed youth receiving mental health services in a juvenile justice facility who need to continue treatment should also have an appointment scheduled in the community upon release. Treatment formats can include individual, group and/or family therapy. Treatment for Major Depression typically includes psychopharmacology and cognitive behavioral interventions that target important areas of youths' lives (*e.g.*, family relationships, peer relationships, academic achievement, substance use). Strategies used may include, cognitive restructuring, problem-solving skills training, social skills training, increase of pleasurable activities, and relaxation skills.

Case Example

Josh, 16, was arrested and charged with robbery. Josh ran away from his mother's home eight months ago. Josh's father committed suicide when Josh was 10 and since that time, Josh has become increasingly oppositional with his mother. Over the past year, Josh has become verbally abusive toward his mother and on two occasions, he physically assaulted her. Since leaving home, Josh has been staying with friends or at the local youth shelter. Josh has been unable to stay in either of these living arrangements for extended periods of time because of his extreme irritability and disruptive behavior. Both his friends and shelter staff usually ask him to leave after several days because of his behavior. Josh refuses to get out of bed before 3:00 p.m., watches television for hours, and says he is too tired to help clean up. Josh rarely eats and tends to keep to himself, even when his friends have parties or there are activities at the youth shelter where he was sleeping. Although Josh rarely talks to anyone, when he does, he uses racial slurs, provokes peers and adults, and often ends up in a physical altercation. For the past four months, the few times Josh got along with his peers was when they were all smoking marijuana. Recently, Josh was asked to leave the youth shelter for the final

time. He felt he had no choice but to rent a motel room or sleep on the streets. Josh decided to rob a taxicab driver to pay for a motel room. Josh was arrested and taken to the local juvenile detention facility, where he had been incarcerated twice before on misdemeanor charges. Since being incarcerated, Josh has spent the majority of his time restricted to his room for provoking peers and attempting to assault staff. Josh says he does not care about the amount of time in "room confinement" he receives. He states he has nothing better to do with his life and that he looks forward to the additional hours of sleep. In fact, his peers overheard him say he wishes he could "go to sleep and never wake up." Josh has never been referred for mental health services, and most juvenile justice professionals are convinced he "enjoys getting into trouble."

Many youth similar to Josh are involved with the juvenile justice system. These youth are often labeled "bad kids" or "difficult kids" and typically given a diagnosis of Conduct Disorder. Given his criminal history and current charge, Josh will likely be sent to a long-term juvenile justice facility. Without an evaluation by a mental health/medical professional and proper treatment, Josh will likely continue his pattern of negative behavior at the next juvenile justice facility. He will likely end up serving the majority of his teenage years confined to his room. Juvenile justice professionals who come into contact with youth who are exhibiting symptoms of Major Depression should bring them to the attention of supervisors and/or refer them to mental health/medical professionals for evaluation.

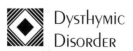 DysThymic Disorder

Dysthymic Disorder (also known as Dysthymia) is a less acute mood disorder than Major Depression but can still have significant nega-

tive consequences for a youth. Although depressive symptoms of Dysthymia are not as severe as those of Major Depression, they are much more chronic in nature. For youth to be diagnosed with Dysthymic Disorder, they need to experience a *depressed* or *irritable* mood most of the day, more days than not, for at least one year (two years in adults) PLUS two of the following (APA, 2000):

- Poor Appetite or Overeating
- Difficulty Sleeping or Excessive Sleeping
- Low Energy or Fatigue
- Low Self-esteem
- Poor Concentration or Difficulty Making Decisions
- Feelings of Hopelessness

Juveniles suffering from Dysthymic Disorder are persistently irritable or depressed and often appear miserable, regardless of what they are doing. They worry much of the time and tend to be critical of themselves. They are frequently preoccupied with their mistakes and failures and often feel they have little to offer others. Youth with this disorder may claim they are bored, tired or uninterested in an activity. Many of these youth are introverted and have difficulty interacting with others. Juvenile offenders with Dysthymic Disorder often describe feeling "pissed off all of the time," or that "everyone gets on my nerves." They become easily annoyed at everything and everyone around them, which can result in significant conflict with peers and staff. Dysthymic youth often complain that no one cares about them and that staff are purposely excluding them or treating them unfairly. Periods of extreme irritability and anger are not uncommon.

Whereas Major Depression represents a *change* from youths' typical functioning, the symptoms of Dysthymic Disorder are *representative* of youths' typical functioning. Individuals with Dysthymic Disorder are often referred to as having a "depressed personality" because their personality and behavior seems they have

80

Juvenile Offenders with Mental Health Disorders: Who Are They and What Do We Do With Them?

always been that way. Dysthymic juveniles often report having the above symptoms of the disorder for "as long as I can remember." Many youth in the juvenile justice system experience periods of irritability or depression, but in order to qualify for a diagnosis of Dysthymic Disorder, youths' symptoms must occur for at least a year. And the symptoms must cause the youth *significant distress* and/or *interfere* with their ability to function in daily activities (*e.g.*, school, home, juvenile justice facility). Dysthymic youths' mood-related symptoms cannot be caused solely by drug and/or alcohol intoxication or withdrawal or be the direct result of a medical condition (*e.g.* hypothyroidism). Dysthymic Disorder is likely to be one of the most misidentified or unidentified diagnoses among adolescents in the juvenile justice system.

Among adolescents, Dysthymic Disorder commonly co-exists with additional psychiatric disorders such as anxiety disorders, Attention-Deficit/Hyperactivity Disorder, Oppositional Defiant Disorder, and Conduct Disorder.

Dysthymic Disorder differs from Major Depression in several ways. Major Depression is usually a much more short-lived, intense type of mood disturbance. Conversely, Dysthymic Disorder is typically a less intense but more chronic form of depression and/or irritability. Dysthymic youth may experience less social withdrawal and sleep/appetite disturbances than youth with Major Depression. These youth also typically do not experience the excessive feelings of guilt and preoccupation with morbid themes associated with Major Depression. However, both Dysthymic Disorder and Major Depression can have significant deleterious effects on youths' functioning and ability to engage effectively with others.

Course of Dysthymic Disorder

Dysthymic Disorder typically lasts for several years. Therefore, most young offenders with Dysthymia do not spontaneously discuss their mental health disorder because their symptoms have become such a typical part of their lives.

These youth often just assume, "It's just the way I am."

The clinical course of Dysthymic Disorder varies among individual youth. Some offenders experience an intense and severe episode of Major Depression in addition to their Dysthymia, often referred to as "double depression." Once the major depressive episode resolves (with or without treatment), the Dysthymic Disorder may still remain. Many juveniles diagnosed with Dysthymia will recover from the illness by the time they reach adulthood. However, a significant percentage of youth diagnosed with Dysthymic Disorder will later experience one or more episodes of Major Depression. After one episode of Major Depression, youth are at risk for continued episodes of Major Depression or Bipolar Disorder (Kovacs, Akiskal, Gatsonis, & Parrone, 1994).

Although it appears to be less severe and incapacitating than Major Depression, Dysthymic Disorder is not a negligible or minor problem. The age of onset for Dysthymic Disorder is usually younger than that for Major Depression, and Dysthymia tends to last a significantly longer time. Dysthymic Disorder can cause a great deal of emotional suffering for juveniles and often interferes with their ability to interact with others (*e.g.*, family, friends, teachers, juvenile justice professionals). In addition, being ill with Dysthymia also places offenders at greater risk for suicidal ideation and a suicide attempt (Kovacs, Goldston, & Gatsonis, 1993). Proper identification and treatment of youth with Dysthymic Disorder can significantly affect these youths' adolescent experiences—as well as possibly prevent the occurrence of other mood disorders (*i.e.*, Major Depression, Bipolar Disorder) as the youth age.

Biological Characteristics of Dysthymia

Similar to Major Depression, Dysthymia also appears to be related to heritable factors. Family members suffering from both Major Depression and Bipolar Disorder are common among individuals diagnosed with Dysthymic Disorder. These rates may even be higher than that for youth diagnosed with Major Depression (Akiskal & Weise, 1992). In addition, significantly more first-degree relatives of Dysthymic individuals are hospitalized for mood disorders in comparison to their counterparts with Major Depression. Adding to this genetic evidence is the finding that identical twins are more likely to share symptoms of Dysthymic Disorder versus fraternal twins.

Stressful life events are also likely to play a role in the development and maintenance of this disorder, but the exact mechanism remains unknown.

Managing Youth with Dysthymic Disorder

Most of the management strategies that are effective with juveniles who have Major Depression are likely to be effective when working with offenders who have Dysthymic Disorder (*see section on Managing Juvenile Offenders with Major Depression*). Youth suspected of having Dysthymic Disorder should be referred to a mental health/medical professional for an evaluation. Antidepressant medication may alleviate some of the youths' symptoms. But engaging these youth in daily activities, encouraging interaction with others (peers and adults), and communicating with these juveniles in a nonjudgmental and accepting manner is also important. Arranging situations where Dysthymic youth can be socially successful can positively influence the way these youths feel about themselves.

In addition, Dysthymic youth may need assistance regarding school-related activities, and communication with school personnel can be critical. As with youth who have Major Depression, using effective behavior management strategies also is essential with offenders suffering from Dysthymic Disorder. Juvenile justice professionals should focus on positively reinforcing appropriate and prosocial behaviors (no matter how small) and provide immediate negative consequences for antisocial, disruptive behaviors.

Case Example

Lawanda, 15, has been incarcerated in a state training school for three months and has four additional months left to serve on her sentence. When Lawanda was four, her mother was placed in a psychiatric hospital for a suicide attempt. Her mother's depression began shortly after the birth of the first of her four children and would come and go without warning. Lawanda was the youngest of her siblings. The state removed all four children from the family home after their mother's suicide attempt, and they all went to live with family members. Lawanda lived with various aunts and cousins, until moving in with her grandmother two years ago.

Lawanda has received several sanctions during her stay at the juvenile justice facility. She attends educational classes at the training school in order to get her GED, but Lawanda hates school and says she finds the work difficult. She repeatedly refers to herself as "stupid" and an "idiot." Lawanda was diagnosed with a learning disorder when she was in the 5th grade and was placed in several special education classes. The teachers in the facility GED program have tried to provide her with extra assistance. But Lawanda becomes angry whenever a teacher corrects her work or makes suggestions as to how she can do things differently. At these times, Lawanda typically demands that everyone leave her alone and refuses to finish her assignments.

Lawanda does not get along well with the other girls at the facility because they think she is too "cranky" and "bossy." Outwardly, Lawanda constantly criticizes her peers, and inwardly, she is constantly criticizing herself. In addition, Lawanda has had the opportunity to be involved with several group activities in her living unit. However, she usually chooses to spend her time alone because "the other girls get on my nerves". Lawanda says she remembers

82

Juvenile Offenders with Mental Health Disorders: Who Are They and What Do We Do With Them?

spending a great deal of time by herself when she was younger. If other kids were around, she would get mad and hit them. She reports feeling this way about other people for as long as she can remember.

Fortunately, Lawanda has not been in a physical fight in more than six months. Most of Lawanda's criminal activity consists of stealing makeup, food from the local grocery store, or clothes. She states that she wants to get her GED. Yet, Lawanda does not know whether she would like to get a job when she is released from the training school. She states that she has no interests or hobbies, so she does not know what kind of work she would do. Because Lawanda is no longer physically assaultive, and she tends to keep to herself, she is not likely to receive much individual attention from staff. Her behavior (including criminal behavior) is not dramatic or serious in appearance. Therefore, she probably will not receive any specialized treatment services. Left untreated, Lawanda's Dysthymia is likely to continue and possibly worsen if she is unemployed after release.

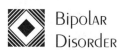 Bipolar Disorder

Juveniles with Bipolar Disorder tend to exhibit significant changes in mood that are typically cyclical in nature. Bipolar Disorder (previously known as Manic Depressive Disorder) refers to a syndrome in which the presence of *mania* typically alternates with symptoms of *depression*. The name "Bipolar" reflects the alternation between the two different *poles* of mood. A description of the *depressed* phase of this disorder was discussed at the beginning of the chapter under Major Depression. The following is a description of the *manic* phase of this disorder.

According to the *DSM-IV-TR* (APA, 2000), in order to meet diagnostic criteria for mania, youth must experience "a period of abnormally and persistently elevated, expansive or irritable mood" that lasts at least one week (or could last any duration if the symptoms are severe enough that psychiatric hospitalization is required). Among youth in the juvenile justice system, manic episodes are typically characterized by an extremely irritable mood more often than an elevated, expansive mood.

Youth with Bipolar disorder must also experience three of the following symptoms (or four of the following if the youths' mood is irritable) persistently or to a significant degree. Similar to symptoms of Major Depression, the following symptoms are typically a change from how juveniles typically behave:

INFLATED SELF-ESTEEM OR GRANDIOSITY

Grandiosity and exaggerated feelings of superiority are common among individuals experiencing a manic episode. Grandiose juvenile offenders often directly challenge authority figures, including juvenile justice professionals. These youth often believe that:

- Juvenile justice facility rules do not apply to them
- They should receive special favors from the staff
- They are "above" the negative consequences given to other youth

These youth do not just have a biased perspective. Manic youth truly hold these beliefs as the "truth."

Manic juveniles may be very outspoken about their dissatisfaction with facility rules and may go to great lengths to try to have them changed. Additionally, juveniles in a manic state may provoke peers who are much larger and tougher than they are. In this state, manic youth typically believe they are able to overpower anyone regardless of their size or status. They may even physically provoke juvenile justice professionals. Even though they are incarcerated, manic juveniles continue to possess an attitude of entitlement because they rigidly hold onto their false beliefs of grandiosity. When receiving sanctions, these youth are often found yelling to staff, "You can't do this to ME."

Grandiosity is much more extreme than the arrogant attitudes seen among some juvenile offenders. During a manic episode, youth may feel extremely important and believe they have special abilities, talents, and knowledge that others do not possess. Manic youth tend to brag and be overly self-confident. They often talk about significant personal achievements in areas where they have no skills or training. They may give peers elaborate advice or specific instructions even though they have no knowledge of a subject. These beliefs can be so extreme that youth become *delusional*, believing things that are completely irrational or illogical. For example, manic youth with delusions may believe they are chosen as a messengers of God, are famous rap stars, or NBA basketball players. Delusional females may believe they are pregnant with the baby of a celebrity, even though they have never met that individual.

DECREASED NEED FOR SLEEP

Youth suffering from Bipolar Disorder may go several nights sleeping only a few hours, or they may go without any sleep at all. Most sleep-deprived individuals would feel tired or lethargic and have difficulty concentrating. Youth experiencing a manic episode, however, continue to have a tremendous amount of energy despite their lack of sleep. This decreased need for sleep is not associated with any type of substance use, such as methamphetamine or cocaine. Evaluations of manic youth should always clarify the juveniles' use of drugs and alcohol because the effects of various types of drugs can mimic manic symptomatology. Youths' report of not sleeping for several days in a row without an accompanying feeling of tiredness is often a classic sign of a manic episode.

MORE TALKATIVE THAN USUAL OR PRESSURED SPEECH

When juveniles are experiencing a manic episode, they may talk very loudly and rapidly. Interrupting them or getting a word in edgewise can be difficult. Youth engaging in this type of pressured speech can talk so quickly that it appears as if they were unable to stop the words from coming out of their mouth—even if that is what they want to occur. Additionally, if they are extremely irritable, these youth can become very argumentative, even over minor or trivial issues. Juvenile offenders with Bipolar Disorder often complain, insult staff, and engage in hostile comments with little provocation. Some manic youth become very dramatic in their speech, overly exaggerating their words or suddenly breaking into song. Manic youth are commonly found talking to others for extended periods of time even though those they are talking to clearly are not interested. In contrast, some manic youth may become hostile and angry in the middle of a pleasant conversation for no apparent reason.

JUMPING FROM ONE SUBJECT TO ANOTHER WITHOUT OBVIOUS CONNECTION OR FEELING LIKE THOUGHTS ARE RACING TOO FAST

Engaging in conversation with youth who are experiencing a manic episode can be difficult. Even when juvenile justice professionals are paying attention and listening to the words of manic youth, the conversation may still make little to no sense at all. The topics may be remotely related, but there is no logical connection between them. This is referred to as *flight of ideas*.

For example:

Fifteen-year-old Cheri had been brought to juvenile detention for not going to school. She was trying to explain to her probation officer why she was so upset. "You don't understand, my mom just called and told me that my boyfriend is hookin' up with another girl. I can't believe that she was wearing those types of jeans. Those jeans have only been worn by

84

Juvenile Offenders with Mental Health Disorders: Who Are They and What Do We Do With Them?

people that live near the water, and I'm so thirsty, I haven't had anything to drink since this morning when they served us that nasty cereal. I can name every single cereal ever made—Frosted Flakes, Rice Krispies, Trix, Fruit Loops, Apple Jacks, Golden Grahams, Honeycomb, Count Chocula, Captain Crunch with Crunchberries, Sugar Pops, Sugar Smacks, Frosted Mini Wheats. I need to get out of here so I can have macaroni and cheese for dinner. I can't believe that I haven't had a TV dinner since I've been locked up. I love that TV show with those funny babies who have televisions in their tummies. Cracks me up because Jackie is pregnant, and soon she'll be going to the laundromat, washing all those socks and cleaning up all those dishes. What time is it? I need to talk to get out of here and meet my friends at Taco Bell."**

Typically, youth experiencing a manic episode believe they are making sense, and they appear to understand what it is they are saying. The abrupt topic changes observed in their speech are likely representative of the type of unorganized thinking processes they are experiencing in their head. Manic youth often describe their thoughts as occurring very quickly. Some juveniles find this situation annoying because their thoughts are occurring too quickly—faster than what they can release out of their mouths. These youth may feel as though they are thinking too many thoughts at one time and have difficulty deciding which ones should be said aloud.

DISTRACTIBILITY
Youth experiencing a manic episode are easily distracted by irrelevant stimuli in the environment. They are frequently drawn to pay attention to everything that is going on around them. For example, background noise, posters on a wall, or an individual walking nearby can

completely throw a manic youth off track. Remaining on one topic of conversation for a significant period of time before something distracts their attention can be difficult for these youth. Juvenile offenders with mania often completely ignore what staff are saying or change the topic of conversation if they think about something of more interest to them. These youth have a hard time discriminating between what is and is not important—everything seems important to them. Manic youth may be listening only half-heartedly when juvenile justice professionals provide them with instructions or explicitly direct them to do something. These juveniles are typically more concerned with what is happening on the other side of the room.

INCREASED ACTIVITY AT WORK, SCHOOL, SOCIALLY
Individuals experiencing a manic episode often have a great deal of energy and are overwhelmed with numerous new ideas. Therefore, they often throw themselves into multiple activities at once. Due to their lack of organization and planning, their actions and plans are typically disorganized and chaotic. They may begin several new tasks simultaneously but leave all of them incomplete as they move onto something new and more interesting. Manic youth involved in the juvenile justice system usually exhibit an increase in the type of activity with which they were previously involved. If offenders were using drugs or alcohol, participating in gang activity, or engaging in vandalism, there may be an increased involvement in these types of activities.

Manic offenders often increase their social activity. They may want to interact with anyone and everyone who is willing to talk with them, which can result in the development of inappropriate relationships. Manic offenders may become involved with individuals much older than themselves, including those who lead dangerous and criminal lifestyles. Because of their intense need for socialization, manic

Mood Disorders: Major Depression, Dysthymic Disorder and Bipolar Disorder

youth may not realize when their social behaviors are inappropriate. For example, they may arrive unannounced at someone's house in the middle of the night or invite strangers to stay in their families' home. Because they want to be around people all of the time, manic juveniles are excited by social interaction and do not think about the consequences of their actions.

Hypersexuality and sexual promiscuity are common among adolescents during a manic episode. This behavior could include engaging in elaborate sexual fantasies, calling sex telephone hotlines, watching large amounts of pornography, experiencing an insatiable appetite for sex with a romantic partner, or desiring to have sex with a variety of partners. Sexual behavior during a manic episode often includes unprotected sex with individuals who could be very harmful to youth in a variety of ways.

Youth diagnosed with Bipolar Disorder may be unaware of their unusual behavior and therefore resistant to any type of mental health treatment.

IMPULSIVE BEHAVIOR

Because they are not thinking about the consequences of their actions, youth in the manic phase of Bipolar Disorder often engage in high-risk activities. Delinquent behavior such as theft, destruction of others' property, and trespassing are not uncommon during a manic episode. Juveniles with no history of criminal involvement might borrow their parents' car during a manic episode and decide to take a cross-country joyride with their best friend. Youth who typically have good judgment may decide to break into their school on the weekend in order to play games on the computers.

During manic episodes, adolescents often place themselves in dangerous, and sometimes deadly, situations. Because they have difficulty appreciating the nature of their behavior, manic

youth often do not think about the ramifications of their actions. Even if they do know the dangers, they feel invincible and indestructible. This feeling is one of the reasons sexual promiscuity, criminal behavior and substance use are common during the manic phase of Bipolar Disorder. Sexual behavior with high-risk partners can be a serious health concern, as youth can be exposed to Sexually Transmitted Diseases and the Human Immunodeficiency Virus (HIV).

When in a manic phase, youth often engage in binge drinking and consume drugs in amounts larger than they are typically used to consuming. They may get into a car and drive significantly over the speed limit, placing their lives and the lives of others in danger. They may engage in serious and dangerous criminal activity, with poor planning and a high likelihood of being injured by potential victims or law enforcement.

Bipolar Disorder should not be confused with the normal, and often intense, mood fluctuations typical of the adolescent years. The emotional instability among youth with Bipolar Disorder is so extreme that it causes significant impairment in these juveniles' ability to function. To be diagnosed with a manic episode, youths' symptoms cannot be caused by drug or alcohol intoxication or withdrawal, and they cannot be the direct effect of a medical condition (*e.g.*, hyperthyroidism). Bipolar Disorder is currently being over-diagnosed among adolescents—including those involved with the juvenile justice system.

Associated Features of Bipolar Disorder

Youth diagnosed with Bipolar Disorder may be unaware of their unusual behavior and therefore resistant to any type of mental health treatment. Although both adults and peers can see the abrupt changes in the juveniles' mood—with shifts from euphoria to anger or depression—the adolescents themselves may be oblivious to their mood fluctuations. At times,

86

Juvenile Offenders with Mental Health Disorders: Who Are They and What Do We Do With Them?

these young offenders may seem similar to Dr. Jeckyl and Mr. Hyde if their moods change frequently enough. While experiencing a manic episode, youth typically refuse to abide by longstanding rules and blatantly defy authority. Their emotional reactions can be extreme; they think in black-and-white terms, and reasoning with them is usually futile.

Some youth with Bipolar Disorder experience psychotic symptoms during either the manic or depressed phase of the illness. They may hear voices of people who are not present, become extremely paranoid, or vigorously hold onto beliefs about themselves that could not possibly be true. Hallucinations and delusions are typically mood congruent. Therefore, if youth are depressed, they typically hear or see negative, pessimistic stimuli (*e.g.*, hearing voices telling them they are bad, deserve to be punished, and/or should kill themselves). Youth in a manic phase may have hallucinations and delusions reflective of how wonderful they believe they are. For example, a female offender may be convinced she is pregnant even though she is still a virgin. A male offender may be convinced that people can read his mind and are trying to steal his ideas because of his incredible intelligence. Due to these types of symptoms, many youth with Bipolar Disorder have been misdiagnosed with Schizophrenia (Carlson, 1990).

Overlapping Symptoms with Other Psychiatric Disorders

Bipolar Disorder is difficult to diagnose among adolescents because many of the symptoms look similar to those of other psychiatric disorders. Distractibility, overactivity, restlessness and impulsivity can be seen among youth with Bipolar Disorder, as well as youth who have been diagnosed with Attention-Deficit/Hyperactivity Disorder (ADHD). In Bipolar Disorder, the impulsivity and overactivity is typically directed toward activities youth find interesting and pleasurable. In contrast, youth with ADHD tend to behave this way regardless of the type of

activity. Extreme irritability, oppositional behavior, belligerence and participation in activities with negative consequences can be present among youth with Bipolar Disorder and youth diagnosed with Conduct Disorder. Bipolar Disorder tends to have an uncontrollable quality to it, with significant changes in mood. Youth with Conduct Disorder, however, typically do not show major changes in mood; their defiance of authority and rule-breaking behavior are more chronic and constant. In addition, youth with ADHD or Conduct Disorder typically do not have some of the other symptoms of Bipolar Disorder (*i.e.*, decreased need for sleep, grandiosity, psychotic symptoms). However, juvenile offenders with Bipolar Disorder can be diagnosed with ADHD and Conduct Disorder in *addition* to their mood disorder. (*Please see Chapters 2 and 5 for additional information on Conduct Disorder and Attention-Deficit/Hyperactivity Disorder.*) Youth who are high on drugs (*e.g.*, cocaine, methamphetamine) can also display symptoms similar to those of mania. This can be a significant diagnostic issue among some juvenile offenders.

Course of Bipolar Disorder

Manic episodes usually begin suddenly and can last anywhere from one week to a few months. Many youth experience episodes of mania immediately before or after an episode of Major Depression. But some adolescents experience symptoms of depression and mania at the same time. The majority of offenders who have one manic episode will continue to have repeated episodes throughout their lifetime. And the episodes are likely to occur more closely together as the youth grow older. About half of the adolescents with Bipolar Disorder will return to their previous level of functioning after a manic episode resolves. But another half may continue to show significant impairment (McClellan & Werry, 1993). Youth with Bipolar Disorder are at increased risk for completed suicide, and this finding is especially true for males in the depressed phase of the disorder.

Mood Disorders: Major Depression, Dysthymic Disorder and Bipolar Disorder

What Causes Bipolar Disorder?

Although the exact cause(s) of Bipolar Disorder is/are not known, heredity clearly plays a significant role (Rice, *et al.*, 1987). Having a close relative, particularly a parent, with Bipolar Disorder significantly increases the chances that juveniles will also suffer from this disorder. Youth at highest risk to develop Bipolar Disorder are those with a history of severe hyperactivity, temper outbursts, unstable mood, and a family history of Bipolar Disorder.

Management of Youth with Bipolar Disorder

REFERRAL

Youth suspected of suffering from Bipolar Disorder should be referred to a mental health/medical professional. If youth meet diagnostic criteria for Bipolar Disorder, the following management strategies can be effective in helping these juveniles continue to participate in facility programming without major disruption to other offenders or major conflict with staff.

PSYCHOTROPIC MEDICATION

Mood Stabilizers (*e.g.*, Lithium®, Depakote®, Tegretol®) are typically prescribed for youth suffering from Bipolar Disorder. Some effects of the medication may be visible within a week, but it may take several weeks for youth to receive the full benefits of the medication. If juveniles are taking Lithium®, their salt and fluid intake should be monitored, because dehydration can cause lithium to reach a toxic level. All youth taking mood-stabilizer medications should be monitored medically (*e.g.*, heart, liver, thyroid) on a regular basis. These medications can potentially cause serious damage to the organs of the body.

Some offenders with Bipolar Disorder do not want to take prescribed medication because they do not want their moods to be stabilized. They enjoy the "high" of the manic phase, including the increased energy and inflated self-esteem. If youth refuse to take their medication

on a consistent basis, juvenile justice professionals should monitor and chart the youths' behavior on and off the medication. Most juvenile offenders with Bipolar Disorder experience significant interpersonal and behavioral difficulties, as well as receive numerous sanctions when they are not taking their medication. Staff should provide youth with objective feedback about how the juveniles' behavior changes in response to the medication. This practice can help offenders realize that although they may subjectively "feel" better not taking their medication, doing so often results in negative and unpleasant consequences.

EDUCATION/CYCLE IDENTIFICATION

Educating youth about their illness is important if they are suffering from Bipolar Disorder. Because juveniles are typically unaware of their rapid shifts in mood and unusual behavior, pointing out these changes them in a non-judgmental manner can be important. A mental health/medical professional should educate young offenders about Bipolar Disorder and the cyclical nature of their illness. Because many youth who have one episode of mania will have another in the future, it is important to help youth identify when they are becoming manic or sliding into depression. This awareness can help them take whatever precautions are necessary to avoid dangerous and destructive behavior.

For example, some females with Bipolar Disorder have engaged in promiscuous sex while manic in the past. These young women may need to stay away from high-risk environments and high-risk individuals if they begin to feel overly excited or full of energy.

Along the same lines, offenders who notice that they are becoming increasingly irritable and getting into verbal altercations may need to spend some time away from others. They may also need to pay special attention to how they are reacting to comments from those around them. Being aware of their tendency to be grandiose can help youth with Bipolar Disorder

88

Juvenile Offenders with Mental Health Disorders: Who Are They and What Do We Do With Them?

maintain more control when they begin to have thoughts regarding their superiority over others. Similar to relapse prevention with substance abusing offenders, the goal is to:

- identify the high-risk situations and behaviors of youth with Bipolar Disorder
- help the youth to avoid those situations and behaviors when the youth begin experiencing changes in their mood

COPING SKILLS
Teaching adaptive coping skills to offenders with Bipolar Disorder is critical. These youth often become irritable with peers and staff, and they can have significant periods of distractibility. Both of these behaviors are likely to interfere with their ability to function in school, as well as interact with peers and staff. Educating youth in adaptive coping skills can occur on an individual basis or in a group. Learning how to cope with and manage their symptoms effectively will help youth with Bipolar Disorder function more successfully in important areas of their lives.

EFFECTIVE BEHAVIOR MANAGEMENT
Offenders with Bipolar Disorder function best in a stable and highly structured environment. Clear directions and expectations with consistent consequences are critical to managing these youths' behavior. Responding quickly to any inappropriate or rule-breaking behavior is essential. *(Please see Chapters 3 and 14 for additional information on effective behavior management.)*

COMMUNICATION WITH SCHOOL PERSONNEL
Because of the erratic nature of the moods and behaviors of youth with Bipolar Disorder, juvenile justice professionals should communicate with school personnel. All adults working with youth who have Bipolar Disorder should respond to rule violations and inappropriate behavior in a consistent and agreed-upon fashion. Efforts should be made to retain these youth in the classroom for as much time as possible.

Communication between the juvenile justice and educational systems is also important because teachers need to be aware when:

- Youth are experiencing psychotic features
- Youth are experiencing suicidal ideation
- Youth are significantly hostile or belligerent

In addition, youth with Bipolar Disorder may require assistance in the classroom if their distractibility is severe.

MENTAL HEALTH SERVICES UPON RELEASE
An appointment for mental health services in the community should be scheduled for youth with Bipolar Disorder if they are scheduled for release from a facility prior to being seen by a mental health professional. Youth with Bipolar Disorder receiving mental health services in a juvenile justice facility who need to continue treatment should also have an appointment scheduled in the community upon release. Treatment typically includes psychopharmacology, psychoeducation for the youth and their families/caregivers, and various skill-building interventions (*e.g.*, anger management, problem-solving skills training, social skills training). Learning to cope with the cyclical nature of Bipolar Disorder, as well as preventing or minimizing relapse into depressive or manic mood states, are critical components of effective mental health treatment for youth with this illness.

Case Example
Lawrence, 16, was brought to the local juvenile detention center after being arrested for stealing a portable compact disc player. Lawrence walked into a WalMart Superstore, took a portable CD player off the shelf, and put on the headphones. He took a CD from the music section of the store and placed it in the portable CD player. He then walked directly out of the store without paying for the CD player or the CD. When he was apprehended outside

Mood Disorders: Major Depression, Dysthymic Disorder and Bipolar Disorder

of the store, Lawrence genuinely appeared shocked that he had done something wrong. He explained to the security guard that he had wanted to hear his favorite song by Eminem, his favorite singer and rapper. Radio stations had recently banned the song. Lawrence said he took the CD and CD player so that he could hear the song whenever he wanted. Lawrence claimed that the law regarding stealing should not apply in this situation because he had a personal relationship with Eminem (which was untrue). He was perplexed as to why he was being arrested.

As the police officer drove him to the detention center, Lawrence talked nonstop about how cool he thought Eminem was. Lawrence said he was going to New York to party with Eminem the following week. He told the officer how he and Eminem are able to communicate telepathically and that whenever the performer does television appearances he sends Lawrence hand signals while he is singing. Lawrence also said he wrote two of the songs off of Eminem's latest CD.

The police officer attempted to get some biographical history from Lawrence, but it was impossible to interrupt him because he was speaking so rapidly. When the officer stated that he did not believe that the youth knew the famous entertainer, Lawrence became very angry and began yelling profanities at the officer. The officer tried to calm Lawrence down. But he became increasingly agitated and attempted to assault the officer while being escorted out of the police car.

The detention center was able to locate Lawrence's mother, who reported that she had not seen her son for the past few days. She said he left the house two nights before around 3:00 a.m. because he was unable to sleep. Lawrence went for a walk and never returned. She reported that before he left home, Lawrence alphabetized his collection of 115 compact discs and all of the books in his bedroom, his sister's bedroom and the living room. He then began alphabetizing the canned foods in the kitchen cuboards when his mother discovered him and told him it was not necessary. Lawrence told his mother that he was full of energy and wanted to "bring order to this f—ed up crazy world." Lawrence's mother thought her son's behavior was odd, but she figured it was just a phase he was going through. He had always misplaced his homework and never cleaned his room, so his mother was pleased he was putting things in order. She did not think his behavior was anything to be concerned about. She was relieved when she received the call from the detention center, as she had been desperately looking for her son for the past two days. Lawrence had never left home like that before and had never had trouble with the law.

This type of youth can easily slip through the cracks of the juvenile justice system because he does not have a mental health or juvenile justice history. He will likely be released to his mother, and his odd (manic) behavior may not even be brought up when his charges are discussed in the courtroom. If Lawrence has Bipolar Disorder, this type of behavior is likely to occur again. However, the next time could have more destructive and/or dangerous results—for Lawrence, as well as others.

Juvenile Offenders with Mental Health Disorders: Who Are They and What Do We Do With Them?

CHAPTER 5

Attention-Deficit/Hyperactivity Disorder (ADHD)

"I love playing guitar, hey what's over there?
That's what my ADHD is like."

Shawn, 17

Marshall, 15, has not been able to sit still since the moment he arrived at the juvenile correctional facility. He is always leaning back in his chair, pacing the floor or tapping his pencil on the desk. Constant reminders about his schoolwork are not effective in helping him get it done, and he rarely, if ever, completes his homework. When Marshall completes a written assignment in his living unit, he typically forgets where he put it. Consequently, he often does not get credit for work he has done. He gets into trouble several times a day. Juvenile justice professionals and teachers are frustrated and tired of reminding him of the rules over and over again.

Robin, 14, never seems to be listening. During group activities, she is always staring out the window watching the birds, butterflies or airplanes. Facility staff describe her as being "out to lunch" and "spacey." She daydreams a great deal at school, and when her teachers remind her to pay attention, Robin becomes irritable and angry.

Many youth involved with juvenile justice experience problems with attention, and many appear impulsive and overly active. All of the following can affect youths' ability to focus their attention and control their behavior:

- Depression
- Anxiety
- Drug and alcohol intoxication

- Drug and alcohol withdrawal
- Trauma
- Abuse/neglect
- Medication side effects
- Medical problems
- Learning Disorders
- Stress
- Fear

Problems with attention and impulsivity also can be related to Attention-Deficit/Hyperactivity Disorder (ADHD). ADHD is one of the most common psychiatric disorders among young people, including juvenile offenders. Whereas 3-7 percent of youth in the general population suffer from ADHD (American Psychological Association, 2000), rates are much higher among youth involved with juvenile justice. Older studies of incarcerated youth have found that 19 percent of juveniles evaluated suffered from ADHD (Davis, Bean, Schumacher, & Stringer, 1991; Halikas, Meller, Morse, & Lyttle, 1990). However, a more recent study of incarcerated youth found that 76 percent of the males and 68 percent of the females met diagnostic criteria for ADHD (Timmons-Mitchell, *et al.*, 1997). In the general population, the disorder is thought to be much more prevalent in males than females, with a ratio of 4:1-9:1. The ratio of males to females among juvenile offenders is not currently known.

ADHD is one of the most common psychiatric disorders among young people, including juvenile offenders.

A sizeable number of youth have been diagnosed with Attention-Deficit/Hyperactivity Disorder (ADHD) disorder over the past ten years. Everyday, more than one million youth take Ritalin®, a psychostimulant medication prescribed for ADHD (Lowe, 1999). Most juvenile justice professionals believe the diagnosis of ADHD is assigned too freely, particularly among the juvenile offender population. There are likely to be some youth in the juvenile justice system who should not have received a diagnosis of ADHD. However, there are probably just as many youth who never received an ADHD diagnosis who should have.

ADHD is a very specific mental health diagnosis with a considerable number of explicit diagnostic criteria. Simply because youth "are

bouncing off the walls," or "never pay attention," does not automatically indicate that they have ADHD.

 ## Diagnostic Criteria for Attention-Deficit/Hyperactivity Disorder

ADHD is not a new mental health disorder. Teachers, doctors, mental health professionals and parents have been concerned about this illness for decades. The disorder has gone through numerous name changes (*i.e.*, Minimal Brain Dysfunction, Hyperkinesis, Hyperactivity, Minimal Brain Damage, Attention Deficit Disorder), but it always has had a similar set of core symptoms. Over the years, there has been a shift in emphasis regarding which aspect of the disorder is primary: *hyperactivity* or *inattention.* The current edition of the *Diagnostic and Statistical Manual of Mental Disorders* (*DSM-IV-TR*; APA, 2000) emphasizes *both* inattention and hyperactivity/impulsivity as core components of this disorder. Youth can suffer from difficulties predominantly in one area or in both areas. The current *DSM* diagnostic criteria were primarily designed for use with children. Therefore, some professionals have questioned whether the same criteria are applicable for evaluating adolescents and adults, both of whom also suffer from this disorder (NIH, 1998).

In order to meet current diagnostic criteria for Attention-Deficit/Hyperactivity Disorder, youth must display a persistent pattern of inattention and/or hyperactivity-impulsivity. This pattern must be more frequent and severe than that of other youth who are the same age or at the same level of development.

Youth who have difficulty with INATTENTION tend to:

- Be easily distracted
- Have difficulty with organization
- Lose things
- Find it difficult to pay attention to one task or activity for a significant period of time

Juvenile Offenders with Mental Health Disorders: Who Are They and What Do We Do With Them?

- Forget things
- Appear as if they were not listening
- Avoid tasks requiring sustained mental effort
- Not follow through on instructions

Juveniles with attention difficulties frequently have a hard time completing chores or responsibilities. These youth are often not purposely engaging in oppositional behavior; they literally forget what it is they are supposed to do. In addition, they may try to avoid written assignments in the classroom (or in a living unit) because paying attention long enough to complete the assignment is too difficult. Juveniles with ADHD frequently misplace their belongings, including both trivial objects and items that are important to them.

Youth who primarily have difficulty with HYPERACTIVITY/IMPULSIVITY tend to:

- Feel extremely restless
- Fidget with their hands or feet
- Move around excessively
- Find it difficult to remain seated for long periods of time
- Have difficulty quietly engaging in play activities
- Talk constantly
- Appear "revved up" and full of energy
- Interrupt others
- Call out answers before a question is finished
- Have difficulty waiting for their turn

Juveniles who are hyperactive/impulsive often touch and take things that do not belong to them. They commonly damage items or knock things over because they are moving around so quickly. Because they have difficulty thinking ahead to the consequences of their behaviors, these youth frequently place themselves in potentially dangerous situations.

According to the *DSM-IV-TR*, there are three types of ADHD:

- Attention-Deficit/Hyperactivity Disorder, Predominantly *Inattentive* Type
- Attention-Deficit/Hyperactivity Disorder, Predominantly *Hyperactive/Impulsive* Type
- Attention-Deficit/Hyperactivity Disorder, Combined Type (if youth exhibit significant symptoms from each of the two areas)

Most youth are inattentive or impulsive at some time or another, but that does not mean they all qualify for a diagnosis of ADHD. Children and adolescents are not expected to follow directions or control their behavior to the same degree as adults. To qualify for a diagnosis of ADHD, juveniles must exhibit *several* problematic behaviors (at least six from one of the above categories) for at least six months. Some of these behaviors must have been evident and causing some impairment before 7 years of age. Also, the youths' behavior has to cause difficulty in two or more settings (*e.g.*, home, school, work, juvenile justice facility, group home). In addition, the youths' behaviors must be causing significant problems in their relationships with others, school, or work. Sometimes, juveniles' difficulties with attention or hyperactivity are due to another mental health disorder, or related to the effects of drugs or alcohol. In these situations, a diagnosis of ADHD is not warranted.

The diagnosis of ADHD is not easy for juveniles to receive when clinicians use the *DSM* in the manner for which it was designed. To determine whether symptoms of ADHD are present to a significant degree and interfering with youths' functioning, a comprehensive mental health evaluation should be conducted. Trained mental health professionals typically gather information from a variety of sources (*e.g.*, youth, family/caretakers, teachers, juvenile justice professionals, previous mental health professionals, medical professionals) and may use psychological tests and behavioral checklists. Juvenile justice professionals can play a critical role during the gathering of information about youths' behavior. Adults who interact closely with youth (*e.g.*, juvenile justice professionals, correctional educators, vocational supervisors, probation/parole officers, recreation staff, mentors, interns, medical professionals) often have important information about juveniles' functioning, and this information should be included in an assessment for ADHD.

Although many juvenile offenders have difficulty paying attention in school and/or are impulsive, most of them do not have ADHD. First, not all juvenile offenders with these problems exhibit a significant number of inattentive or hyperactive symptoms; they may demonstrate only a few. Second, for youth who do have several problematic behaviors, most do not exhibit them to such an extreme that they interfere with the juveniles' ability to function in important areas of their lives. Third, most young offenders do not experience impairment from these behaviors before 7 years of age. Instead, many youth began to have difficulties with inattention, restlessness or impulsivity during later childhood or their early teenage years. Fourth, symptoms of inattention and hyperactivity can be caused by a variety of factors other than ADHD (*e.g.*, high levels of stress, traumatic experiences, physical or sexual abuse, parental neglect, drug or alcohol use, anxiety, medical disorders). So while a significant number of juvenile offenders exhibit problems in the areas of attention and impulsivity, only a subset of them truly meet diagnostic criteria for ADHD. However, for those youth with attention and impulsivity problems due to factors other than ADHD, treatment services may still be necessary. Intervention strategies should be specifically responsive to these juveniles' underlying issues (*e.g.*, substance use, trauma).

There is no single psychological, medical or neurological test to identify ADHD. The diagnosis of this disorder is made after a comprehensive evaluation is completed. Evaluations for ADHD may include some or all of the following:

- Interviews with several individuals who have interacted with/observed the youth
- Psychological tests
- Behavioral checklists/rating scales
- Medical tests
- Neurological exam

Mental health professionals should assess whether the constellation of symptoms necessary for the ADHD syndrome is present, while at the same time rule out other possible explanations for the youths' symptoms. Clinicians should pay special attention to the assessment of co-existing psychiatric disorders (*e.g.*, anxiety disorders, mood disorders, Conduct Disorder, learning disorders, substance use disorders) because having these disorders in addition to ADHD can significantly influence treatment strategies for juveniles. An assessment for ADHD can take anywhere from several hours to several days to complete.

Unfortunately, there are some medical and mental health professionals who do not conduct comprehensive evaluations, yet diagnose youth with ADHD. These professionals may only speak with juveniles and possibly their parents/caretakers during an assessment. They may spend only a brief amount of time gathering information. In addition, they may pay little attention to co-existing psychiatric disorders and/or conditions other than ADHD that might explain the youths' problematic behavior. Because of this practice, some youth in the juvenile justice system have been diagnosed with ADHD (and receive treatment for it), even though they do not have the disorder. Moreover, these juveniles may actually suffer from another psychiatric disorder that has gone undetected and typically untreated.

There may also be a subset of older adolescent offenders who were evaluated and accurately identified as having ADHD when they were younger but who no longer exhibit symptoms of the disorder. Some of these youth may have developed adaptive coping skills to manage their difficulties with attention and/or

94

Juvenile Offenders with Mental Health Disorders: Who Are They and What Do We Do With Them?

hyperactivity. Or, some may have literally outgrown the most troublesome ADHD symptoms. A mental health diagnosis can influence placement and intervention decisions within the juvenile justice system. Therefore, re-evaluation of youth diagnosed with ADHD who are not exhibiting mental health symptoms should occur among adolescents every few years—particularly if they initially received a diagnosis of ADHD prior to puberty.

Conversely, a sizeable number of youth in the juvenile justice system are suffering from ADHD, but they have never been evaluated and diagnosed with the disorder. A variety of reasons might account for this situation, including:

- Families/caretakers may not have had access to medical/mental health care

- Families/caretakers may not have been able to afford comprehensive evaluations for ADHD

- Families/caretakers/teachers have different tolerance levels with regard to behaviors typical of ADHD

- Families/caretakers do not want to experience the stigma associated with visiting a mental health professional

- Families/caretakers have had negative personal experiences with mental health services, so they do not think the services will be helpful to their children

Hyperactivity may be viewed as "excess energy" by one family/caretaker/teacher and "pathological behavior" by another. Only individuals viewing juveniles' behavior as abnormal or bothersome consider referring youth for mental health evaluations or health care services.

 ## What Exactly is Attention-Deficit/ Hyperactivity Disorder?

To participate successfully in society, individuals need to control and regulate their behavior. As we develop through childhood and adolescence, we learn which behaviors are appropriate to certain times, places and situations. Youth with ADHD seem to have a deficit in relation to controlling and regulating their behavior. Because of this, ADHD can be considered a "behavioral inhibition disorder" (Barkley, 1995). Based on what is currently known about the syndrome, many of the behaviors displayed by youth with ADHD relate to a core problem with the ability to inhibit their behavior. These youth appear hyperactive because they constantly respond to everything and everyone around them. In situations where most youth would restrain themselves, juveniles with ADHD do not. They often have trouble exhibiting behavioral control in situations where constraint is required. Therefore, their actions are often displayed more loudly, more quickly and more powerfully than those of their peers.

Problems paying attention for a sustained period of time are also likely to be related to a behavioral inhibition deficit among youth with ADHD. When engaging in a task or participating in a conversation, juveniles with ADHD are often distracted by other stimuli in their surroundings. These youth may see a different activity in which they want to take part, or they may see someone else with whom they would rather converse. Non-ADHD youth are also aware of these distractions in the environment. But non-ADHD peers inhibit the desire to join a different activity or interact with a new person they think will be more interesting. Non-ADHD youth continue to focus on the task at hand or the person with whom they were already involved. Refraining from acting on impulse takes tremendous effort for juveniles with ADHD. In this situation, they would need to inhibit their desire to walk over and join a new activity. Or they would need to restrain themselves from walking away from one conversation to participate in another that appears more interesting to them.

Mental health/medical professionals used to think that youth with ADHD were overwhelmed because of a deficit in discriminating important from nonimportant information. Professionals believed these juveniles had a "filtering" problem: that they did not know *what* to pay attention to at a particular time. Professionals now believe that youth with ADHD and youth without ADHD pay attention to exactly the same things. But youth with ADHD do not pay attention as *long* because they get bored and move on to something more stimulating (Barkley, 1995). Juveniles with ADHD can be referred to as "stimulation seekers" because these youth are always looking for something new, fun and interesting to see, touch and do. If something is not exciting and stimulating in the current moment, they are typically not interested in doing it. Youth with ADHD are extremely focused on "right now."

 ## Associated Features of Attention-Deficit/Hyperactivity Disorder

Juveniles with ADHD are more likely to have a variety of health problems and physical impairments in comparison to their peers without ADHD. Mothers of youth with ADHD are more likely to have experienced complications during pregnancy and the birth of their children (*e.g.*, toxemia, fetal distress, long labor, postmature delivery). Additionally, youth with this disorder typically have more medical difficulties immediately after birth and during infancy (Hartsough & Lambert, 1985). These youth are more likely to experience delays in developmental milestones (*e.g.*, crawling, talking, bowel control), as well as problems with speech development. Poor general health and chronic health problems are not unusual among youth with ADHD.

Juveniles with ADHD tend to be involved in various accidents, sometimes resulting in injury. Plus, these youth often have poor motor coordination, which can affect their ability to write, use computers, and engage in particular sport and recreational activities. Sleep problems can occur as well. A number of juveniles with ADHD have difficulty falling asleep, awaken several times during the night, and are unusually tired in the morning.

Juveniles with ADHD can be self-centered, bossy and demanding. They want what they want, when they want it—and they typically want it *now*. They frequently:

- Have difficulty waiting for things
- Cut in line
- Take something that is not theirs
- Shout out answers when juvenile justice professionals/teachers are asking questions of a large group

Youth with ADHD are easily frustrated and may become upset if their needs are not met immediately. These youth often intrude upon the conversations and activities of others. They may monopolize conversations and then not listen when someone else begins to talk. Because of these behaviors, youth with ADHD can have difficulty getting along with peers their own age. Juvenile justice professionals and teachers may find these youth rude, obnoxious or annoying. Rejection by peers and adults is common and can lead to feelings of low self-esteem as well as depression. Unfortunately, most juveniles with ADHD have little insight into what they are doing that pushes people away.

Some youth with ADHD move physically all of the time. They might fidget with things on a desk, kick their feet, lean back in a chair, or continually get out of their seat. When placed in their room in a living unit, they may ask to come out over and over again. These youth have a hard time adjusting their behavior so that it fits with what is expected. Slowing down or relaxing is hard for them—it is as if they had *too much* behavior. Most juveniles know to stay quiet when watching a movie with others or to stay seated in a classroom. But youth with ADHD are unable to stop themselves from doing these things. The problem is not that they do not know what is expected of them or that they deliberately break the rules; they are often unable to restrain their behavior.

Because of their impulsivity, juveniles with ADHD rarely think before they act. If they want

Juvenile Offenders with Mental Health Disorders: Who Are They and What Do We Do With Them?

to do or say something—they just do it—without thinking about the ramifications of their actions. Because they give little thought to possible negative consequences, these youth may commit crimes even with the likelihood of placing themselves in a dangerous situations or being apprehended. Their impulsive nature can result in multiple arrests, numerous sanctions during incarceration, and/or physical assaults by peers.

These juveniles not only frequently *act* before thinking through a situation but also often *react* before thinking through a situation. Juvenile offenders with ADHD may immediately become angry or upset over something someone said or did to them. If peers brush up against them, youth with ADHD may automatically assume that their peers are trying to disrespect them (or are looking for fight)—instead of realizing that the behavior was an accident. When asked to go to their room in a juvenile justice facility, these youth may become upset; they may yell and scream that they are being unfairly punished. These juveniles may not realize that everyone on the unit was also asked to go to their room due to staff changing shifts. What appears to be emotional immaturity is typically an emotional reaction that occurs so quickly that juveniles do not have time to look at the facts of a situation. Even though juveniles with ADHD frequently feel bad about their inappropriate reactions, those around the youth may avoid them after a few negative experiences.

Juveniles with ADHD are very present-focused and concerned with what is happening *right now.* They often have an inaccurate understanding of the concepts *time* and *future.* Minutes spent on an uninteresting or boring activity can seem like an eternity to youth with ADHD. These juveniles live in the moment and are constantly moving on to the next thing that is of interest to them. Because they react to things so quickly, these youth typically do not take the time to look at what they could learn from past experiences and past mistakes; they do what feels good now. Given their emphasis on the

present, warnings about future consequences mean little to them. In addition, a complete focus on what is going on in the moment can result in the following behaviors among youth with ADHD:

- Difficulty following a rigid schedule
- Arriving late to appointments and activities
- Forgetting when they are supposed to make a phone call (*e.g.,* to family members, probation/parole officers)
- Not keeping their word or promises
- Not completing assignments by agreed upon times

Even when youth with ADHD contract with juvenile justice professionals to accomplish a task by a specified time in order to get a treat, they often do not follow through. These youth tend to get caught up in whatever they are doing in the moment and lose track of time. Supervising juvenile offenders with ADHD can be a challenge. These youth often need several reminders to do what is instructed or to follow facility rules. Adults (*e.g.,* juvenile justice professionals, teachers, recreation staff, vocational supervisors) can become frustrated, annoyed and sometimes angry when working with young offenders with ADHD.

Not surprisingly, the extreme focus on what is occurring in the current moment makes it difficult for juveniles with ADHD to delay gratification to achieve long-term goals. The threat of arrest and incarceration is usually not a major deterrent for these youth. And receiving additional sanctions during incarceration also does not mean much to these youth—particularly in comparison to the stimulating activity in which they are involving themselves. Their lack of interest in setting goals and making future plans often leads juvenile justice professionals and teachers to view these youth as irresponsible, unreliable, lazy and apathetic about their future. Even when they do make plans and set goals, these juveniles often have difficulty achieving them. Between the view adults hold

Attention-Deficit/Hyperactivity Disorder (ADHD)

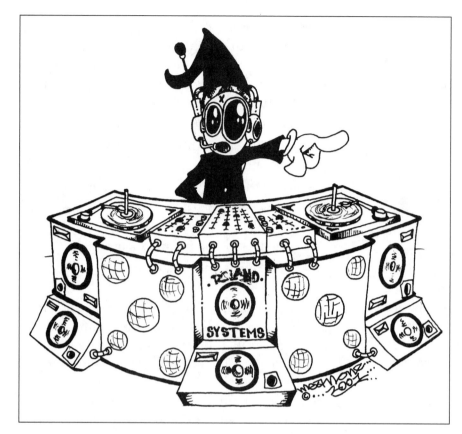

can be confusing for adults interacting with youth who have ADHD because one day the juveniles are able to accomplish several tasks successfully with little to no reminders. The next day, ten reminders do not seem to be enough to keep the youth on track. Juveniles with ADHD appear to be working only when they "feel like it." But their involvement usually has more to do with their level of interest in specific tasks and what else is going on around them.

Juveniles with ADHD are particularly affected by situational circumstances, and as situations change, so does their behavior. Behavioral consistency is rare among these youth because they are so affected by their environment (*e.g.*, with whom they are interacting, what the juveniles are asked to do, how many other people are in a room with them). This lack of consistency can also make the diagnosis of ADHD more challenging. Juveniles with ADHD can be calm and focused while interacting with an adult on a one-on-one basis (*e.g.*, physician, nurse, mental health professional, clergy, intern), especially when the interaction is structured. But the same youths may be loud and excessively active the moment they return to a living unit or classroom—especially if several of their peers are around and/or the environment is unstructured. Juvenile justice professionals may feel exhausted and frustrated after working a full shift with youth who have ADHD. Consequently, they may ask another staff member to take these youth out of a unit for a brief period of time. This "break" often enables staff members to attend to their other responsibilities. When the youth with ADHD are returned to the living unit, they are often accompanied by an

of them and their view of themselves, juvenile offenders with ADHD often end up feeling hopeless and doomed to failure.

School can be a very frustrating place for youth with ADHD. Most juveniles with this disorder are not lacking in intelligence, and many have at least average IQs. The demands of the typical classroom, however, are often too much for these youth. Consequently, juveniles with ADHD may be placed in special education classes due to problems with learning or behavior. A significant number of these youth have been held back at least one grade or have been suspended or expelled. Many will drop out of high school before graduating.

Juveniles with ADHD are capable of completing school tasks, assignments and activities accurately and efficiently if they are interested in them. If they are not interested in certain assignments or tasks, however, they may have difficulty sticking with them until completion. These youth are likely to be distracted by more engaging events occurring around them. This

98

Juvenile Offenders with Mental Health Disorders: Who Are They and What Do We Do With Them?

adult who reports that the youth were calm, friendly and focused. This report can add considerable frustration to juvenile justice professionals' already-aggravated mood.

 ## Course of Attention-Deficit/ Hyperactivity Disorder

Many juvenile offenders with ADHD exhibited symptoms of inattention or hyperactivity/ impulsivity at a very young age, some as early as preschool. Most youth with ADHD, however, come to the attention of medical/mental health professionals once they enter elementary school and the demands in the classroom (academic and behavioral) increase. About 20-30 percent of youth "outgrow" this disorder by adolescence, but the rest continue to experience these behaviors throughout their teenage years and some even into adulthood. Problems with paying attention usually continue. But the hyperactive characteristics of the illness may dissipate as adolescents become increasingly aware of what is acceptable and nonacceptable public behavior. Rather than running around and climbing on things, hyperactive symptoms are more likely to manifest internally (*e.g.*, inner feelings of restlessness and jumpiness) once youth reach adolescence. However, some juveniles may continue to be fidgety and unable to sit still for long periods of time, especially during activities that are not very interesting.

The mood changes occurring in adolescence may be intensified among youths with ADHD, and small conflicts may erupt into major explosive outbursts. During their teenage years, juveniles are faced with increasingly difficult decisions about their lifestyle, health, friends, sexuality and so forth. Youth with ADHD may not make the healthiest decisions. These juveniles are focused on the moment and not considering the possible ramifications of their actions. Therefore, adolescents with ADHD may engage in a variety of high-risk, and potentially life-threatening, behaviors. For example, youth with ADHD begin using drugs and alcohol

earlier than their peers without ADHD. These youth are also more likely to receive speeding tickets and get into automobile accidents (Barkley, 1995). When juveniles with ADHD are focused on the excitement of the moment, they are less likely to think about the potential dangers and negative consequences associated with:

- Unprotected sex
- Delinquent activity
- Running away from home

Suicidal behavior is also more common among adolescents with ADHD in comparison to non-ADHD peers. Because their impulsivity increases these juveniles' suicide risk, juvenile justice professionals should take all talk of suicide seriously and have these youth immediately evaluated.

 ## Co-Existing Mental Health Disorders

Almost half of all youth who have ADHD also have another psychiatric disorder, and this is particularly true among youth involved with the juvenile justice system. Many juvenile offenders suffer from two or more psychiatric disorders in addition to ADHD.

The most common psychiatric disorders that co-exist with ADHD are Oppositional Defiant Disorder and Conduct Disorder. Juveniles with ADHD can be stubborn, argumentative and annoying. They may lie, steal and run away from home. Some youth with ADHD verbally attack others, and they may become involved in physical altercations. By late adolescence, up to one-half of all youth with ADHD develop a persistent pattern of behavior that includes delinquent activities and the violation of the rights of people around them. Juveniles suffering from both ADHD and Conduct Disorder have more severe psychiatric problems, more aggression, and more problems with substance abuse than youth with Conduct Disorder without ADHD (Riggs, Leon, Mikulich, & Pottle, 1998).

(Please see Chapter 3 for additional information on Oppositional Defiant Disorder and Conduct Disorder.)

ADHD co-exists with a variety of other psychiatric disorders as well. Up to one-third of youth with ADHD suffer from an anxiety disorder, and up to one-third suffer from a mood disorder (Biederman & Steingard, 1989). The combination of ADHD and a mood disorder can significantly increase juveniles' risk for suicide. In addition, learning disorders, substance abuse disorders and communication disorders can co-occur with ADHD.

Juvenile offenders with ADHD often suffer from a variety of mental health symptoms in addition to their trouble with attention and impulsivity. A common cluster of psychiatric difficulties seen among incarcerated juveniles is ADHD, Conduct Disorder, one of the learning disorders, and a substance abuse disorder. Some of these juveniles may also suffer from Posttraumatic Stress Disorder or a mood disorder such as Major Depression or Dysthymic Disorder. Not surprisingly, as the number of youths' psychiatric diagnoses increases, so does the extent of the youths' difficulties. Strategies to manage juveniles with ADHD need to take into account the complexity of the juveniles' behavior.

 ## What Causes Attention-Deficit/ Hyperactivity Disorder?

Most youth with ADHD have some type of abnormal brain development. The orbital-frontal part of the brain is located at the front of the brain and connects with the caudate nucleus and the limbic system. This part of the brain is responsible for the *executive* functions. It helps us control our behavior so that we can behave appropriately in society. The front portion of the brain and its connections help us:

- Pay attention when we want to focus
- Stop talking when asked to do so or when someone else is speaking
- Not take things that do not belong to us
- Not hit people when we are angry

This part of the brain also plays a large role in helping us control our emotions. It helps us remain calm and complete our responsibilities if we become overly excited or upset. In addition, the front part of the brain facilitates our adherence to rules, as well as thoughts about future goals.

One of the most popular current theories about ADHD is that these juveniles have less activity in the orbital-frontal part of their brains. Studies using electroencephalographs (EEGs) and positron emission tomography (PET) have shown that these youth have:

- less electrical activity,
- less blood flow, and
- less brain activity in the front part of the brain and throughout its connections (Barkley, 1995).

Additionally, when juveniles with ADHD are given stimulant medication (one of the most common treatments for ADHD), their brains look similar to their non-ADHD peers. This type of medication helps youth with ADHD focus and behave more appropriately. It is believed that juveniles with ADHD have *less* activity occurring in the part of the brain that controls attention and regulates behavior. Therefore, their brains have *less* control, so the youth pay attention to *more* things and engage in *more* behaviors. Although this theory about ADHD has received support, more study is needed to truly understand the disorder.

ADHD runs in families, and there is likely to be some type of genetic component to the disorder. Siblings of youth with ADHD have two to three times the risk of also having ADHD, and this risk is even higher when the siblings are twins. One study found that 79 percent of identical twins and 32 percent of fraternal twins had ADHD if their twin had already been diagnosed with the disorder (Gillis, Gilger, Pennington, & Defries, 1992). The rate among nonrelated youth is 3–5 percent. A considerable number of parents of youth with ADHD also have ADHD themselves, although the disorder may never have been formally diagnosed. Although heredity plays a major role in the development of this disorder, the mechanism for passing the illness is not yet known. Youth with ADHD possibly inherit a predisposition to have problems with the front part of the brain and its connections. Or a particular gene or set of genes may be passed from one generation to the next.

ADHD does not appear to be caused by "bad parenting." Families of youth with ADHD tend to report increased levels of stress, marital problems, feelings of parental inadequacy, and social isolation (Edwards, Schulz, & Long, 1995). However, these factors may be related to raising youth who have ADHD, and possibly other co-morbid psychiatric disorders, as well as parental mental illness (including, but not limited to, ADHD). Mothers of juveniles with ADHD often display more controlling behavior and less positive emotions when interacting with their children in comparison to mothers of non-ADHD youth. These behaviors may be a response to interacting with youth who experience difficulty paying attention, remaining on task, and behaving appropriately. Mothers of ADHD youth give fewer demands and display more positive emotions when their children are taking stimulant medication.

Controversy continues regarding the influence of specific foods, preservatives and artificial colorings on symptoms of ADHD. These substances are not likely to *cause* the disorder. But many parents of youth with ADHD report a worsening of symptoms among their children after the consumption of these substances. A subset of juveniles with ADHD may be more sensitive to specific foods and chemicals than others. Some studies have shown that eliminating particular foods, preservatives or artificial colorings in the diets of youth with ADHD improves youths' symptoms (Boris & Mandel, 1994; Weiss, 1982). Yet other studies have shown that these substances do not improve youths' symptoms (Kavale & Forness, 1983; Rosen, *et al.*, 1988). Removing specific foods, preserva-

tives and artificial colorings should not be the sole treatment for youth with ADHD. However, science has demonstrated a link between what individuals eat and their physical and mental health. Therefore, if juveniles' symptoms are exacerbated when certain substances are included in their diets, there appears to be no harm (and a possible benefit) in removing them.

 ## Managing Juvenile Offenders with Attention-Deficit/Hyperactivity Disorder

One of the keys in managing youth with Attention-Deficit/Hyperactivity Disorder is remembering that much of their off-task and/or disruptive behavior is related to the way their brains have developed. In general, much of their negative behavior is typically not a result of disrespect, laziness, or intentional provocation of staff and peers (although it may look that way). There is a subset of juvenile offenders with ADHD, however, who do purposefully avoid responsibility, disobey rules and incite those around them. Many of these particular youth have co-existing Oppositional Defiant Disorder or Conduct Disorder. Determining which behaviors stem from the youths' ADHD and inability to control their behavior, and which behaviors are deliberate and volitional can be difficult. Among youth in the juvenile justice system specifically, both factors may be playing a role. Juvenile justice professionals need to investigate problematic situations closely and not automatically assume that juveniles are acting in a purposeful manner when they engage in negative behaviors. While under juvenile justice supervision, many youth with ADHD receive multiple sanctions for behaviors that may not be completely under their control.

Juvenile offenders should be held accountable for their behavior, and youth diagnosed with ADHD are no exception. Suffering from ADHD is not an "excuse" to engage in inappropriate or rule-violating behavior. It is also not an excuse for youth to avoid engaging in mandatory activities or tasks that may not be of interest to them. Juvenile justice professionals need to be aware of which juveniles are suffering from ADHD. This way, staff can use specific management strategies to help these juveniles function more successfully and have the living unit run more smoothly and safely. The following management strategies apply to most juvenile offenders but are critical for staff working with juvenile offenders who have ADHD. Although these approaches may take a little more time initially, they result in saving juvenile justice professionals a great deal of time in the end.

Referral to Mental Health/ Medical Professional

Juveniles should be referred to a medical/ mental health professional for an evaluation if the youths' impulsivity, overly active behavior or inattention is interfering with their ability to function successfully—in a living unit, classroom or work setting. Adults who interact with these youth on a regular basis (e.g., juvenile justice professionals, teachers, vocational supervisors, recreational staff) should provide information about the juveniles' behavior to the clinician conducting the evaluation. If possible, clinicians should also obtain information from youths' parents/caretakers. Due to conflicting schedules, it is often difficult for professionals to provide information to clinicians face to face. If phone contact is not feasible, staff members may want to give clinicians a one-page summary of the types of behaviors the youth in question have been exhibiting. Staff should also identify what management strategies have and have not been successful with the youth. Clinicians may ask juvenile justice professionals and teachers to complete brief rating scales or checklists describing various aspects of the juveniles' behavior. These tools typically require less than ten minutes to complete and usually assess how often youth are restless, fidgety,

loud and so forth. Input from adults who interact with the youth in various situations and settings is critical in helping clinicians make accurate psychiatric diagnoses. This input helps evaluators determine whether youth are suffering from ADHD, experiencing another psychiatric disorder, or reacting to situational factors.

Highly Structured Environment

Because youth with ADHD have trouble remaining focused and regulating their behavior, providing them with clear expectations and rules is critical. All policies and behavioral expectations should be concise and easy to understand. They should be explained to juveniles verbally, as well as written down. Providing a copy of rules and expectations for youth to post in their room can be helpful for juveniles with ADHD. Many of these juveniles forget what was previously discussed. In addition, a fixed routine will help juveniles with ADHD stay on track. Posting the youths' morning routine or daily routine in their room so that they can check off tasks upon completion may be necessary. This practice can help youth with ADHD monitor their own behavior; it also will likely reduce the number of questions that are often posed to juvenile justice professionals over and over again (e.g., "What is happening next?" "What am I supposed to do now?"). The more predictable the youths' environment, the better the youth know what is expected of them. If there will be any major changes (e.g., new schedule, different daily routine, new staff member, new classroom), juveniles should be told in advance, whenever possible. Juvenile justice professionals should provide specific information regarding the change(s) that will be occurring, as well as review what behaviors are expected of the youth.

By their very nature, juvenile justice facilities are typically highly structured environments with clear expectations. Therefore, some youth with ADHD function *better* while incarcerated than they do in the community. Some juveniles are even able to reduce the amount of

102

Juvenile Offenders with Mental Health Disorders: Who Are They and What Do We Do With Them?

medication they take for ADHD while residing in a juvenile justice facility because the degree of structure provided is so high. Many youth with ADHD, however, will need to continue their current dose of medication to be able to comply with facility rules, as well as the strict demands on their behavior.

Effective Behavior Management

Self-control is difficult for juveniles with ADHD. These youth often heavily rely on the external environment to help them manage their behavior. Therefore, juvenile justice professionals should be clear about which behaviors result in which consequences. Staff need to respond immediately and consistently to both positive and negative behaviors, so that youth can make the connection between their behavior and resulting consequences. If juveniles engage in behavior that is clearly against the rules, they should receive a sanction. Negative consequences should occur as soon as possible after a problematic behavior occurs, and juvenile justice professionals should explain to youth exactly what they did wrong.

Juvenile justice professionals should respond similarly when youth engage in positive behavior. For example, suppose juveniles complete an assignment, adhere to all rules during an activity, and the like. These youth should receive some type of positive consequence (e.g., verbal praise, points in a token economy system) as soon as possible after engaging in the prosocial behavior. If too much time elapses between youths' behavior and the resulting consequence (negative or positive), youth with ADHD will not make a connection between the two. Juveniles with ADHD live in the moment, and their concept of time is not as accurate as that of youth without ADHD. Providing sanctions or incentives related to consequences occurring in the distant future are not likely to be effective with this population of juveniles.

Many juvenile offenders with ADHD received vague and inconsistent discipline in the past, particularly in their family/caregiving environments. Therefore, receiving consistent consequences for negative behavior is critical. If kicking peers is against facility rules and results in a particular sanction, youth should receive that sanction each and every time they kick peers. Where the youth engages in the behavior (e.g., the cafeteria, a living unit, their room with a roommate, a classroom, the gymnasium, the visiting area) should not matter. Consistent consequences and predictability are key to managing juvenile offenders with ADHD.

Consistency can be a challenge in a juvenile justice facility when there is flux in the everyday environment. For example:

- Youth typically spend a portion of the day in school and another portion in a living unit
- Youth may transfer from an intake unit to a living unit
- Youth may be reassigned from one living unit to another living unit
- Youth may be transferred from one juvenile facility to another facility.

Even when juveniles remain in one location, they interact with a variety of adults throughout a 24-hour period—including juvenile justice and educational personnel who have different personalities and management styles. All staff should be providing youth who have ADHD with the *same* consequences for the *same* behaviors. This consistency is unlikely to occur without clear communication among all professionals who interact with the youth. Once juveniles with ADHD experience success in a particular living unit, classroom or work situation, caution should be exercised before moving these youth to another setting. In the new setting, they will be required to learn a new set of expectations and interact with a new group of staff members. Juveniles with ADHD will likely need time to readjust, and their behavior may again become problematic.

When staff are choosing consequences with which to reward and punish juveniles with ADHD, it is important to make certain that they

Attention-Deficit/Hyperactivity Disorder (ADHD)

are meaningful to the youth. Most juveniles in juvenile justice facilities desire extra points within a "level" system, extra time on the telephone, snack food and so forth. To use the most effective incentives with youth who have ADHD, juvenile justice professionals should ask youth what specifically motivates them. Although exploring what motivates youth is important for all juveniles, staff may be particularly surprised at what activities and tasks youth with ADHD find enjoyable. Due to their difficulty in delaying gratification, most youth with ADHD prefer smaller, immediate rewards in comparison to larger, but delayed, rewards. Having a multitude of small, immediate reinforcers that can be used with these youth is critical for all juvenile justice professionals.

Most incarcerated youth, particularly those with ADHD, find one-on-one time with adult figures (*e.g.*, juvenile justice professionals, teachers, facility supervisors, volunteers, recreational staff, clergy) very rewarding. Whether talking briefly to adults without major distractions or helping them accomplish a task or chore (*e.g.*, folding towels, filing papers, putting books away, preparing food), most juvenile offenders with ADHD find private time with an adult pleasurable and meaningful. In addition, these youth often *enjoy* activities typically viewed by staff as sanctions and punishments. For example, chores (*e.g.*, cleaning bathrooms, doing laundry, mopping floors) are often assigned to young offenders in response to negative behavior. In contrast, many youth with ADHD want to engage in these behaviors because they give the youth something to occupy their minds and bodies. Therefore, chores should be treated as a reward for positive behavior among these particular youth.

Discovering what negative consequences are most effective for these youth is just as important as identifying reinforcers. The threat of losing points on a "level" system may mean nothing to juveniles with ADHD. Removing these juveniles from treatment groups or recreational activities may be exactly what the youth

want to happen. Having to spend time alone in their room may be torture for some youth with ADHD but relaxing and calming for others.

Because juvenile offenders with ADHD are a heterogeneous group of youngsters, juvenile justice professionals should take the time to find out what motivates particular youth. This effort increases the effectiveness of behavior management strategies and treatment plans. Although facility staff may think they do not have the time to do this, they will undoubtedly spend the same amount of time (if not more) reacting/responding to the youths' noncompliant behavior. It is always better to invest the time initially, so that staff can be more strategic in their interactions with youth. Involving youth with ADHD in the development of their own treatment plans offers an ideal opportunity to gather information about what motivates particular juveniles. Moreover, when juveniles are involved in treatment planning, they are less likely to challenge negative consequences once a plan is put into action. *(Please see Chapters 3 and 14 for additional information on effective behavior management.)*

Positive and Simple Instructions

Juvenile offenders with ADHD do not respond to long-winded lectures or threats. Juvenile justice professionals should give instructions that are brief and to the point. They may need to repeat these instructions aloud to ensure that the youth heard correctly what was said. Directives about what is expected of youth should be specific and concrete. Telling juveniles with ADHD to behave "appropriately" or to keep their anger "under control" is too vague for them to understand. When juvenile justice professionals are specific and concrete in their instructions, both staff and the youth are better able to assess whether or not the youth engaged in expected behaviors. "Appropriate" can mean various things to different individuals and juveniles may think their behavior is appropriate, even though the staff do not. If youth are given a negative consequence in this circumstance, they will feel unfairly sanctioned.

104

Juvenile Offenders with Mental Health Disorders: Who Are They and What Do We Do With Them?

Clearly defined behaviors are also important so that juvenile justice professionals can easily recognize and reinforce when juveniles with ADHD engage in positive behavior. Unambiguous instructions and concrete behavioral expectations also facilitate consistency from shift to shift because juveniles and a variety of staff members all know exactly what behaviors are being targeted.

Youth with ADHD should always be told what *to* do, instead of what *not* to do. Instructing juveniles to speak quietly is more effective than telling them to stop yelling. Likewise, directing youth to keep their hands to themselves during treatment groups is more effective than telling youth to stop touching and poking their peers. If juveniles with ADHD are solely told what they *should not* be doing, they do not receive the benefit of learning what adaptive behavior they *should* be doing instead. Each time youths' behavior is corrected, they have an opportunity to learn how to do something different—and more prosocial—the next time they are in a similar situation.

Juvenile justice professionals should give juvenile offenders with ADHD one instruction at a time. Unfortunately, some staff give the following type of instructions: "Go to your room, make your bed, and then wipe down your sink. Once you do that, you can call your cousin, but you have to be finished with your call in the next 15 minutes so you can help set up for dinner." Youth with ADHD are likely to go into their room, make their bed and then become distracted by something else in their room. They may start looking out the window, pick up a book, or begin conversing with peers in the next room through a vent. Or youth with ADHD may be so excited about calling their cousin after making their bed, they may immediately go to the phone to make the call. In this situation, juveniles might talk for 20 minutes, completely oblivious to the 10-minute time limit for personal phone calls. To juvenile justice professionals, these youth may appear to have deliberately:

- Not cleaned their sink
- Avoided helping set up for dinner
- Violated the time limit for the phone

Often, youth with ADHD just forget what they are supposed to do. Providing these youth with one instruction at a time makes it more likely the juveniles will complete what is asked of them. Once youth with ADHD have completed an initial task, the next instruction should be provided. If this is not possible due to staffing patterns or time constraints, multiple instructions can quickly be written down and given to youth. Juvenile justice professionals can ask youth with ADHD to check off each task after completing it. These youth should understand that they will not receive an incentive until all items are checked off.

When too many instructions are given at once, juveniles with ADHD are set up to fail. Also, juvenile justice professionals often become frustrated and annoyed. Providing specific, succinct instructions for small, definable behaviors may require additional staff time. But if this time is not provided on the front end, staff will be spending extra time with these youth:

- engaging in power struggles, or
- providing and enforcing sanctions for the youth not following directives.

Frequent and Immediate Feedback

Because of their short attention span, juveniles with ADHD need continuous feedback on their behavior. Telling youth how much staff appreciate their help cleaning up the living unit *as* they are cleaning the living unit is effective—rather than commenting on the juveniles' behavior at the end of the day. If they are behaving inappropriately in a group situation, staff should inform juveniles with ADHD about what the youth are doing that is unacceptable during the group. Staff should not wait until the group is over. If juveniles are quietly working on school assignments, staff should comment on the youths' positive behavior in the moment, instead of waiting until the assignments are completed, if they are completed. This immediate feedback helps youth with ADHD understand what type of behavior juvenile justice professionals expect of them and when the youth are actually performing the behavior correctly.

Providing frequent and immediate feedback requires juvenile justice professionals to take the time to pay attention to youth with ADHD when they are doing well—not just when the youth is engaging in problematic behavior. This type of monitoring and feedback can be can be challenging given the numerous duties assigned to most juvenile justice professionals, but it helps youth with ADHD experience success. It also can improve the relationship between these juveniles and the staff because there are more opportunities for positive interactions. Although all juvenile offenders can benefit from immediate feedback on their behavior, juveniles with ADHD need it much more frequently. This feedback should be brief and to the point, as these youth will tune out any long-winded conversations.

There is a subset of youth with ADHD who have severe symptoms of the disorder. If staff were to provide immediate feedback to these youth ever time they were not on task, it would occupy all of the staff members' time. If youth with severe ADHD are having difficulty maintaining appropriate behavior for even short periods of time, staff may need to readjust their behavioral expectations of those particular juveniles. This is especially true if the non-compliant behavior is not intrusive or dangerous (*e.g.*, foot tapping, making minor noises, jumping up and down).

Improving Social Skills and Anger Management

Youth with ADHD often have difficulties with social relationships, academic achievement, and the appropriate expression of their emotions. Many of these have few friends because their peers can find them irritating and obnoxious. Juveniles with ADHD can benefit from groups,

tutoring and activities that assist them in these areas. These youth frequently need basic education on how to interact with their peers in a way that does not annoy or irritate them. They need to learn how to listen to others, take turns and not be too bossy or demanding. Role-playing can be effective with youth who have ADHD. Juvenile justice professionals can play the role of the youth, and the youth can play the role of a peer or staff member. When juveniles with ADHD are on the receiving end of someone who is bossy, demanding or intrusive, these youth can become more aware of how their behavior affects others. Juvenile justice professionals can then role-play more adaptive and prosocial ways of interacting with others and then have the youth with ADHD practice these new skills. Feedback regarding the juveniles' portrayal of new skills is critical. These types of role-playing should be done respectfully and supportively. The goal is for the young offenders to learn new ways of socializing, not to embarrass or shame them.

Juvenile offenders with ADHD often have difficulty controlling their anger because they react so quickly and impulsively to incidents that occur. They do not take the time to think about a situation and evaluate the best way to respond. Exhibiting explosive moods or displaying temper tantrums is not unusual. Juveniles with ADHD can benefit from learning how to identify their anger when they first begin to feel it. Then, they can think about what they should do next instead of reacting automatically (*e.g.*, "STOP-THINK-ACT"). Learning to be more *proactive* with regard to their emotions—and less *reactive*—is critical. Not thinking through difficult situations before reacting to them emotionally often results in negative sanctions for juveniles with ADHD, as well as a loss of social relationships.

Opportunities for Recreation

Juvenile offenders with ADHD need a prosocial outlet to dispel some of their excess energy. Allowing these youth to run around or speak

Juvenile Offenders with Mental Health Disorders: Who Are They and What Do We Do With Them?

louder than usual when playing outside can be a helpful release. The limitations and constraints placed upon them outdoors are less than in a living unit or classroom/vocational environment. Negative sanctions for youth with ADHD should not include removing standard recreational exercise made available to other juveniles in a facility. Recreational activities not only can help discharge energy but also can provide youth with ADHD an opportunity to interact with peers in a less formal and more relaxed environment. The social demands on a basketball court or grass field are typically not as high as inside a juvenile justice facility.

Help Youth Experience Success

It is important for juvenile justice professionals to reward youths' small successes if they expect youth to make significant changes in their behavior. Youth with ADHD often feel inadequate and embarrassed when they are unable to manage their behavior, attention and emotions in the same manner as peers. Frequent positive reinforcement can help counteract these feelings. Successful functioning is more likely when juveniles with ADHD engage in activities by themselves or with one other peer, versus interacting with a large number of youth. Juveniles with ADHD can become distracted and disruptive in groups. The more people around them, the harder it is for these youth to pay attention to a task at hand. Some facilities have found the *buddy system* helpful. Staff ask prosocial, responsible peers to help the youth with ADHD complete assignments and/or specific tasks. This type of buddy system can be beneficial to both sets of juveniles.

Every effort should be made to help juveniles with ADHD experience success during group activities. Some juvenile justice facilities mandate that youth attend treatment groups 60-90 minutes in length, often without a break. This amount of time is too lengthy to keep the attention of most juvenile offenders, but it is nearly impossible for youth with ADHD. These juveniles often have difficulty controlling their behavior or paying attention during a prolonged group activity.

Therefore, juvenile justice professionals should allow these youth to take a short break and then return to the group. After a quick drink of water or trip to the bathroom, many youth with ADHD can sit through the remainder of a group session without problems. Too many juvenile offenders with ADHD are removed from treatment groups due to unrealistic expectations regarding their behavior. This sanction typically results in these juveniles having less access to important, and often much-needed, treatment interventions (*e.g.,* anger management, social skills, victim empathy). When working with juvenile offenders, staff should provide short breaks routinely during any educational or treatment group that lasts more than 30 minutes. If it is not feasible to allow youth to leave a room (*i.e.,* safety, security or staffing reasons), juvenile justice professionals can ask the juveniles to stand up and stretch or do jumping jacks. Or staff can just allow the youth to talk informally with each other for a few moments. This brief period of "downtime" in the middle of a treatment or educational group can result in the remainder of the group session running more smoothly and productively.

To keep them motivated and working toward treatment goals, juveniles with ADHD need to experience success on a regular basis. When possible, activities and assignments should be broken down into smaller sections so that youth with ADHD can experience a sense of completion. Many juvenile justice facilities use a "level" system, where youth earn "points" for good behavior. When using this type of system, staff may need to evaluate the behavior of youth with ADHD at the end of each shift versus at the end of the day (or the end of the week). Juveniles with ADHD typically forget their positive accomplishments if they later receive sanctions for negative behavior. Positive behavior exhibited by youth early in the day should not be overshadowed or negated by negative

Attention-Deficit/Hyperactivity Disorder (ADHD)

interactions or negative behaviors in the evening.

Make It More Interesting

Youth with ADHD are attracted to things that are novel and interesting. They typically have a great deal of difficulty when they are bored or uninterested in a task or activity. When asking these juveniles to complete lengthy assignments or duties, juvenile justice professionals may need to develop creative ways to keep the youth motivated. Turning mundane tasks or chores into games or contests can have a profound impact on motivating juveniles with ADHD to participate in the activities. Similarly, small modifications made to standard classroom assignments can significantly increase these youths' motivation to complete them.

When residing at a juvenile justice facility, juveniles can spend a significant amount of time in their room (*e.g.*, while awaiting court, during shift change, during free time). Most juvenile offenders are able to relax or even take a nap when placed in their rooms during the day. Many youth with ADHD, however, become overly active and are unable to remain in their room for a significant period of time. These youth may:

- Continuously knock or bang on their doors

- Repeatedly press their intercom buttons

- Make several trivial requests of staff

- Annoy peers by talking to them through walls or air ducts

This type of behavior is often due to these youth being bored and unable to occupy themselves. The individual rooms in juvenile justice facilities are typically bare, with few items to look at or play with in the rooms. When juveniles with ADHD have items in their rooms that are of interest to them, they are less likely to be disruptive when required to remain there for an extended period of time. Depending on the rules of a specific facility, young offenders may be able to hang their own artwork, pictures from

magazines, or photographs from home. Allowing them to have a magazine or a book that is of interest to them can provide these youth with something constructive to do. The goal is to provide juveniles with ADHD with something to look at and pay attention to in the room. Otherwise, they will search out staff and peers to help occupy their minds.

Communication with School/ Vocational Personnel

Many youth in juvenile justice settings participate in some type of academic programming or vocational training. Although juveniles with ADHD can have difficulty in a living unit, they typically have just as many, if not more, difficulties in a classroom or work setting. To be successful at schoolwork or vocational tasks, juveniles must be able to remain focused on a task at hand and keep their behavior under control. A school or work setting can be torture for youth who are impulsive and/or unable to pay attention for extended periods of time. This situation is particularly true if assignments or tasks are uninteresting and repetitive, and there is not an opportunity for frequent breaks.

Juvenile justice professionals and school/ vocational personnel should communicate regularly with each other about youth with ADHD. Discussing which management strategies have been effective with particular youth and which strategies have not been effective can benefit all involved parties. After significant challenges with specific youths, some staff members may have discovered creative strategies and incentives that motivate these youth and keep them on task. This information should be passed on to other professionals interacting with the youth, as these staff members are likely to also be facing similar challenges. This way, not everyone has to struggle and try to reinvent the wheel. Because consistency is critical when working with juvenile offenders who have ADHD, these youth should receive the same consequences each time they engage in a behavior—regardless of whether it occurs in

108

Juvenile Offenders with Mental Health Disorders: Who Are They and What Do We Do With Them?

a classroom, work site or living unit. Such consistency can be difficult to maintain in large facilities. However, this is a goal to which all staff should strive. Consistency can be accomplished only with frequent communication between the various professionals interacting with the youth.

Psychotropic Medication

Psychostimulants (*e.g.*, Ritalin®, Dexedrine®, Adderall®) are typically prescribed for youth with ADHD, and many youth suffering from this disorder demonstrate beneficial effects from the medication. Psychostimulants usually remain in the body for only a short period of time, so most youth with ADHD require multiple doses of the medication on a daily basis. Newer forms of these medications, however, have recently become available (*i.e.*, single-dose-per-day, sustained release, long-duration) resulting in some youth only needing to take one pill per day. Positive effects of stimulant medication can typically be seen within a few days or less. Although these medications are stimulants, they do not make youth with ADHD *more* hyperactive. It is believed that this type of medication stimulates the part of the brain that helps focus attention and regulates behavior, so that youth become more calm and able to focus.

Psychostimulants can help decrease youths' impulsivity, restlessness and disruptive behavior, as well as increase their ability to pay attention and focus for longer periods of time. These medications can also help youth with ADHD behave more cooperatively with adults and peers, which can positively influence their social relationships. Psychotropic medication should never be the *sole* treatment for ADHD in the case of most juvenile offenders. Because these youth usually have difficulties in multiple arenas, medication should not take the place of the other types of management strategies discussed.

Although psychostimulants can help juveniles with ADHD pay attention better and control their behavior, these youth typically require additional treatment services (*e.g.*, individually tailored behavior modification strategies, academic assistance, social-skills training, anger management). Taking psychostimulant medication on a regular basis helps juveniles with ADHD sit still and pay attention long enough to participate in and benefit from, much-needed psychosocial interventions. Some youth with ADHD are able to decrease their psychostimulant medication, or discontinue it altogether, when placed in a long-term juvenile justice facility. The high level of structure and consistency provided by many facilities can help some of these juveniles manage their impulsive and hyperactive behavior without medication—particularly if their symptoms are mild. However, if these youth

> The high level of structure and consistency provided by many facilities can help some of these juveniles manage their impulsive and hyperactive behavior without medication—particularly if their symptoms are mild.

continue to experience significant problems with attention, they may need to continue taking medication regardless of a structured setting.

Due to the short amount of time stimulant medication remains in the body, observing a "rebound" effect when juveniles' medication begins to wear off is not uncommon. When a dose of medication is wearing off, youth may become restless, loud, irritable and overly active. This behavior can appear to juvenile justice professionals as if the youths' medication has stopped working, or the youth were returning to their pre-medicated state. This reoccurrence of symptoms can occur if the times of youths' doses of medication are spread too far apart, or if youth refuse to take a dose of their medication. This dynamic commonly occurs when juveniles with ADHD who have regularly been taking psychostimulants do not have their medication with them when they are incarcerated. These youths' troublesome behaviors will typically decrease once stimulant medication is restarted, or dosing of the medication becomes more frequent. However, if juveniles with ADHD are taking psychostimulant medication and their behavior continues to worsen, an investigation is necessary. In this situation, juveniles may be:

- Sporadically refusing to take their medication

- Pretending to swallow their medication, but they are actually spitting it out

- Misdiagnosed with ADHD (*i.e.*, their difficulties are related to another mental health disorder)

Regardless of the reason, a referral to a mental health/medical professional is warranted.

There is some concern over the abuse potential of psychostimulants, particularly Ritalin®. Among the majority of youth with ADHD, abuse of psychostimulants is rare. However, caution should be used when this medication is prescribed to juveniles with ADHD who also have Conduct Disorder and/or a history of substance abuse (a common combination among youth involved with the juvenile justice system). Rather than abuse it themselves, juvenile offenders with ADHD may sell or trade their medication to peers without the disorder who want to get "high." Non-ADHD youth may snort or inject Ritalin® for strong stimulant/amphetamine effects. Parents, various family members and other caretakers of juvenile offenders with ADHD have been known to steal youths' Ritalin® to take it themselves. Some of these individuals are probably attempting to get "high." But some may find that the medication helps them to better control their own attention and behavior because ADHD runs in families. As with all psychotropic

medication, the distribution and storage of psychostimulants should be closely monitored.

Tricyclic antidepressants (*e.g.*, Tofranil®, Pamelor®,) may be prescribed for youth who have both ADHD and a mood disorder, such as Major Depression. Youth can accidentally or intentionally overdose on this type of medication, so it should be monitored closely, especially among this impulsive population. Wellbutrin®, an atypical antidepressant, is also sometimes prescribed for youth with ADHD, particularly if they are aggressive and/or have issues related to substance abuse. This medication does not have the potential overdose dangers of the tricyclic antidepressants. Wellbutrin®, is often as effective as the psychostimulants, but because it lacks an amphetamine-like effect, the abuse potential is much lower (Riggs, Leon, Mikulich, & Pottle, 1998).

Juveniles with ADHD may not be accurate reporters of how well their medication is working. Therefore, input about youths' behavior on and off medication should be solicited from juvenile justice professionals and teachers. This helps to obtain a more accurate impression of whether a particular medication (or a specific dose of medication) is effective for an individual youth.

Mental Health Services Upon Release

An appointment for mental health services in the community should be scheduled for youth with ADHD if they are scheduled for release from a facility prior to being seen by a mental health professional. Juveniles with ADHD receiving mental health services in a juvenile justice facility who need to continue treatment should also have an appointment scheduled in the community upon release. Treatment formats can include individual, group and/or family therapy. Treatment for ADHD typically includes psychopharmacology, psychoeducation and cognitive behavioral interventions that target important areas of youths' lives (*e.g.*, family relationships, peer relationships, academic achievement). Substance use issues are

110

Juvenile Offenders with Mental Health Disorders: Who Are They and What Do We Do With Them?

also addressed when indicated, as many juvenile offenders with ADHD are attracted to substances to self-medicate (*e.g.*, marijuana). Strategies used may include behavior management training for parents/caregivers, problem-solving skills training, social skills training, anger management training, and academic assistance.

Effectively managing juvenile offenders with ADHD requires a *team* approach. Supervising one or several offenders with ADHD can be exhausting and frustrating for juvenile justice professionals. Care should be taken so that particular staff members do not assume total responsibility for all of the youth with ADHD. This dynamic often occurs when certain juvenile justice professionals work particularly well with youth who have special needs. Preventing these gifted staff members from being overburdened with most or all of the juveniles on a living unit who have a mental health disorder (or behavior problems) is important. Supervising a diverse group of youth (ADHD and non-ADHD) helps staff members and the ADHD youth gain exposure to pro-social behaviors from a variety of juveniles.

Although working with juveniles who have ADHD can be emotionally and physically draining, these youth are also some of the most emotionally rewarding youth that juvenile justice professionals supervise. Youth with ADHD are usually very creative and social. Their zest for life, desire to interact with others, and commitment to hobbies of interest to them can be infectious and fun to observe.

Case Example

Robert, 14, has been arrested three times for trespassing and was recently arrested for theft. Most of his trespassing charges are related to being on school grounds in the evening with his 13-year-old neighbor, Ryan. Most of the time, Robert and Ryan are just poking around the school buildings and not engaging in any delinquent activity. However, when Robert was appre-

hended during his most recent evening visit on school grounds, he was carrying some sports equipment from the school gymnasium. This resulted in an arrest for theft. Robert said he "just wanted to borrow a soccer ball and some orange cones," so he could "practice his soccer skills at home." He seemed surprised when the police arrested him. Robert lives with his mother, stepfather and 6-year-old sister. Robert's mother describes him as "hyperactive since the day he was born." She remembers him climbing out of his crib and constantly trying to touch things that were out of his reach. Robert has broken several bones while playing sports and is always covered with bruises due to skateboarding and bicycle accidents. Robert describes school as "lame" and "boring." He was placed in special education classes during the third grade because of problems completing assignments and disruptive behavior in the classroom. Robert has always found it hard to pay attention in class and tends to daydream while the teacher is talking. He is always tapping a pen or pencil on the desk and makes clicking noises with his mouth while his teachers are lecturing. Robert typically asks to go to the bathroom or get a drink of water a minimum of three times in each of his 45-minute classes. His teachers usually do not let him go.

When Robert gets bored, he likes to poke and taunt his peers. He often pulls the hair of the girls sitting in front of him at school or yells offensive and racist comments at peers walking down the street, "just to get a reaction." Although he has never physically assaulted anyone, Robert was beaten up several times in elementary school by classmates. Robert's peers describe him as "weird," "annoying," "geeky," and "obnoxious." Robert says it is hard for him to relax and that he feels "amped all of the time." He is well-skilled in Nintendo, loves to go to action-adventure movies, and

enjoys talking about and drawing pictures of UFO's. Unfortunately, Robert has few friends with whom he can share these activities.

His special education teachers find him bright and friendly, but his behavior can be frustrating for them. Robert needs to be told to do things over and over again in the classroom, and he often interrupts adults when they are giving him instructions. Robert's mother and stepfather are beginning to feel hopeless about their son's behavior, particularly his sneaking out at night to spend time on school property. Attempts at punishment by grounding him or taking away his video games have had minimal effect on his behavior. In addition, recent threats to send Robert to a special camp for "out of control" teenagers also seemed to have little effect. Robert will remain in juvenile detention until his court date, and his parents hope his incarceration experience will be enough to motivate him to change his behavior.

Because Robert's difficulties appear related to (not necessarily caused by) his ADHD, incarceration alone will have minimal impact on his delinquent behavior. In addition, his problems related to school and his interpersonal relationships are also likely to continue without appropriate treatment. Robert clearly needs to be held accountable for his trespassing and stealing behavior. But he should also be provided with special services (*e.g.*, medication, and his parents given training on behavior management) to help manage his mental health disorder.

112

Juvenile Offenders with Mental Health Disorders: Who Are They and What Do We Do With Them?

CHAPTER 6

Posttraumatic Stress Disorder (PTSD)

"This last year, my dad was shot, and my cousin was shot. And now my best friend was shot. What can you do? People die. That's just the way it is."

Jamal, 17

Sarina, 13, was difficult for juvenile justice professionals to manage. She always seemed upset about something. Sarina would often become extremely angry or depressed for days at a time, making it difficult for her to remain in a classroom. Juvenile justice professionals described Sarina as being "keyed up" and hypersensitive to everything around her. She constantly focused and commented on what everyone around her was doing. This behavior was annoying to staff and peers, and the other girls on the unit often ostracized her. Sarina refused to interact with any of the male staff and frequently accused them of looking at her in "sex-crazed" ways or of trying to "feel her up." Although she presented herself as popular and sexually promiscuous, she had few friends and was terrified to talk to boys. She felt damaged and disgusted about the way she looked and could not imagine why any boy would be attracted to her. She even carved the words "ugly" and "trash" on her skin. Sarina was molested by her stepfather from the ages of 6 to 12. She was also raped by a 16-year-old neighbor when she was 11.

An extraordinarily high number of juvenile offenders have experienced traumatic experiences at some point in their lives. Numbers as high as 73 percent for males and 76 percent for female juvenile offenders have been reported (Steiner, Garcia, & Matthews, 1997; Cauffman, Feldman, Waterman, & Steiner, 1998). Although the numbers for both genders is extremely high, female offenders are much more likely to develop Posttraumatic Stress Disorder (PTSD) versus their male counterparts (Cauffman, *et al*, 1998; Giaconia, Reinherz, Silverman, Pakiz, Frost, & Cohen, 1995). Some juvenile offenders have witnessed or directly experienced more traumatic incidents by the age of 15 than most adults will in a lifetime. Reported experiences of incarcerated juveniles include, but are not limited to:

- Seeing a parent murdered (sometimes by the youths' other parent)

113

- Watching a parent overdose on drugs
- Discovering a parent who has committed suicide
- Being shot
- Shooting a peer on purpose
- Shooting a close friend or sibling by accident
- Being involved in a serious motor vehicle accident
- Learning about the unexpected death of a close friend or family member (often while the youth were incarcerated)
- Witnessing a drive-by shooting
- Having their best friend shot and then dying in the youths' arms
- Being severely beaten by gang members
- Being forced to participate in Satanic rituals by parents
- Being forced to have an abortion
- Having a miscarriage
- Being sold into the pornography industry by parents
- Being physically abused
- Experiencing severe parental neglect
- Experiencing sexual victimization/rape by family members
- Experiencing sexual victimization/rape by strangers
- Living in a refugee camp before relocating to the United States
- Experiencing suicides of close friends
- Being homeless
- Prostituting their bodies
- Watching family members kill and mutilate the youths' pet
- Being released from a juvenile justice facility and finding their family had relocated with no forwarding address
- Being told they have HIV
- Being locked in a trunk for hours or days
- Being forced to eat feces
- Being forced to eat vomit
- Burning down their family home with their parents and siblings inside
- Being locked in a closet with a dead parent, after watching their parent be murdered
- Being in a car with siblings that is driven off of a cliff by a parent, and being the sole survivor

Even perpetrators of serious and violent crimes can develop Posttraumatic Stress Disorder when traumatized by their own behavior. Many youth involved with the juvenile justice system have grown up in environments characterized by poverty, domestic violence, and widespread drug and alcohol use. These experiences can result in significant distress and trauma-related symptoms (Martinez & Richters, 1993). Some juvenile offenders have experienced one specific traumatic event, while others have been traumatized repeatedly for months or years. Exposure to traumatic events can result in a variety of negative behavioral, emotional and cognitive effects for youth (Giaconia, et al., 1995). For some juveniles, the effects of trauma are so severe that they interfere with the youths' ability to function in daily activities.

Posttraumatic Stress Disorder (PTSD) is one of the most common anxiety disorders among youth in the juvenile justice system. Researchers estimate that 6 percent of adolescents in the general population meet the criteria for Posttraumatic Stress Disorder at some time in their lives (Giaconia, 1995). In comparison, a recent study found that almost one-third (32 percent) of a group of incarcerated juveniles were currently experiencing Posttraumatic Stress Disorder (Steiner, et al., 1997). This percentage was even higher among incarcerated females, with almost *half* of the girls currently suffering from the disorder (Cauffman, et al., 1998). Despite the prevalence of chaos and violence in the lives of juvenile offenders, not all of them develop PTSD.

114

Juvenile Offenders with Mental Health Disorders: Who Are They and What Do We Do With Them?

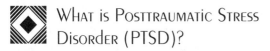

What is Posttraumatic Stress Disorder (PTSD)?

Posttraumatic Stress Disorder (PTSD) is a mental health disorder characterized by (APA, 2000) as:

- Exposure to a traumatic event
- Re-experience of the trauma
- Avoidance of things associated with the trauma
- Emotional numbing
- Increased arousal

A *traumatic* event is typically an incident in which youth experience, witness, or are involved in the actual or threatened death or serious injury of themselves or someone else. At the time of a traumatic incident, juveniles typically experience intense horror, fear or helplessness. These experiences are often sudden, unexpected and out of the range of experiences of most people. Offender reports of horrific experiences such as being shot, witnessing the murder of a family member, being raped, and the like, clearly fit the above description of a traumatic experience. However, even prolonged exposure to just hearing about traumatic events (e.g., shootings, stabbings) in youths' neighborhoods can be enough to constitute a traumatic experience and result in untoward effects for young people (Horowitz, Weine, & Jekel, 1995). Some juvenile offenders are raised in communities in which stabbings, beatings and shootings are frequent occurrences, and hearing about these events is commonplace.

Re-experiencing the Trauma

Juvenile offenders with Posttraumatic Stress Disorder typically continue to re-experience a traumatic event that occurred. Youth may have distressing, and even horrifying, dreams about the stressful incident. These nightmares can be very intense, and these youth can feel as if they are experiencing the traumatic event all over again. Some juveniles are not able to stop thinking about a distressing event when they

are awake. Thoughts about a traumatic incident might pop into their minds during school, recreational activities, or in the midst of a conversation with friends. Youth with Posttraumatic Stress Disorder often try to keep themselves constantly occupied so as to avoid thinking about these disturbing thoughts. Incarcerated juveniles with this disorder often experience these types of intrusive thoughts while they are alone in their room. Prolonged room confinement and/or bedtime can be particularly difficult for them. If youth with Posttraumatic Stress Disorder are exposed to something that reminds them of a traumatic event, they may become very angry, upset, and/or anxious. These youths' behavior and personality can change, sometimes drastically, around "anniversary" dates of a traumatic event.

Some youth will have actual flashbacks of a distressing event they experienced. They may act or feel like the horrible incident is happening all over again in the present moment. For some juveniles, flashbacks are more common when they are intoxicated/high and their inhibitions are lowered. For others, this type of experience mostly occurs when the youth are completely sober. Flashbacks are often triggered by something that reminds the juveniles of a traumatic event (*e.g.*, smells, sounds, people). This reliving of the trauma can be frightening and upsetting because the youth usually experience the same disturbing thoughts and emotions as when the event initially occurred.

Flashbacks can be quite confusing for juvenile justice professionals to understand, particularly when a youth is experiencing them in the moment. For example, some young offenders who suffer from Posttraumatic Stress Disorder have been victims of serious gang beatings. If staff need to physically restrain these youth, this action could trigger memories of the beatings. During a "take down," these juveniles may literally feel as if the previous beatings were happening to them all over again. Consequently, they may fight off the staff as if they were enemies. Most offenders decrease their aggressive and assaultive behavior while being physically restrained by staff. But some youth with Posttraumatic Stress Disorder will actually become more assaultive and react to the staffs' restraint with increased anger, agitation and all out swinging, biting and kicking. Staff are usually taken aback by the youths' increased aggression because of its extreme nature. These juveniles seem to be reacting to a completely different situation. But this behavior makes perfect sense to juveniles suffering from flashbacks. They are misinterpreting their current circumstance, perceiving the staff as enemies who want to beat them. These youth believe that they need to fight for their life. It is not unusual for female juvenile offenders who have been raped to respond in the above manner when physically restrained by staff. These young women may become extremely frightened and upset, terrified that they are being raped again.

Many juvenile justice professionals are unaware of the types of behaviors, statements, or situations that can trigger youth to re-experience traumatic events. Many female juvenile offenders (and an increasing number of male juvenile offenders) have histories of being sexually victimized by someone in their household late at night. Some of these juveniles become anxious and fearful when staff walk past their doors to do a generic "room check" during the evening or overnight shift. This action can remind these youth of times when a perpetrator came to their bedroom door to sexually abuse them after family members went to sleep. Some sexually abused female juvenile offenders with PTSD have reported that hearing the voice of male staff members outside of their door at night—or having someone physically knock on their door once the lights have gone out—is particularly frightening. These experiences with staff can result in sleepless nights, anger and feelings of wanting to physically hurt themselves on the part of these youth. Juvenile justice professionals typically have no idea their behavior is having this type of influence on the young women.

Avoidance

Most juvenile offenders with Posttraumatic Stress Disorder attempt to avoid any reminders of a traumatic event they have experienced. Youth may not want to talk about what happened to them when asked about the incident. Some may not even remember exactly what happened to them, or they may forget relevant details. When juveniles are not forthcoming with information related to traumatic events, juvenile justice professionals often believe these youth are trying to cover something up. This belief is especially likely when a traumatic incident is associated with criminal behavior (e.g., shooting, stabbing, rape, beating). However, some traumatized juveniles may truly forget some of the details of a distressing incident because it is too painful or overwhelming for them to remember.

Juvenile offenders with Posttraumatic Stress Disorder also may avoid people or places that remind them of a traumatic incident. Some youth will avoid interacting with peers from a certain racial group because someone from that racial background is related to their trauma (e.g., shot by an Asian-American gang member, raped by a Caucasian neighbor, mugged at gunpoint by an African-American peer). If a traumatic incident occurred in a certain neighborhood, youth with Posttraumatic Stress Disorder may avoid going back to that neighborhood—as well as avoid associating with anyone who resides or hangs out in that particular area.

The following is an example of a youth who avoids things reminding him of a traumatic incident:

Brian, 15, was recently diagnosed with Posttraumatic Stress Disorder. Over a year ago, Brian had come home from school to find his mother lying dead on the living room couch. His favorite punk rock compact disc was still playing on the stereo. His mother had overdosed on heroin. The young man continued to live in the same apartment with his stepfather and older sister. Even one year after his mother's death, Brian refused to sit on the couch where his mother died. He also had difficulty spending more than a few minutes in the living room. Brian tried to spend as much time away from the family apartment as possible. When he did come home, he would spend most of his time in his bedroom or the kitchen. This youth became extremely agitated when he heard punk music on the radio or when he would go out with his friends to clubs where punk bands played. Brian took down all of his posters of punk bands and gave away most of his compact discs explaining to friends that he was "bored with this kind of music." Any time his sister or stepfather talked about the youth's deceased mother, the young man became agitated and angry; he would typically find a way to change the subject or leave the room.

Some female offenders who have been physically and/or sexually victimized by males avoid interacting with male staff. These youth often feel safer developing relationships with female staff members. Some of these young women may have extreme emotional reactions to particular male staff, even when there is no apparent provocation. It is possible that certain male staff may remind these young women of a past abuser. Although their reactions may not make sense to an observer, these youths' emotional reactions make sense to them. They are a protective mechanism to avoid being victimized and hurt again.

Sometimes the avoidance behavior of juveniles with PTSD is more subtle. These youth may lose interest in once enjoyable activities and people. They often describe feeling "different" from those around them and as if they cannot "relate" to their peers anymore. Juveniles with PTSD are not necessarily sad all of the time, although some youth with the disorder do experience feelings of depression. Instead, these youth have a restricted range of emotions. They may not experience much joy, and they may also not experience much sadness. Some youth with Posttraumatic Stress Disorder say they are afraid that if they allowed themselves to experience their emotions, it would be too

overwhelming. They are scared they would not be able to handle such strong feelings. Others juveniles say that it is hard for them to feel anything at all. They describe being emotionally "numb," as if nothing really affected them one way or another. They might not get as excited about events that their peers look forward to (e.g., family visits, movie night, pizza parties, release date). Because of the terrible things that have happened to them, these youth often believe it is better not to get their hopes up. This way, they can avoid being disappointed and hurt yet again.

Many juveniles with PTSD report that they are unable to trust anyone, even those closest to them. They protect themselves emotionally and do all they can to avoid feeling emotionally or physically vulnerable. These youth commonly keep interpersonal relationships on a superficial level, and they may become uncomfortable if they begin to truly care about someone—or someone begins to truly care about them. If juvenile offenders with PTSD begin to feel attached to a particular staff member, they may start to engage in behaviors that push that person away. These youth may withdraw socially and try to avoid interacting with that individual. Or, they may become irritable and angry during interactions with that staff member. This behavior can be confusing, frustrating and disappointing for juvenile justice professionals, particularly when they have been building relationships with specific youth over time.

Juveniles with PTSD frequently have difficulty discussing long-term plans and goals (Terr, 1991), something required in many juvenile justice programs. Due to the traumatic experiences they went through, these youth typically feel unsure of what the future holds for them. Many juvenile offenders with PTSD question whether they will be alive to carry out their long-term goals because they are not sure they will live past the age of 21. These youth often describe the world as unpredictable and say that bad things could "take you out" at any moment.

Posttraumatic Stress Disorder (PTSD)

They are usually pessimistic about their own lives and often doubt that they will ever truly be happy (Martinez & Richters, 1993).

A sense of a foreshortened future is not restricted to juvenile offenders with PTSD. Other youth involved with the juvenile justice system also hold similar beliefs due to the reality of these youths' lifestyles and the communities in which many of them live. A significant number of juvenile offenders have family members and peers who died before the age of 21, and serious violence may be commonplace in their neighborhoods. When evaluated by mental health professionals, a subset of these youth will clearly meet the diagnostic criteria for PTSD due to experiencing negative symptoms or behavior in relation to this type of lifestyle. Another subset of these youth will not meet diagnostic criteria for the disorder because they have adapted to their violent lifestyles and violent communities. However, there is a subset of juvenile offenders who have adapted to a chronically violent and dangerous household or community, and who also suffer from symptoms of PTSD.

Increased Arousal

Posttraumatic Stress Disorder is an *anxiety* disorder, so youth diagnosed with this illness often experience physiological symptoms typical of individuals who suffer from high levels of anxiety. Juveniles may complain of feeling "revved up," "tense," or "on edge" much of the time. Youth with PTSD typically have not experienced these symptoms of increased arousal before experiencing a traumatic event. But the symptoms can persist months, and even years, after a traumatic event occurs.

Many juvenile offenders with PTSD report that they cannot fall asleep at night. Or, if they can fall asleep, they find it difficult to remain asleep until morning, often awakening several times during the night. These youth often describe being flooded with negative thoughts as soon as their head hits the pillow and being unable to "turn off" their thinking so that they

can fall asleep. At times, intrusive memories and thoughts about a traumatic event keep them awake for hours—particularly if juveniles are frightened and do not feel safe in their surroundings. If youth have been physically and/or sexually victimized, sharing a room with a roommate they do not know can be frightening. This situation is particularly true if the youths' roommate is known to have a history of violent and/or sexual offending. Bedtime at juvenile justice facilities can be very difficult for youth with PTSD, especially once the lights are lowered or turned off completely. Some youth with PTSD try to engage with staff when it is time to go to bed as an attempt to avoid having to go into their room at night (*e.g.*, asking repeated questions, requesting to do "one more thing," refusing to go into their room, starting an argument with staff).

Some youth with PTSD report that they have sleep difficulties only when incarcerated. While there are many reasons why juveniles may experience problems sleeping in a juvenile justice facility (*e.g.*, uncomfortable bed, cold temperature, fear of roommate, noise), their problems may be directly related to symptoms of anxiety. Many of these youth believe they do not have problems sleeping "on the outs." However, staff should clarify whether the youth are able to fall asleep outside of a facility without any mind-altering substances. Many juvenile offenders with PTSD drink alcohol or smoke marijuana before they go to sleep when residing in the community, and they rarely go to bed completely sober. When this is the case, the juveniles' sleep problems are likely to be more serious and longstanding than the youth report.

Attention and concentration difficulties are common among juveniles suffering from PTSD. These youth may find it difficult to focus on one thing for a significant period, particularly in an academic environment. Severe difficulties with attention and concentration can lead some mental health/medical professionals to mistakenly believe these youth have Attention-Deficit/

118

Juvenile Offenders with Mental Health Disorders: Who Are They and What Do We Do With Them?

Hyperactivity Disorder (ADHD). Juveniles with PTSD may be distracted because of intrusive thoughts or memories of a traumatic event, which is very different than the distractibility seen in youth with ADHD. Even youth with PTSD who rarely, if ever, consciously think about the trauma they experienced, can suffer from concentration problems. Some youth with PTSD have difficulty paying attention because they are focusing on details that are not relevant to a task at hand. In fact, many of these youth are *overly* attentive (hypervigilant)

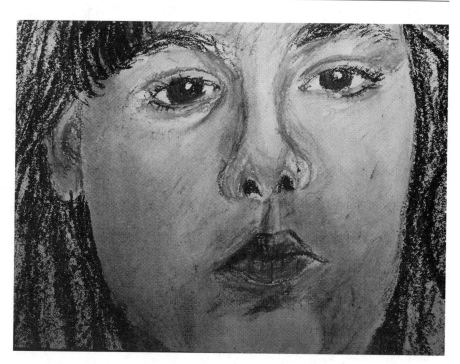

regarding their surroundings. These juveniles often know exactly who is doing what, to whom, where, and in what manner this differs from what occurred the day before.

For example, juveniles with PTSD attending an anger management group may be carefully observing other group members instead of focusing on the topic being discussed and the skills being taught. These youth may be concentrating on which group members are becoming irritable and who is remaining calm. Juveniles with PTSD tend to be always on their guard and cautious when interacting with others. After experiencing a trauma, youth want to feel safe in their environment. Being watchful of what goes on around them and of what others are doing is one way juveniles with PTSD attempt to help themselves feel safe.

Youth with PTSD walk around feeling revved up and tense much of the time. They may jump at loud noises and are easily startled if staff comes up behind them unexpectedly. In addition, juvenile offenders with PTSD are often irritable and easily upset. They may have unexplained outbursts of anger and/or may overreact to even slight provocation from staff or peers. Extreme anger and aggression are not

uncommon among this population. Some youth with this disorder may be so frightened by their angry emotions that they react in the opposite manner, responding passively to threatening situations (Terr, 1991). Some youth with PTSD fluctuate between strong anger and passive resignation. Due to their irritability and anger, as well as difficulty in controlling their impulses (Steiner, *et al.*, 1997), these youth often receive multiple sanctions in juvenile justice facilities due to negative, and sometimes dangerous, behavior.

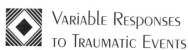 VARIABLE RESPONSES
TO TRAUMATIC EVENTS

Although a significant number of juvenile offenders have experienced traumatic events, not all of these youth develop PTSD. After a traumatic incident occurs (*e.g.*, witnessing a murder, being raped, being in a serious motor vehicle accident) juveniles commonly experience significant distress (Pynoos, 1992). They may go through several cognitive and behavioral changes for days, weeks or months after the traumatic event. Some youth are affected for years after a traumatic event. However, not all changes in thinking or behavior are pathological. The human mind and body needs to process and cope with overwhelming emotions associated with traumatic stressors. The diagnosis of PTSD is given only when youth are experiencing symptoms from each of the three areas: re-experiencing the trauma, avoidance and increased arousal. The symptoms must be present at least four weeks after the traumatic stressor occurs, *and* the symptoms must cause clinically significant distress or functional impairment in important areas of youths' lives (*e.g.*, school, work, interpersonal relationships; APA, 2000). Many individuals with PTSD experience a complete recovery from their symptoms within three months of a traumatic event; however, others continue to suffer for many years (APA, 2000; Giaconia, *et al.*, 1995).

Individual youths cope with stress and trauma in their own unique way. Why some youth develop PTSD while other youth do not is unknown—even when they have experienced similar stressful events. Juvenile offenders who have experienced numerous horrific events but appear to be functioning adequately can be perplexing for staff. This situation is especially true when other youth have significant symptoms of PTSD, even though they report experiencing a much lower level of trauma. Some juvenile offenders have experienced so many traumas in their lives that additional traumatic incidents do not seem to affect them strongly.

For example:

Patrick, 17, was locked up in juvenile detention when he was informed that his close friend had been stabbed and killed outside of their local hangout. Staff were concerned that the young man would become suicidal and/or react with extreme aggression. Patrick took the news calmly, and there was no observable difference in his behavior over the next three weeks. When a mental health professional talked with him, he stated that two other close friends had died in the past six months and that his father had committed suicide the previous year. He said, "You just get used to this s—t, and soon it doesn't bother you any more. There ain't nothin' you can do about it." Patrick's behavior in the living unit and in the school remained satisfactory, and there appeared to be no change in his relationships with staff or peers.

Patrick's reaction is not usual among juvenile offenders. However, some youth may react with extreme anger and helplessness after hearing about the death of a close friend. These types of feelings can lead to aggressive outbursts and/or a serious suicide attempt.

Each juvenile has his or her own individual coping style. Some youth want to talk about traumatic events they have experienced, and "getting it out" helps them to process and integrate the terrible thing(s) that have happened to them. Other youth deny that a traumatic event is negatively affecting them. They may refuse to talk to anybody about what happened, as well as avoid anything related to the event. There is no *right* way to deal with traumatic stressors. There is a great deal of variation among youth with regard to the way they manage their emotions and survive stressful situations. Talking about a trauma may be beneficial for some youth, while expressing how they feel about a trauma through artwork may be more effective for others. Some juveniles minimize the effect of a trauma and do nothing in particular to "deal with it." Little is known about youth who have been exposed to severe traumas but who do not demonstrate any associated symptomatology; however, it is estimated that 10-20 percent of these youth will experience negative effects years later (Putnam, 1997).

There is no set time when juveniles should be "over" a traumatic event. Youth commonly experience nightmares, fear, anxiety, anger, problems with concentration, or other responses to trauma for days, weeks or even

Juvenile Offenders with Mental Health Disorders: Who Are They and What Do We Do With Them?

months after exposure to an extreme stressor. Such responses are normal (Marmar, 1991). Some youth become rebellious and even engage in antisocial acts after a severely traumatic experience (Pynoos and Eth, 1984). These symptoms eventually resolve for most youth but can later resurface when reminders of the trauma are present (*e.g.*, anniversary dates, exposure to people or things that remind them of the event, talking about the event with juvenile justice professionals or mental health professionals individually or in a treatment group). For some juveniles, memories of a traumatic event remain with them throughout adulthood. If youth are suffering from PTSD after someone dies, it can interfere with the natural grief process. In addition, youth may not be able to experience the normal set of grief reactions if a victim is killed in a traumatic and/or violent manner. Memories of the deceased can be painful, disgusting and frightening. If youth try to avoid thinking about what happened because it is too painful and disturbing, they may have a more difficult time moving through the mourning process.

The impact of trauma on juveniles is probably due to a combination of a variety of factors, including those related to the youth, the youths' family, and the nature of the trauma itself (Steiner, *et al.*, 1997; Warner & Weist, 1996; Fitzpatrick & Boldizar, 1993). The following factors can all affect how youth cope with a traumatic experience:

- Age
- Developmental level
- Genetics
- Temperament
- Exposure to previous trauma
- How the youth interpret what happened
- The presence of a psychiatric disorder

In addition, family support, parental income, which caretakers reside in the youths' household, and the presence of a significant relationship with an adult figure can play a role. The nature of a traumatic experience can also affect how youth handle stressful incidents, including:

- Whether the youth were victims versus witnesses of the event
- How long the trauma lasted
- How close the youth were to getting hurt or killed themselves
- Whether the perpetrator was a stranger or family member
- How attached the youth were to the victim
- Whether the event was sudden and unexpected

Although the disorder typically manifests itself soon after a stressful event occurs, symptoms of PTSD may not become evident for months to years. The diagnosis of PTSD is given when juveniles are suffering significant, acute symptoms of arousal, avoidance and re-experiencing a traumatic event. These symptoms must interfere with the youths' ability to function in school, work, relationships or other important areas of their lives. Even if they do not meet the full criteria for PTSD, however, juveniles who have experienced significant traumatic events are still at high risk for:

- Academic problems
- Poor health
- Suicidal ideation
- Suicide attempts

(Giaconia, *et al.*, 1995)

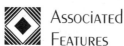 Associated Features

Juvenile offenders with PTSD often experience a variety of problems associated with the disorder that affect several important areas of their lives. For example, many of these youth have significant difficulty regulating their emotions. These juveniles may experience severe mood swings, sometimes becoming angry and hostile with minimal provocation. Impulsivity is also not uncommon among juvenile offenders with PTSD. Some of these youth feel constantly threatened, as if everyone were "out to get them." This can result in juveniles responding to annoying or irritating situations/individuals in an aggressive or argumentative manner. Because they have difficulty with affect modulation, once juvenile offenders with PTSD become angry or emotionally upset, they often find it difficult to calm themselves.

Stomachaches, headaches, and vague muscle or joint pain commonly occur among youth with anxiety disorders, including PTSD. Juvenile offenders, particularly male offenders who are concerned about looking tough and macho, may be reluctant to report feelings of anxiety or fear related to traumatic incidents.

A number of juvenile offenders report feeling guilty that their best friends were shot instead of them.

For some of these youth, their anxiety manifests itself in more physical, health-related symptoms.

Feelings of guilt and shame often accompany PTSD. Juvenile offenders may suffer from "survivor guilt," wondering why they were not killed or hurt as badly as someone else. A number of juvenile offenders report feeling guilty that their best friends were shot instead of them. Or they report feeling guilty over younger siblings receiving more physical and/ or sexual abuse than they themselves experienced. Some of these youth feel guilty for not being able to "save" or "protect" their friends or family members when terrible things happened to them. Incarcerated juvenile offenders, in particular, may lament over their belief that had they not been locked up, they might have been able to do something to prevent tragedies in the community. Many youth who have been sexually abused report feelings of shame, as if they

were damaged in some way. Some female sexual abuse victims feel "dirty" and "bad," as if they did something to provoke the unwanted sexual activity. Male juvenile offenders who have been molested by men or older boys can feel guilt around experiencing sexual activity with someone of the same sex—with some youth wondering whether they are homosexual. Depending on their beliefs about homosexuality, this may result in feelings of guilt and shame and can lead these juveniles to question their own sexual orientation.

Some youth with PTSD experience episodes of *dissociation*. When experiencing something incredibly painful and overwhelming, the mind can try to separate the experience from consciousness. For example, traumatic experiences can sometimes be so overwhelming that juveniles cannot tolerate the pain—physically and/ or emotionally—of what is occurring (*e.g.*, female youth being raped by a male adult, male youth being beaten up by several gang members). It is as if their minds shut down, so as not to process the terrible things that are happening. Some female juvenile offenders have reported that while they were being sexually victimized, they tried to "disconnect" from their body. This way, they did not have to emotionally experience the pain their physical bodies were going through. These young women sometimes describe this type of situation as if they were "watching themselves from above."

Even after traumatic incidents are over, juveniles with PTSD may still experience symptoms of dissociation. In the past, this reaction was their bodies' way of helping the youth survive, and it served as a coping mechanism during periods of extreme stress. For some juveniles, this way of coping can become so automatic that whenever they are faced with a highly charged or stressful situation, their mind begins to shut down. When dissociating, youth may have a blank stare on their faces and look as if they are "spacing out." They can actually lose track of time (*e.g.*, be unable to recall what happened for several minutes or hours).

Feelings of *derealization* can also occur, in which youth feel that the world around is unreal and unfamiliar. They may feel detached from their peers and/or as if they are walking around in a dream-like state. This is much more serious and intense than a youth just "spacing out."

Investigators are currently evaluating the neurological impact of early and severe trauma. It has been suggested that this type of trauma can result in significantly altering youths' ability to respond to future stressful events. (*Please see Chapter 15 for additional information about exposure to trauma and the developing brain.*)

Some juvenile offenders with PTSD engage in self-injurious behavior, such as cutting or carving their bodies. A number of youth engaging in self-injurious behavior are attempting to end periods of dissociation or derealization. The physical sensation of cutting or scratching their skin, as well as seeing their blood, can help bring dissociating youths' attention back to their present surroundings. High levels of anxiety and tension are common among juveniles with PTSD, and some of these youth report that mutilating their bodies is calming and helps to "ground" them. Many self-injurious youth with PTSD state that the physical pain of cutting is easier to deal with than their emotional pain. For some of these juveniles, the physical pain actually helps release some of the emotional pain. (*Please see Chapter 12 for more information on self-injurious behavior.*)

Unfortunately, identifying which juvenile offenders are suffering from PTSD is difficult, and many of these youth remain undiagnosed. Some of these juveniles have never told anyone about their significant symptoms of anxiety. In an environment such as a juvenile justice facility, youth typically want to appear strong, tough and in control. There can be a great deal of stigma attached to being "mentally ill," and juveniles typically do not want their peers to see them as weak, vulnerable or "crazy." Some youth with PTSD perceive *themselves* as "going crazy." They know that something is wrong with them, but they still do not want anyone else to find out

about it. They cannot understand why they are unable to stop thinking or dreaming about horrible things that happened to them in the past— or of violent things that they have done to others.

Youth who dissociate typically do not understand why they are unable to account for certain periods of time. Some of these youth are concerned that there is something wrong with their brain. Juveniles with PTSD often do not know why they feel tense or on edge much of the time. They may feel as if they cannot control their angry reactions, even when making a conscious effort to do so. From the outside, these youth can appear strong and tough to juvenile justice professionals and peers, but inside, these youth often feel frightened and uneasy. They may be unable to shake a general sense of feeling "different" from those around them, as if they were broken in some way. Sometimes juveniles with PTSD are aware of how they avoid certain places, situations or people. But they may not link their apprehension and avoidance behavior to previous traumatic events.

Many juvenile offenders (and individuals with PTSD in general) do not want to talk about traumatic incidents they have experienced, even when directly asked. Some of these youth do not see the point in discussing agonizing issues that happened in the past. These youth often feel it is a waste of time because nothing can undo what has occurred. In addition, they do not want to re-expose themselves to the painful emotions they have already experienced. Some youth minimize traumatic events and deny that they are having negative effects on their emotions or behavior. Other juveniles will not discuss traumatic events so as to avoid having criminal charges filed (against peers, family members, or themselves) if the traumatic events were associated with illegal activity.

Depending on what youth have witnessed or the incidents in which they were directly involved, retribution (from individuals inside a juvenile justice facility and/or from individuals in the community when youth are released) can be a realistic fear if these youth speak of their experiences. Refugee youth who have emigrated from other countries may be fearful of the political ramifications of disclosing the torture and trauma they witnessed or experienced. In addition, juveniles who have been severely physically or sexually abused by parental figures may be aware of the possible consequences of reporting such abuse. A social service agency may investigate their parents/caretakers and possibly require the youth and/or their siblings to live separately from their parental figures. Fear of retribution from family members or a desire to keep the family unit together can prevent many abused juveniles from revealing horrible things that have happened to them.

 ## Management Strategies When Working With Youth Who Have PTSD

Youth suffering from PTSD have typically been affected cognitively, emotionally and behaviorally by traumatic events. Juveniles with PTSD are at higher risk for having a variety of additional mental health issues. Researchers have found an increased rate of severe emotional-behavioral problems, interpersonal difficulties and suicidal behavior (*e.g.*, suicidal ideation, actual suicide attempts) among youth with PTSD versus nontraumatized peers (Giaconia *et al.*, 1995). The youth with PTSD also had higher rates of Major Depression, phobic disorders, and drug and alcohol dependence. Juveniles with PTSD may use drugs and alcohol as an attempt to shut out intrusive memories of what happened. Or these youth may use substances to help reduce their symptoms of anxiety and increased arousal.

Symptoms of this illness also can lead to additional negative outcomes in the future. Juveniles' beliefs can be shaped by traumatic experiences, and they may never fully trust anyone again. This distrust can significantly impact the quantity and quality of their interpersonal relationships throughout adolescence

and into adulthood. These youth are at increased risk for job instability, additional psychiatric disorders, chronic medical illness, weakened social support systems, and suicide attempts as they grow older (Davidson, Hughes, Blazer, & George, 1991). Youth with PTSD also can develop a phobic avoidance of particular things that remind them of a trauma they experienced, which can place limits on their lifestyle. Avoidance behavior can interfere with their ability to physically go to certain geographical areas or interact with specific individuals. For example, several juveniles who had been severely beaten while at school refused to return to the schools in which the incidents occurred. And they found being on the grounds of other schools extremely stressful and anxiety-provoking.

The psychological treatment of juvenile offenders with PTSD is often challenging and complex. Youth suffering from this illness should receive mental health treatment for a significant period of time by mental health professionals trained in the effects of trauma. Effective psychotherapy for PTSD typically includes a variety of cognitive-behavioral strategies (*e.g.*, slowly exposing youth to trauma-related stimuli, confronting negative beliefs, relaxation training, distraction). Eye Movement Desensitization and Reprocessing (EMDR) focuses on stimulating the brain to facilitate processing and healing of traumatic events. Treatment outcomes for EMDR are promising, but more research is needed to state its clinical effectiveness.

This type of individual treatment is typically not available within most juvenile justice facilities. Therefore, long-term recovery from PTSD may not be possible until youth are released from a facility and obtain psychological services in the community. That being said, the following strategies are suggested to help decrease the severity of youths' symptoms during incarceration. Juvenile justice professionals can play a critical role in whether juveniles' symptoms of PTSD diminish during their incarceration, or

124

Juvenile Offenders with Mental Health Disorders: Who Are They and What Do We Do With Them?

whether the symptoms are exacerbated. They can:

- Listen and provide support
- Let the youth set the pace
- Be aware of time limitations
- Refer youth to a mental health/medical professional
- Educate youth about the effects of trauma
- Provide psychotropic medication (based on medical supervision)
- Encourage various modes of emotional expression
- Be aware of their own issues
- Be alert to physical complaints
- Be direct about reporting requirements
- Teach coping skills
- Be aware of triggers
- Refer to mental health services upon release

One misconception about trauma is that a youth must *talk* about what happened to them in order to prevent any negative impact from an incident. Some mental health and juvenile justice professionals are eager to have youth open up and talk about the horrible things these juveniles have experienced. These adults usually believe that bringing trauma out into the open and re-experiencing emotions attached to an event will result in therapeutic and healing outcomes for youth. Although this practice may be helpful for some, it is not for others.

Why certain juveniles are profoundly affected by traumatic experiences whereas other youth appear to have few to no symptoms following a trauma is not clear. Juveniles' ability to cope with traumatic experiences is probably due to a combination of factors related to:

- An individual youth
- The youths' family environment
- The specifics of the traumatic experience

Currently, there is no reliable way to predict which particular juveniles will:

- Develop significant mental health symptoms
- Develop a serious psychiatric disorder that persists for years
- Require little to no intervention

(Saywitz, Mannarino, Berliner & Cohen, 2000)

Intervention, including talking about a traumatic event, is clearly needed for youth who are experiencing acute symptoms of PTSD (*e.g.*, flashbacks and nightmares, avoidance behavior, increased arousal) if these symptoms are interfering with the youths' ability to function and/or causing them significant distress. However, some juvenile offenders who have experienced trauma function adequately in living units and in school. If these youth state that they do not want to talk about traumatic

---

Using denial and avoidance may be helpful for some juveniles to deal with the terrible things that have happened to them.

---

events from their past, it may not be helpful to have them do so.

Coercing youth to talk about traumatic incidents after they have made it clear they do not want to do so can sometimes do more harm than good (Berliner, 2000). Even though most adults think they are doing the right thing by forcing youth "out of denial," this practice can actually result in some youth being re-traumatized. Individual youth cope in a variety of different ways. Using denial and avoidance may be helpful for some juveniles to deal with the terrible things that have happened to them. Offering youth the opportunity to talk about traumatic events can be helpful but insisting that they do most likely will not.

Various juvenile justice facilities have different policies regarding how much personal interaction should occur between staff and juveniles. These differences may be a function of philosophy, resources, type of juvenile justice program and so forth. For example, in some facilities, line staff are solely responsible for custody and control. These staff members are typically expected to automatically refer youth to a caseworker, counselor or psychologist if they are experiencing difficulties related to personal issues. In facilities where no mental health professionals are present, line staff may be expected to provide informal counseling to the youth, in addition to carrying out security-related tasks. There are also facilities in which the expectation is not clearly distinguished. In this situation, some line staff choose to engage with youth around personal issues, while other staff prefer to focus more on security issues.

Moreover, if mental health professionals are available to staff in this type of situation, they may only refer those youth who are too clinically complex for the staff to handle. The following recommendations are designed to be relevant for juvenile justice professionals in a variety of roles; however, not all of them will be appropriate for every staff member. When talking with youth suffering from PTSD, juvenile justice professionals should adhere to the expectations and policies of their particular facilities—as well as engage in discussions with traumatized youth only to the degree to which staff are comfortable.

Juvenile justice professionals should not attempt to do "therapy" with youth who have PTSD. The psychological treatment of juvenile offenders with this illness is usually a complicated, involved and often long-term process. When done incorrectly, it can result in juveniles experiencing additional distress and severely affect possible long-term resolution of trauma. Because they are not trained in the psychological treatment of traumatized youth, juvenile justice professionals should focus on *identifying* and *referring* youth with PTSD to appropriately trained mental health professionals. In addition, being empathic and supportive with these juveniles is critical for staff. A concerned and caring attitude from juvenile justice professionals can significantly impact whether juveniles' symptoms of PTSD decrease or intensify during incarceration.

Not all juvenile offenders who have experienced significant traumatic events suffer from the full-blown symptom pattern of PTSD. However, if youth are experiencing acute distress related to a particular trauma, they are likely to benefit from the following management strategies. These strategies are not instructions on how to conduct therapy. Instead, they are suggestions related to how juvenile justice professionals can most effectively interact with youth who are experiencing difficulties associated with traumatic events.

Listen and Provide Support

Being able to talk about what happened to them, in their own words, can be extremely helpful for juveniles with PTSD. Juvenile justice professionals can bring up the issue of a traumatic incident in a calm and caring manner, but they should then establish whether youth want to discuss it. If not, staff should let these juveniles know that staff will be available if the youth decide they would like to talk about the incident at a later time. Once they begin to trust staff, juveniles may mention a comment in passing about something painful that has happened to them. As they are folding laundry or playing a game of checkers with staff, these youth might make comments such as, "Yeah, my sister was killed like that girl on TV," or "I know what it's like to almost die." When staff ask these youth to elaborate, the juveniles often state they do not want to talk about the incident. In these situations, youth are often "feeling the staff out" to see:

- Whether staff will be shocked by what the juveniles say

- Whether staff will be disgusted by what the juveniles say

- Whether staff will reject the youth after hearing what the juveniles say

126

Juvenile Offenders with Mental Health Disorders: Who Are They and What Do We Do With Them?

- Whether staff care enough to follow up on what the juveniles say

Sometimes youth think they want to talk about a traumatic event, but once they begin to say something aloud about it, they change their mind. Juvenile justice professionals should encourage youth to talk about the incident with a mental health or juvenile justice professional at a later time if the youth begin to feel more comfortable. Policies should be established so that there is always a professional available with whom distressed juveniles can talk.

Let the Youth Set the Pace

Juvenile justice professionals should allow youth to set the pace regarding what they are willing to discuss. Juveniles disclose personal information at the rate with which they are comfortable. Staff should not press youth to reveal too much too quickly because pressuring youth to discuss painful information when they are not ready can be re-traumatizing. Juvenile justice professionals also should not accuse youth of being in denial. Instead, staff should find ways of helping juveniles feel safe, such as developing trusting relationships with adults to whom they can slowly uncover painful experiences.

Be Aware of Time Limitations

Juveniles commonly mention intimate, personal or painful information to juvenile justice professionals moments before staff are about to take a break, leave for the day, or depart for a vacation. As a group of offenders is about to proceed to the gymnasium or sit down for lunch, youth with PTSD might approach a staff member announcing that they are ready to talk about the bad things that happened to them. Some traumatized youth may finally open up to juvenile justice professionals days, or even hours, before the youth are being released to the community. Juvenile justice professionals should not allow youth to *open* themselves and become vulnerable if there is not enough time to *close* them again. Once they begin talking about painful things that have happened, these

youth may be flooded with feelings once buried deep inside. They need time to process and integrate these emotions. Staff should not allow juveniles to disclose traumatic experiences and then leave them alone. Youth with PTSD will typically be left feeling anxious, upset, or angry—unaware of what to do with these strong, and sometimes overwhelming, emotions. When emotionally overwhelmed, juvenile offenders can become oppositional or aggressive and may be at higher risk for self-injurious and suicidal behavior. If youth bring up these types of issues at an inopportune time, juvenile justice professionals should:

- Reinforce youth for their willingness to discuss painful material

- Explain the particular time constraints

- Commit to a future time when the staff member (or a mental health professional) will continue the discussion with the youth

- Follow-through with all commitments made to the youth

Refer to a Mental Health/ Medical Professional

Juveniles experiencing *acute* symptoms of PTSD should be referred to a mental health/medical professional for evaluation and intervention. Individual or group therapy may be needed and/or psychotropic medication may be prescribed. Juvenile justice professionals and mental health/medical professionals should work collaboratively, integrating their areas of expertise and experience with particular youth to develop individualized treatment plans and effective management strategies. The trust and rapport that develops between juvenile justice professionals and youth with PTSD is crucial to positive treatment outcomes. This trusting bond is an important adjunct to the services provided by mental health/medical professionals. Just because youth have experienced a traumatic event, however, does not mean that they should automatically be referred to a mental health professional. Currently, most juvenile justice facilities do not have the mental health resources to accommodate the high number of referrals that response would bring about. However, youth should be referred if:

- They are experiencing symptoms related to a trauma
- They are distressed by trauma-related symptoms
- Trauma-related symptoms are interfering with the youths' ability to function

If treatment for PTSD occurs while a youth is incarcerated, staff should expect the youth's behavior to change (often for the worse) during different phases of treatment. Because the juvenile's overall function may decrease, staff often think that the treatment for PTSD is not working. Staff should discuss their observations and concerns with the treatment/trauma provider. This helps determine if the youth's reaction is a normal part of the treatment process or if the treatment is having negative affects on the youth.

Educate About the Effects of Trauma

Most juvenile offenders are unaware of how traumatic events can impact their thoughts, emotions and behavior. Sleep difficulties, increased anxiety and irritability commonly occur after individuals experience traumatic events. Juvenile justice professionals should explain to youth that experiencing strong negative emotions and intrusive memories in response to significant stressors is natural and to be expected. These juveniles should be reassured that they are not "going crazy." These youth also need to understand that their minds are probably trying to process and integrate the horrible thing(s) that they have witnessed or that have happened to them. Wanting to avoid certain things or feeling differently from their peers is common. Staff can play an important role in normalizing experiences related to stress and trauma. Their listening and support is crucial for youth to even consider allowing trauma out. Stress reactions typically diminish over time,

but working with a mental health professional may be necessary if youth are suffering from serious symptoms— particularly if they last for a month or more.

Provide Psychotropic Medication

There is no one type of medication that is always used to treat PTSD. However, the selective serotonin reuptake inhibitors (SSRIs, *e.g.*, Prozac®, Zoloft®, Paxil®) are often tried first. The SSRIs' typically target symptoms of both anxiety and depression. Anti-anxiety medication such as Buspar® is also sometimes used. Clonidine® can be helpful for youth with PTSD who have significant hyperarousal symptoms, including angry outbursts. Because they tend to have fewer side effects, the SSRIs are usually the most commonly used medication among juvenile offenders with PTSD. However, medication typically only alleviates the symptoms of the disorder, and cognitive-behavioral strategies are still often required for the disorder to truly resolve.

Encourage Various Modes of Emotional Expression

Some juvenile offenders want to communicate how they are feeling, but they are not comfortable expressing strong emotions verbally. Juvenile justice professionals can encourage youth with PTSD to use a variety of methods to express feelings related to traumatic events. Recording their thoughts and feelings in a journal, as art work, in a letter, as poetry, or in a rap song has been valuable for a variety of juvenile offenders. These activities not only can allow for emotional expression but also can be less threatening than a one-on-one conversation. Juvenile justice professionals can offer to look at what youth have written or created but that should not be the goal of the activity. The goal is the youths' natural expression of emotions.

Be Aware of Their Own Issues

Juvenile justice professionals need to be aware of their own comfort level when talking with youth about painful subjects. Discussing traumatic issues can be difficult for all staff. However, some staff may have their own unresolved issues related to traumatic events (*e.g.*, death, physical/sexual abuse, violence) and listening to juveniles discuss disturbing memories can be particularly difficult for those individuals. In these situations, some juvenile justice professionals may respond to youth by discouraging them from talking about upsetting events. Others may be able to relate to the youths' pain and become overly involved with their suffering. Juvenile justice professionals should be aware of interpersonal boundaries and maintain a separation between their own issues and those belonging to traumatized youth. Maintaining this separation is not always easy. If they believe their own personal issues are affecting their relationship with specific youth, staff should connect the juveniles with other staff members who can be more objective about the youths' experiences. Discussing these types of challenging situations with supervisors can be helpful for staff.

Be Alert to Physical Complaints

Some youth manifest their anxiety in physical symptoms. Juveniles with PTSD might continually report some type of physical complaint (*e.g.*, headache, stomachache, vague muscle/joint pain). These youth may make multiple requests to see a doctor or nurse. Juvenile justice professionals should take youths' bodily complaints seriously, and communicate with medical personnel. This can help to determine whether youths' bodily symptoms are related to anxiety, another psychiatric disorder, or a physical illness.

Be Direct About Reporting Requirements

Most staff in the juvenile justice system are legally mandated to report incidences of child abuse/neglect or illegal activity of which they become aware. This mandate should be made clear to all juveniles. If youth begin to disclose personal information, juvenile justice professionals should explain up front:

- What type of information can remain confidential (if any)
- What type of information cannot remain confidential
- Who will likely receive information if confidentiality must be broken

Certain information may need to be reported to legal authorities, social service agencies, and/or to supervisors and various juvenile justice professionals.

Teach Coping Skills

If youth with PTSD have difficulty managing their anger or feelings of depression, juvenile justice professionals can help them develop coping strategies specifically related to these emotions. Cognitive-behavioral skill-building approaches (*e.g.*, anger management, problem-solving skills training) can be particularly helpful. Most youth attend a variety of educational and rehabilitation groups while residing in juvenile justice facilities. Juvenile justice professionals can help reinforce youth when they use the positive coping skills they have learned while in the program.

Be Aware of Triggers

Juveniles with PTSD may have particular difficulty with their thinking, moods or behavior when confronted with stimuli reminding them of a traumatic event. Anniversary dates of a traumatic event, staff members that remind them of perpetrators, particular smells or sounds, and the like can *trigger* youths' distress. Juvenile justice professionals should talk with youth who have PTSD about potential triggers and help them cope with situations in which those triggers are present. Staff should provide additional support to youth when they are faced with triggers of traumatic events.

Refer to Mental Health Services Upon Release

An appointment for mental health services in the community should be scheduled for youth with PTSD if they are scheduled for release from a facility prior to being seen by a mental health professional. Juveniles with PTSD receiving mental health services in a juvenile justice facility who need to continue treatment should also have an appointment scheduled in the community upon release. These juveniles should be informed that working through the effects of significant trauma is often a long-term, sometimes life-long, process. This is one of the reasons it is critical to secure therapeutic services for the youth in the community. Locat-

---

TREATMENT for PTSD CAN include GRADUAL EXPOSURE TO TRAUMA-RELATED STIMULI, RELAXATION TRAINING, BEHAVIOR MODIFICATION, ANGER MANAGEMENT, PROBLEM-SOLVING SKILLS TRAINING, AND PSYCHOTROPIC MEDICATION.

---

ing mental health professionals who are trained and have experience working with adolescents who have encountered traumatic events is important. Treatment for PTSD can include gradual exposure to trauma-related stimuli, relaxation training, behavior modification, anger management, problem-solving skills training, and psychotropic medication. Links to community resources should be made and an appointment scheduled *before* youth are released from a facility.

COPING WITH FLASHBACKS

Juvenile offenders with PTSD may be anxious and frightened if they are having intrusive memories, nightmares or flashbacks. They may feel as if a terrible past experience is happening to them all over again. The following approaches can help youth cope with flashbacks:

- Educate youth about "re-experiencing" symptoms and how they are a common occurrence for individuals who have experienced trauma. Although re-experiencing a trauma can be uncomfortable and often upsetting, it is one of the ways juveniles' minds try to heal from traumatic experiences.

- Help youth identify triggers of re-experiencing symptoms. Because they typically think their intrusive thoughts, nightmares and flashbacks occur randomly, many juveniles are often frightened that they will re-experience a trauma when they least expect it. Re-experiencing symptoms often occur in response to particular triggers, and juvenile justice professionals can help youth identify which triggers are strongest for them (*e.g.*, certain days, times, smells, sounds, people, places). Asking juveniles to write down what is happening or what they are thinking *right before* they re-experience a trauma can help provide insight into what prompts their episodes. This can also help youth feel like they have more control over what is happening to them.

- Explain that intrusive memories and painful thoughts about traumatic experiences are more likely to occur during times when youths' minds are less busy (*e.g.*, alone in their room, daydreaming in school, trying to fall asleep). Providing juveniles with prosocial activities or tasks (*e.g.*, books, nondemanding assignments) can be helpful in keeping youths' minds occupied while they are alone in their room for a significant period of time. The goal is not to provide extra incentives to juveniles because they are suffering from symptoms of PTSD. Instead, the goal is to decrease their distress and the negative effects re-experiencing symptoms have on their emotions and behavior. Decreasing re-experiencing symptoms can positively influence youths' ability to function, which is also likely to benefit a living unit as a whole.

- Help youth develop several ways to distract themselves when they begin to have intrusive thoughts and memories of a traumatic event. Giving them simple activities or tasks to accomplish can help juveniles with PTSD, if they cannot get a traumatic incident out of their minds. Examples of distracting strategies include counting the tiles on the ceiling, doing crossword puzzles, counting backwards from 100 by 7's, drawing, reading, listening to music, writing a letter, reciting the lyrics to a rap song, or looking at a picture of their girlfriend/boyfriend.

- Restructure youths' thoughts about a traumatic event. If youth are unable to decrease their intrusive memories, juvenile justice professionals may be able to help them modify what they remember. Or staff can help the youth interpret what they remember so that it is not as frightening.

For example:

Christine, an incarcerated juvenile who was raped by an older cousin, became anxious every night in her room when it was time to go to sleep. She would typically refuse to go to her room, often getting into significant power struggles with staff. Once in her room, Christine would lie awake for hours or would repeatedly ring her intercom buzzer as an attempt to interact with staff. When she tried to fall asleep, she kept thinking that she heard a male coming into her room, walking up to her bed, preparing to rape her. She was unable to stop these thoughts. Christine truly believed that she

heard someone entering her room and standing in the dark next to her bed each night. She felt as if what happened with her cousin were happening to her all over again. Christine had often spoken of her close relationship with her grandfather before he died. Staff asked the young woman if she would be willing to imagine that the sounds she heard at night were the spirit of her grandfather coming to tuck her into bed, instead of being her cousin (who was currently in prison). At first she was to imagine the new thoughts. However, after several weeks, Christine was able to modify her thinking and able to sleep in peace. Sometimes, she even reported that she could smell the smoke from her grandfather's pipe in the room.

- Help youth remain focused on the "here and now." If they become aware that youth are having flashbacks, staff should help the youth concentrate on the present moment. Staff members should repeat the youths' name to them and remind the juveniles where they are—emphasizing that the youth are safe. Staff should identify themselves, their role at the facility, and their relationship to the juveniles.

Youth with PTSD can be taught to calm themselves if they begin to have flashbacks. These youth should engage in deep breathing exercises and think certain thoughts such as:

- "This is not real"
- "That staff member is not my stepfather"
- "I am not really hearing gunshots"
- "I cannot really hear my mother's cries of pain"
- "This is just my mind trying to process what happened to me"
- "I am safe right now"

Juvenile offenders with PTSD require formal mental health treatment if they are experiencing acute symptoms of the illness. These symptoms must cause the youth significant distress and/or interfere with the youths' functioning in daily activities. The most beneficial types of interventions for youth with PTSD are those that educate them about typical responses to trauma. Intervention approaches should use cognitive-behavioral skill-based strategies that focus on specific symptoms of re-experiencing traumatic events, avoidance behaviors, and hyperarousal (Lipovsky, 1991; Saywitz *et al*, 2000). Mental health professionals trained in these types of interventions have a variety of strategies they can employ with youth over time. Most juvenile offenders with PTSD have other emotional-behavioral difficulties as well, so individualized, multi-faceted, and long-term mental health treatment is usually necessary. Given the current mental health resources within most juvenile justice facilities, this type of treatment is typically not available while youth are incarcerated. Consequently, mental health/medical staff and juvenile justice professionals should work together to:

- Educate youth with PTSD about their symptoms

- Help decrease the youths' psychological distress

- Facilitate successful functioning while youth are residing within a facility

- Arrange for additional (and more intense) mental health treatment upon youths' release to the community, when indicated

Case Example

Fernando, 16, had been held for several weeks in a detention facility awaiting his court date. He was becoming increasingly frustrated. Fernando just wanted to know whether he was going to be released or was going to be "sent up" to one of the state training schools. He had been in detention before, but this time was different. He was anxious, on edge and had angry outbursts in reaction to minor incidents. He had difficulty falling asleep at night and once he did fall asleep, he often had terrible nightmares. Even though Fernando knew some of the other boys in his unit, he mostly kept to himself, which was completely out of character for him. If nothing else, he previously enjoyed harassing some of the weaker, more vulnerable youth. During past detention stays, Fernando would parade around the unit as if he owned the place. This time around, he seemed more reserved, almost unsure of himself. His athletic prowess disappeared, and he often refused to participate during daily opportunities for physical recreation. His anxiety did not appear to be related to possibly being sentenced to a training school. He had been detained on a robbery charge and thought he had a 50 percent chance of beating it. Plus, several of his cousins and friends were already residing at various training schools across the state. He admitted that it would help him stay sober if he remained incarcerated.

When a staff member entered the living unit to begin his shift, Fernando could smell the scent of french fries on him. When Fernando asked about the smell, the staff member stated he had just eaten at McDonald's and that his uneaten french fries were in his coat pocket. When he pulled them out and offered some to Fernando, the youth turned white, began to shake and walked quickly down to his room without saying a word. Because the juvenile's response was so unusual, the staff asked Fernando about it later that night. Fernando told the staff about an incident that had occurred at McDonald's about two months previously. The youth had taken his six-year-old brother to McDonald's for some food, and Fernando was "jumped" by several boys from a different neighborhood while in the parking lot. The boys severely

Juvenile Offenders with Mental Health Disorders: Who Are They and What Do We Do With Them?

beat him, repeatedly punching and kicking him. One boy grabbed a baseball bat and cracked it against Fernando's shoulders, legs and head. Fernando was terrified during the assault, but he could do nothing to defend himself. As he was being beaten, Fernando could smell the scent of McDonald's french fries and could hear his younger brother's tiny voice in the background screaming "Nando, Nando, Nando." Fernando never reported the incident to the authorities, but when he told his friends what happened, they tracked down the group of boys and retaliated. Fernando ended up with a mild concussion and some bumps, bruises, cuts, and a swollen lip and eye. Fernando's alcohol and marijuana consumption increased for days and weeks after the incident. He said it was to dull the pain of his injuries. However, even after he recovered physically, Fernando's substance use remained high. Fernando stopped going to school and began constantly fighting with his mother and her boyfriend.

Fernando's stay in detention was the first time he had been continuously sober since the beating in the McDonald's parking lot. He was, all of a sudden, plagued with anxiety that would not subside. He did not trust anyone and lacked confidence in his ability to defend himself if his peers began harassing him. Whenever he tried to sleep, he would hear his younger brother yelling , "Nando, Nando, Nando," and he could not get the voice out of his head. Over the weekend, one of the other boys had to be physically restrained by several male staff. Fernando could not watch or listen to what was going on. He began sweating and feeling as if he were going to pass out. He refused to play baseball during recreation time because he could not handle seeing all of the baseball bats. It kept reminding him of the bat the boys used when they beat him. Fernando would leave the room if a McDonald's commercial came on while he and his peers watched television. When the staff member came onto the unit smelling of McDonald's french fries, Fernando panicked. Had the staff member not followed up on the youth's odd response, juvenile justice professionals would have never known about the incident in Fernando's past. And they would have been unable to help him cope with it, as well as refer him to the appropriate mental health/medical professionals.

CHAPTER 7

Developmental Disorders: Mental Retardation, Learning Disorders and Fetal Alcohol Syndrome

"Some kids just don't get it. You can tell them something over and over and over. It's like their brain is never going to get it. Never."

Juvenile Probation Officer

Mario, 17, spends much of his time looking at pictures of dinosaurs or watching music videos. His speech and behavior seem more like those of a 10-year old. He has been in special education classes at school, but he has been removed from his classrooms numerous times due to disruptive behavior. Facility staff are easily frustrated with Mario because he needs constant reminders to complete even the simplest of tasks in the unit.

Marcie, 16, hates school. She often refuses to go to the classroom at the juvenile justice facility because "it's boring." She was in special education classes throughout junior high, but she completely dropped out of school in the tenth grade. Although she says the schoolwork at the facility is "easy" for her, she has difficulty completing any of her class assignments. She enjoys reading, but it takes her an extensive period of time to complete a book. She frequently mixes up words and letters, regardless of whether she is reading silently or aloud.

The term *developmental disorder* can be used to describe a number of childhood and adolescent disorders, and various states, agencies, and professionals use this term differently. In this chapter, the term *developmental disorder* is used to describe syndromes that:

- Arise early in child development
- Are related to brain functioning
- Are not primarily due to environmental causes
- Are relatively pervasive across many situations

134

Juvenile Offenders with Mental Health Disorders: Who Are They and What Do We Do With Them?

- Affect youths' ability to function successfully
- Are persistent throughout development

Although many disorders may fit this description, this chapter focuses on the most common developmental disorders among juvenile offenders: Mental Retardation, Fetal Alcohol Syndrome and the various learning disorders.

Youth with cognitive impairments enter and reside in juvenile justice facilities at high rates (Leone & Meisel, 1997). Cognition includes the ability to think about things, process information and make decisions. Not surprisingly, juveniles' cognitive functioning can greatly affect their ability to adjust and participate in programming and treatment. To be successful in facilities, youth need to be able to understand what is expected of them and what consequences (positive and negative) are associated with which particular behaviors.

Identifying youth with developmental disorders within juvenile justice can be challenging. Some youth with cognitive impairment have been previously identified and evaluated by mental health and/or educational professionals. For some of these youth, the associated information has been communicated to the juvenile justice system. For others, relevant information from mental health/educational evaluations has not been communicated. Additionally, a number of youth with cognitive limitations who are involved with the juvenile justice system have never been identified or evaluated for developmental disorders, and their difficulties remain undetected.

Youth with developmental disorders may not be able to comprehend information in the same manner as their same-age peers. Juvenile offenders commonly disobey staff directives. However, there is a significant difference between youth intentionally choosing not to follow instructions versus youth not understanding the instructions in the first place. Staff should be aware of youths' level of cognitive functioning and how cognitive limitations can

affect youths' behavior. Youth with developmental disorders can be challenging to manage in juvenile justice facilities. But they can also be some of the most engaging and rewarding youth with whom juvenile justice professionals will ever work.

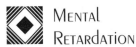 ## Mental Retardation

Juveniles with Mental Retardation have significantly sub-average intellectual functioning, as well as deficits in several areas of adaptive functioning (APA, 2000). The diagnosis of Mental Retardation is typically based on youths' Intelligence Quotient (IQ), as well as measures of their current level of adaptive functioning. Most youth have IQs in the Average Range (90-109). Youth with Mental Retardation have IQs that are significantly lower. Mental Retardation ranges in severity from mild to profound.

MILD Mental Retardation	IQ of 50-55 to Approximately 70
MODERATE Mental Retardation	IQ of 35-40 to 50-55
SEVERE Mental Retardation	IQ of 20-25 to 35-40
PROFOUND Mental Retardation	IQ below 20 or 25

Approximately 13 percent of juvenile offenders are mentally retarded (Casey & Keilitz, 1990). The majority of these youth probably falls into the mild range of Mental Retardation and typically function at about a sixth-grade level. Youth at the higher end of the mild range may be able to function adequately in a juvenile justice facility with additional guidance and supervision. This situation is particularly true when juvenile justice professionals are aware of the youths' cognitive limitations and make programmatic accommodations as necessary.

Youth in the moderate range of Mental Retardation usually function close to a second-grade level and need a tremendous amount of adult supervision and support. Even with additional assistance and structure, these juveniles often have a difficult time adjusting to a correctional environment. The majority of youth in the severe and profound range of Mental Retardation reside with their families or in specialized residential facilities. However, a few severely retarded youth have ended up behind the walls of juvenile justice facilities. Housing and supervising youth in the more serious ranges of Mental Retardation creates significant problems for these juveniles and the facility as a whole.

Youths' IQs (or IQ-equivalents) are typically determined from individually administered, standardized intelligence tests that are given by professionals trained in testing cognitive abilities. IQ tests commonly used with adolescents include the Wechsler Intelligence Scale for Children-Third Edition (WISC-III), the Wechsler Adult Intelligence Scale-Revised (WAIS-R), and the Stanford Binet Intelligence Scale-Fourth Edition.

In addition to low IQs, youth with Mental Retardation have difficulty adapting or coping with basic life functions. These youth are not able to behave as independently as one would expect given their chronological age. They may have problems taking care of themselves (e.g., hygiene, meals, clothes) and may have difficulties with communication, social skills, academic skills or keeping themselves safe.

Juveniles with Mental Retardation comprise a heterogeneous group of youngsters. Some youth with Mental Retardation are very gentle, compliant and dependent on adults. Others are aggressive, impulsive and oppositional. And some youth display a combination of these behaviors. Juvenile offenders with Mental Retardation can become hostile or aggressive when they are having difficulty communicating their wants and needs to those around them. These youth may not always understand the rules of a juvenile justice facility or how certain consequences are related to specific behaviors. Most juvenile offenders who self-injure are not

mentally retarded, but some youth with Mental Retardation bang their heads against walls and doors or slap their face and other parts of their bodies. Supervising juveniles with Mental Retardation can be frustrating for juvenile justice professionals, particularly when they do not understand the motivation underlying these youths' behavior. Determining whether juveniles' negative behavior is purposefully oppositional or whether it is associated with the youths' cognitive limitations can be difficult.

A number of youth with Mental Retardation have trouble successfully participating in the rehabilitation or treatment programs provided within the juvenile justice system. A large component of many juvenile justice treatment programs is helping offenders gain insight into their behavior. Youth are often encouraged to identify their offense cycle, recognize when they are becoming angry, and develop empathy for their victims. Frequently, there is a focus on setting goals, as well as understanding the link between the juveniles' thoughts, feelings and behavior.

Youth with significantly low IQs may not be able to participate fully in treatment that is cognitive in nature. They may be unable to think abstractly or gain insight into why they behave as they do. Cognitively, these youth may not be capable of truly understanding other peoples' perspectives.

For example, sex offenders with IQs in the mentally retarded range may regularly attend sex offender treatment groups that are cognitive in nature. Because most juvenile offenders do not have cognitive impairments, treatment material is usually presented at a level above the abilities of mentally retarded youth. During treatment groups, these particular youth may not have the ability to gain insight into their own deviant behavior and, instead, focus on the sexually stimulating conversation of their peers (e.g., hearing the word penis, listening to repeated stories containing sexual themes). Clearly, given these circumstances, sex offender treatment groups are not likely to decrease

136

Juvenile Offenders with Mental Health Disorders: Who Are They and What Do We Do With Them?

these developmentally delayed youths' inappropriate sexual behavior. Rehabilitation/treatment groups that are cognitive in nature work well for most offenders because they have the cognitive skills with which to participate. However, this type of approach is not always the best approach for youth with severe cognitive impairments. Some agencies have developed special facilities or living units exclusively for juvenile offenders who are intellectually impaired. Programming is modified in these special facilities/living units so that youth with cognitive limitations have an increased chance of being successful.

Many youth with Mental Retardation experience interpersonal difficulties during incarceration. Most of these juveniles do not understand the peer culture within juvenile justice facilities and are often teased because their interests and behaviors may be childlike and immature. Mentally retarded juveniles are also likely to be victimized by peers. Due to their low intellectual functioning, these youth frequently have poor judgment and are unable to distinguish whom they should and should not trust. Peers commonly "set up" cognitively impaired youth so that they are left to take the blame for something they have not done.

In addition, mentally retarded youth also can be physically or sexually victimized if they are not appropriately supervised. Although some peers will try to exploit cognitively limited youth, others will do the opposite and provide extra support for mentally retarded juveniles. Higher functioning peers may take lower functioning youth "under their wing"—as a means of providing protection or as a way to help the mentally retarded youth adjust to the environment. This dynamic usually proves rewarding for all juveniles involved. There is no one cause of Mental Retardation, and this disorder is probably the end result of a variety of etiological factors. Events occurring prior to birth can play a role in the development of Mental Retardation, including:

- Maternal alcohol consumption
- Exposure to toxins
- Chromosomal changes
- Gene abnormalities

Premature birth also has been linked to Mental Retardation. Once a baby is born, poor postnatal care, infections and trauma can play a role in the development of this disorder. In addition, environmental factors (*e.g.*, significant deprivation of socialization and stimulation) have been shown to be related to Mental Retardation, as has the presence of a mental health disorder (*e.g.*, Autistic Disorder or another pervasive developmental disorder). The specific cause of cognitive impairment remains unknown for a large number of youth who have been diagnosed with Mental Retardation (APA, 2000).

 LEARNING DISORDERS

A significant number of youth involved with the juvenile justice system suffer from one or more learning disorders, also known as learning disabilities. Juveniles with learning disorders tend to have difficulty accurately interpreting information they see or hear because of problems integrating information from the various parts of the brain. A comprehensive review of the literature concluded that around 36 percent of juvenile offenders have learning disorders (Casey and Keilitz, 1990), although this percentage is likely to be an underestimate. Because the symptoms of these disorders are subtler than those of Mental Retardation, many youth with learning disorders have never been formally evaluated. Consequently, their learning difficulties remain unidentified.

A learning disorder is diagnosed when youths' achievement on individually administered, standardized tests (in reading, mathematics or written expression) is substantially below what would be expected, given the youths' intelligence, age and schooling. The learning problems must significantly interfere with juveniles' schoolwork or other daily activities that require reading, writing or mathematical skills (APA, 2000). To diagnose youth with a learning disorder, clinicians typically administer IQ tests to measure juveniles' overall level of intellectual functioning. Youth are also given specific academic-related (*i.e.*, reading, writing, mathematics) tests. Regardless of youths' IQ, one would expect similar performance on both types of tests. Juveniles with an average level of intellectual functioning (*i.e.*, average IQ) should perform in the average (or close to average) range on academic tests. When this is not the case and youth score significantly lower on school-based tests, youth are likely to receive a learning disorder diagnosis. Learning disorders are not reflective of how smart juveniles are. Youths' IQs may be in the average, below average, or even genius range. But they can still have a learning disorder if their academic scores are significantly lower than what would be expected, given their overall level of intellectual functioning.

Some states have strict standards about which youth are eligible for special education services. Even when they have learning problems (and experience difficulties in relation to them), juveniles may not necessarily qualify for special education services. When learning disordered youth do not receive special services in school, their poor educational functioning is usually attributed to a poor attitude and a lack of motivation.

Juvenile offenders may be diagnosed with any (or a combination) of the following learning disorders:

- *Reading Disorder*—A Reading Disorder is the most common of the learning disorders and is usually known as Dyslexia. Any aspect of youths' reading ability can be affected. The accuracy of their reading may be poor, they may read very slowly, or they may not be able to comprehend what it is that they read. Youth with a Reading Disorder may add or omit certain letters or complete words. They may also have difficulty connecting the letters of the alphabet with specific sounds, making it hard to sound out words they do not immediately recognize.

- *Mathematics Disorder*—Youth with a Mathematics Disorder can have a variety of difficulties with numbers and mathematical skills. These juveniles may have a hard time understanding mathematical concepts or translating mathematical word problems into numerical symbols. They may forget to do important mathematical operations, such as carry a number, or not pay attention to whether addition or subtraction is required for a task. It is often hard for these youth to remember what steps are required to solve mathematical problems or to learn and remember multiplication tables. Many juvenile offenders with a Mathematics Disorder have a Reading Disorder or a Disorder of Written Expression as well.

- *Disorder of Written Expression*—Youth with a Disorder of Written Expression tend to have significant difficulty with grammar, punctuation and spelling. Their handwriting skills are often significantly poor. These youth tend to make many errors when asked to copy down what is being said or when asked to spontaneously write a story. Disorder of Written Expression commonly co-exists with a Reading Disorder or a Mathematics Disorder.

Some youth in the juvenile justice system display difficulties in reading, mathematics or written expression, but they do not necessarily have a learning disorder. A learning disorder is diagnosed only when youths' academic difficulties are significantly below what would be expected, given their age and overall level of intellectual functioning. Furthermore, these difficulties must considerably interfere with juveniles' schoolwork or other daily activities that require academic skills. Young offenders' poor performance on academic tests may be related to the youth not learning the material in the first place (due to missing school or attending classes in an inadequate school system) or solely to emotional factors. In these cases, a learning disorder should not be diagnosed.

The exact cause(s) of learning disorders currently remains unknown. However, research has shown that a variety of factors can play a role in the development of learning disorders, including:

- In utero exposure to tobacco, alcohol, or other drugs
- Complications during pregnancy or delivery
- Genetic factors
- Environmental toxins (*e.g.*, lead poisoning)
- Incidents after birth (*e.g.*, nutritional deprivation, head injuries, child abuse)

Some research has shown that the brains of individuals with learning disorders appear structurally different from those without learning disorders. Additional research is needed to better understand how brain structures and brain functioning are related to the problems experienced by learning-disabled individuals (NIMH, 1993).

Associated Features

Problems related to information processing are common among juveniles with learning disorders. These youth are often bright and have good ideas. In fact, a number of juveniles with learning disorders have at least average intelligence and may even know many of the answers required of them. However, transferring what is in their brains onto a piece of paper can be difficult and trying. This situation is especially true when these juveniles are given short time periods in which to complete assignments. Some youth with learning disorders have difficulty learning information solely by hearing it aloud and actually need to see information in

written form. Other youth have difficulty translating their thoughts into language; they know what they want to communicate, but when they open their mouth to speak, the message is not exactly what they intended.

Juveniles with learning disorders are usually able to repeat what they have heard someone saying, but they may not comprehend the message in the way the speaker intended it. Some messages seem to be modified when translated in the brains of youth with learning disorders, which can be frustrating for juveniles and the adults interacting with them. Not surprisingly, incidents of miscommunication are commonplace when juvenile justice professionals work with these youth.

Information processing difficulties can interfere with youths' ability to be successful within interpersonal relationships, and many juvenile offenders with learning disorders have poor social skills. These youth often do not understand the "give and take" of relationships with other people and can be slow to pick up on subtle social cues. Youth with learning disorders may misinterpret what peers or adults are saying to them and may attribute hostile intent to neutral statements. Their interpersonal style can inadvertently irritate or offend others.

Due to problems related to school and social relationships, many juveniles with learning disorders have a negative view of themselves. They often feel stupid and do not understand why schoolwork is so difficult for them. They also do not understand why they continue to have interpersonal difficulties with others. Throughout the years, adults may have accused these youth of being "lazy" or "not applying themselves." By the time they reach adolescence, many juveniles with learning disorders are tired of struggling academically. They may stop trying to achieve in school, and a high percentage will drop out before high school graduation. Because school is such an integral part of childhood and adolescence, repeated failure in the academic setting can result in these juveniles feeling discouraged and demoralized.

For many juvenile offenders with learning disorders, school is a challenging and unpleasant experience. If their learning disorders have never been identified, these youth are likely to feel angry and frustrated when unable to complete their academic work as expected. Even when diagnosed with a learning disorder, many of these youth do not understand why they work more slowly than their peers—or why they continue to receive poor grades, regardless of how much they study. To avoid feeling bad about themselves, these juveniles often try to avoid difficult classroom situations.

For instance, juveniles with learning disorders may try to convince their parents to let them stay home from school (*e.g.*, feign illness). Or they may begin to skip certain classes without parental permission in order to avoid the challenges of academic work. In addition, youth with learning disorders may become disruptive, oppositional or aggressive toward teachers or peers in order to be removed from the classroom, if even for a short period of time. The more time these juveniles spend outside of the classroom, the more they miss out on learning critical information. This typically results in their falling further behind in their schoolwork. As the youth fall increasingly behind, the classroom (and often school itself) becomes an arena full of anxiety, frustration, conflict and unpleasant experiences.

After awhile, learning-disordered youth may begin to avoid school altogether, missing all of their classes for days or weeks at a time. When these youth are away from school, they are likely spending time with other juveniles who have left school without permission (and who also probably have learning disorders). With so much unoccupied time on their hands, these young people commonly engage in delinquent behavior (*e.g.*, drugs and alcohol, criminal activity). School suspension or expulsion can be the final consequence for youth who have been repeatedly truant, disruptive or aggressive in the classroom. Ironically, for many juveniles with a learning disorder, this result is not viewed as a negative consequence. These youth may even be relieved that they have to remain out of the school environment they find so aversive.

In addition to their academic difficulties, many juveniles with learning disorders also suffer from mental health disorders such as:

- Major Depression
- Dysthymic Disorder
- Attention-Deficit/Hyperactivity Disorder
- Conduct Disorder
- Oppositional Defiant Disorder

With each additional diagnosis, youths are likely to have increased difficulties. These difficulties can manifest in several important areas of their lives (*e.g.*, school, family, peers, work)

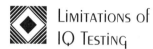

Limitations of IQ Testing

The diagnoses of Mental Retardation and learning disorders rely heavily on evaluating youths' cognitive functioning. One of the most common ways to measure youths' intellectual functioning is to *individually* administer standardized IQ tests. Juveniles should only receive IQ testing from clinicians with specific training and experience in these types of tests. Youths' IQs are not necessarily the absolute measure of their level of intellectual functioning. Currently, there is no way to look inside juveniles' brains to determine youths' exact intellectual capacity. Even if this could be done, what determines "intelligence?" That being said, the most commonly used IQ tests of today are typically accepted as an adequate measure of youths' cognitive capacity. Scores on these tests have been shown to be fairly stable over time, and they are good predictors of future learning and academic success. These tests are designed to take into account both verbal and nonverbal abilities. During an IQ test, youth are usually asked verbal questions related to vocabulary, abstract reasoning and comprehension. They are also asked to complete tasks that are not related to verbal skills but that tap into youths' visual-spatial skills. Numerous

140

Juvenile Offenders with Mental Health Disorders: Who Are They and What Do We Do With Them?

subtests, measuring different areas of cognitive functioning, are given in order to obtain a comprehensive view of youths' cognitive functioning and abilities. However, some experts argue that there are additional realms of functioning that need to be assessed in order to determine juveniles' true level of intelligence (*e.g.*, emotional intelligence; Gardner, 1993; Goleman, 1995). In addition, these tests do not measure creativity, motivation or study skills.

Juvenile offenders' IQ scores may be an underestimate of their intellectual functioning. This situation can occur despite appropriate tests being given and trained professionals administering them. The following is a list (albeit not exhaustive) of possible issues that could negatively influence juvenile offenders' performance during an IQ testing session. Some of these factors can have a direct influence on the juveniles' test-taking behavior, while others are more indirect.

- Sleep-deprived from staying up late the night before
- High on drugs or alcohol during the testing session
- Hungry because did not eat anything before the testing session
- Anxious in testing environment
- English is not the youths' primary language
- Hungover from partying the night before
- Discomfort with the examiner
- Youths' culture does not emphasize speed or trying to do tasks as quickly as possible (can affect timed subtests)
- Experiencing hallucinations
- Visual impairment/needs glasses
- Hearing impairment
- Does not want to do well on the test because others will expect more of youth
- Does not want "evidence" to prove that they are not smart

- Would rather not try on the test versus fail at it
- Unmotivated because they do not see the relevance of the test
- Fear doing well on the test will affect their juvenile justice disposition
- Oppositional attitude toward authority figures
- Distracted by problems at home
- Depressed mood (unmotivated or slowed thinking/behavior)
- Attention-Deficit/Hyperactivity Disorder (difficulty paying attention or sitting still during the testing session)

Professionals who administer IQ tests (or any tests assessing cognitive functioning) to juvenile offenders should be aware of these issues and do all they can to diminish their influence on youths' performance. If examiners believe resulting IQs are an underestimate of juveniles' cognitive ability, they should state this in their reports—as well as what their conclusion is based upon. If such statements are present in the reporting of IQs, juvenile justice professionals must be cautious of focusing on specific IQ numbers when making decisions regarding programming and disposition. Once IQs are recorded in juvenile justice paperwork, they are often automatically transferred from one file to another. Because youths' IQ can influence important decisions within several different systems, this type of information must be as accurately communicated as possible.

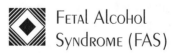 Fetal Alcohol Syndrome (FAS)

Fetal Alcohol Syndrome (FAS) is a form of permanent brain damage caused by maternal consumption of alcohol during pregnancy. However, not all youth who are exposed to alcohol in utero have Fetal Alcohol Syndrome. The amount of damage to a developing child, if any, depends on a variety of factors, including:

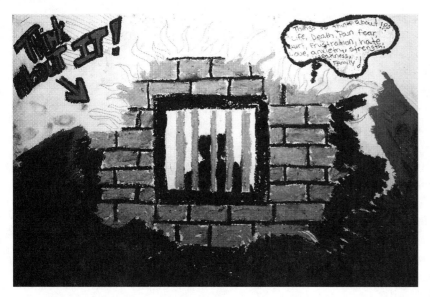

against providing an alcohol-related diagnosis when all of the criteria for Fetal Alcohol Syndrome are not present (Aase, Jones, & Clarren, 1995).

The diagnosis of Fetal Alcohol Syndrome typically focuses on the following factors (Astley & Clarren, 1999):

Brain—Youth with Fetal Alcohol Syndrome have brain damage. The actual structure of juveniles' brains may have been affected, and certain areas of their brains may have developed abnormally. Or youth with FAS may suffer from neurological problems such as seizures, difficulty with coordination or problems with their hearing or vision. Many of these juveniles have severe learning and behavioral problems that cannot be explained by environmental or genetic factors. These learning and behavioral problems also usually do not improve with typical types of intervention or treatment. Attention-Deficit/Hyperactivity Disorder, Mental Retardation, learning disorders, speech and language problems, impulsivity, and deficits in reasoning and judgment commonly occur in youth with Fetal Alcohol Syndrome.

Face—Certain facial features are characteristic of juveniles with Fetal Alcohol Syndrome. These youth tend to have small heads, flat faces, shorter distances between their lower and upper eyelids, and thin upper lips. The area between their upper lips and nostrils tends to be smooth or has minimal ridges in comparison to other youth. Because various ethnic groups have different facial features (*e.g.*, flatter noses, thicker or thinner lips), taking into account cultural factors when observing facial features of youth with FAS is important. The facial features of youth with FAS tend to be most pronounced during childhood and are less obvious during adolescence.

Body Size—Some juveniles with FAS are fairly small. They often weigh less, and some

- How much alcohol a mother drinks during her pregnancy
- When she drank the alcohol
- The mother's metabolism
- The child's metabolism
- What part of the brain is developing when the alcohol is ingested
- Genetic influences
- Whether the child was exposed to any other toxins or substances that can cause birth defects

Some mothers are unaware that they are pregnant when they ingest alcohol and immediately discontinue their drinking once their pregnancy is discovered. For some juveniles, the damage may already have been done.

Fetal Alcohol Syndrome is a recognized medical diagnosis and is determined when a variety of specific factors are present. A comprehensive evaluation involving a variety of health and mental health professionals is necessary to make an accurate FAS diagnosis.

Fetal Alcohol Effects (FAE) is a term that has also been used to describe youth with cognitive and behavioral problems due to alcohol exposure in utero. However, these juveniles do not meet all of the criteria required to receive the diagnosis of FAS. Although the term FAE is widely used, some experts in the field caution are shorter in height, in comparison to same-age peers. Many youth with FAS experience growth spurts during puberty, which can result in more normal physical growth during the adolescent years.

Alcohol Exposure—The diagnosis of FAS is specific to in utero *alcohol* exposure. If youths' mother absolutely did not consume alcohol during pregnancy, the diagnosis of FAS should not be given. The juveniles' cognitive and behavioral impairments are probably due to something else.

A number of youth in the juvenile justice system were exposed to trauma or toxins in utero. Some mothers of juvenile offenders have used drugs such as methamphetamine, marijuana, cocaine or heroin during part or all of their pregnancy. Some youth involved with juvenile justice were born with chromosomal abnormalities and/or experienced complications during their birth. Each of these factors can potentially have serious negative effects on a developing child, including cognitive and behavioral difficulties similar to those seen in FAS.

Associated Features

No two youth with FAS look or behave alike. The brain of each individual juvenile is different, and the level of brain damage among youth with this disorder can be minute to substantial. Most juveniles with FAS have some school-related difficulties. Even if their IQ is in the average range, these youth tend to think concretely and have difficulty problem-solving in difficult situations. They frequently have poor memories and can forget to complete even simple tasks. These youth may be impulsive, overly active, and/or violate the personal space of others. In addition, making logical connections between events is hard for many juveniles with FAS. Therefore, when they receive negative consequences for rule violations, these youth often do not understand the relationship between their behavior and the sanctions given.

Many youth with FAS have poor social skills. Even though they may appear to be listening to what others are saying, they have difficulty truly tracking what is being said. They may even have difficulty tracking what they themselves are saying. Youth with FAS can be very talkative, even to the point of monopolizing conversations. They may digress to tangential topics or change the topic of conversation altogether, midstream. Many of these youth have poor social judgment, which can get them into a variety of troublesome situations.

For example, juveniles with FAS may not comprehend the importance of listening to directives from juvenile justice professionals and, thus, may not consistently respond to staff instructions. Or these youth may belligerently argue with gang members who are more than twice their size. Adults and peers may become frustrated or annoyed by juveniles with FAS because they sometimes display mood swings with little provocation. They may alternate between being gentle and friendly and then hostile and rude. There is a great deal of variation among the temperaments of these youth. Some juveniles with FAS are dependent and loving, while others are aloof and oppositional.

Youth with FAS are at high risk for physical, emotional and sexual victimization in juvenile justice settings. Because of their poor social judgment, they may be confused as to who their friends are and who their enemies are. Peers can easily persuade these youth to engage in delinquent behavior. Some youth with FAS may be attracted to gang or pseudo-gang membership because these types of groups typically offer structure and a clear social hierarchy. In addition, some of these groups are made up of other youth who are also having problems in school, as well as difficulty getting along with adult figures. Because youth with FAS are often naïve and gullible, these types of social groups can exploit these juveniles—as well as set them up to take the blame for the delinquent behavior of others.

One of the most challenging aspects for juvenile justice professionals working with juvenile offenders with FAS is the unpredict-

Developmental Disorders: Mental Retardation, Learning Disorders and Fetal Alcohol Syndrome

ability of these youths' behavior. One day, juveniles with FAS may be able to follow directives, complete all assigned tasks and interact appropriately with peers. The next day, the same juveniles may have difficulty completing basic tasks, fail to follow instructions from staff, and may get into a fight with their roommate. Because these youth were able to accomplish certain behaviors the day before, staff know that those particular skills are in the juveniles' behavioral repertoire. Concluding that the youth must be *choosing* to act in this negative manner is natural for staff. Juvenile justice professionals commonly view juvenile offenders with FAS as manipulative and oppositional. However, part of these youths' brains have been damaged by alcohol. Depending on the extent and location of this damage, their brains may not work exactly the same two days in a row. More often than not, these juveniles *cannot* do what is asked of them versus *choosing* not to do it. Clearly, there will be times when youth with FAS do not want to do something and intentionally defy authority. However, juvenile justice professionals should explore the situation fully and not assume automatically that FAS youth are being purposely oppositional.

Some youth with FAS have never received a formal diagnosis because they have never been evaluated by a mental health/medical professional. Even if they have received an evaluation, because some of these youth do not exhibit *major* impairment in one particular area (*e.g.*, attention, impulsivity, language, reading), clinicians may have overlooked their difficulties. However, these youth may have *minor* difficulties in *many* areas, making successful functioning difficult. Juvenile justice professionals are more likely to attribute FAS youths' non-compliant behavior to willful manipulation when these juveniles have not received a formal FAS diagnosis—or received specialized intervention services in the past. This dynamic is common when youth with FAS are incarcerated, especially when the juveniles are of at least average intelligence.

 ## Managing Juvenile Offenders with Developmental Disorders

Most young offenders with developmental disorders (*e.g.*, Mental Retardation, learning disorders, Fetal Alcohol Syndrome) have the capacity for success in either academic or vocational programs. These youth can become productive and full participants in society. Juvenile justice professionals should identify the strengths of cognitively impaired juveniles—and help build on these strengths.

Juveniles with developmental disorders respond best in highly structured settings where there is consistency and routine. They need clear expectations and swift consequences for positive and negative behavior. Well-run juvenile justice facilities tend to already have this type of structure in place. However, periods of change and transition (no matter how small) can be particularly difficult for these youth to handle. They may become dependent on certain staff members or attached to particular sleeping rooms in a living unit. Youth with developmental disorders may become upset if there is a change in the daily schedule, new staff members in a unit, or a move to different sleeping quarters. Depending on the severity of youths' cognitive impairment, much of their organizational skills may be dependent on external cues and directives. When changes in the external environment occur, these juveniles can become disorganized and confused. This often results in anger, frustration, anxiety or withdrawal.

The following intervention strategies can be helpful for juvenile justice professionals when working with a variety of different youth with developmental disorders. Depending on youths' level of cognitive impairment, staff may want to use some or all of the following approaches. Some juvenile offenders with learning disorders function adequately in a structured juvenile justice facility and only experience difficulties in the academic arena. Other youth with learning disorders may have difficulty with language

144

Juvenile Offenders with Mental Health Disorders: Who Are They and What Do We Do With Them?

processing and social skills, which affects their behavior on a larger scale. Youth with Mental Retardation and/or FAS typically have more serious cognitive impairments. These impairments can result in youth having difficulty functioning successfully in several areas of programming within a juvenile justice facility. Further, some youth with severe Mental Retardation or FAS will not be able to function at all in a juvenile correctional environment. If this is the case, these youth should be transferred to a program specifically designed for this population of youth.

Although the recommended management strategies may initially seem overwhelming, they are not intended to be used simultaneously with all youth who have developmental disorders. They are suggested ways of responding that can be used when cognitively impaired youth appear to have problems complying with the expectations and rules of juvenile justice facilities. These management strategies are most helpful for youth who seem to not "get it" when juvenile justice professionals repeatedly explain things to them. They are also particularly beneficial for juveniles with developmental disorders who are having problems adjusting to a facility in general and/or continually receiving negative sanctions.

Structure, Structure, Structure

Juvenile offenders with developmental disorders function best in highly structured environments. If an environment is predictable, it reduces the number and types of cognitive demands placed on the brains of these youth. Having juveniles with developmental disorders follow the same routine on a daily basis is best. Having consistent staff members (*e.g.*, juvenile justice professionals, teachers) is also helpful. This type of consistency provides juveniles who have developmental disorders with the external cues necessary to be successful in daily activities. It also decreases the likelihood these youth will become confused or frustrated. Due to the structured nature of most juvenile justice

settings, many higher-functioning cognitively impaired youth can conduct themselves adequately in well-run juvenile facilities.

Extra Supervision

Increased monitoring is typically required for youth with significant cognitive impairment. Because these juveniles often have difficulty with impulsivity, problem-solving and judgment, they commonly involve themselves in risky situations. Juvenile justice professionals must be vigilant about victimization. Unsophisticated social skills and low IQs can result in cognitively impaired youth being physically, emotionally or sexually victimized by peers. All youth in juvenile justice facilities should be given a clear message from staff that no form of teasing or victimization will be tolerated.

Extra Support During Periods of Transition or Change

Because youth with developmental disorders function best in predictable environments with routine and consistency, these youth may experience difficulty during periods of transition or change. Depending on the level of juveniles' impairment, even minor transitions or changes (*e.g.*, change of classrooms, lunch an hour later than usual, cancellation of movie night, cancellation of a recreational activity, bedtime change) can result in confusion for them.

Larger transitions or changes (*e.g.*, assignment to a new primary staff member, change of living units, transfer to a treatment program, staff vacations, release from a juvenile justice facility) can result in major distress for juveniles with developmental disorders. Providing these youth with several warnings before transitions or changes occur (*e.g.*, "Ten more minutes until bedtime," "Lunch will be after your fifth-period class today instead of your fourth-period class") can be helpful. Planning ahead for larger transitions and changes can reduce the likelihood of these youth experiencing problems when actual transitions/changes occur. Providing juveniles

Developmental Disorders: Mental Retardation, Learning Disorders and Fetal Alcohol Syndrome

who have developmental disorders with calendars can assist them in tracking how many days are left before changes or transitions occur. This strategy can also decrease the number of times these youth will continually ask staff questions related to upcoming changes (*e.g.*, "How many days until I leave?" "When will my staff be back from vacation?"). Youth can be directed to look at their calendars and count the number of days themselves. Much of the anxiety experienced by juveniles with developmental disorders is related to not knowing what is going to happen next. Their environment becomes increasingly more predictable with additional external cues.

> Youth with developmental disorders function most successfully when there are clear behavioral expectations and swift consequences (positive and negative) in response to their behaviors.

Clear Expectations

As they enter juvenile justice facilities, youth receive information about the expectations and rules of a program. Youth with developmental disorders may need to have these rules and expectations written down and posted in their room if they have difficulty remembering them. If juveniles have significant cognitive impairment, pictures from magazines may be needed to help the youth fully grasp certain concepts (*e.g.*, two youth fighting with a big X over it, individuals brushing their teeth as a reminder of hygiene issues). Because they frequently have to reiterate program rules as new youth arrive in a unit, juvenile justice professionals may have a tendency to go over the information fairly quickly. Staff should make sure that this information is not only heard but also understood by juveniles with developmental disorders. Even when this occurs, staff will still probably have to go over the program rules and

expectations again on a periodic basis with particular youth—especially if staff are working with juvenile offenders who are cognitively impaired.

Effective Behavior Management

Youth with developmental disorders function most successfully when there are clear behavioral expectations and swift consequences (positive and negative) in response to their behaviors. Some token economy programs (such as point systems or level systems) may not provide feedback immediately enough for juveniles who are cognitively impaired. These youth may not be able to wait until the end of the day to find out whether they received all of their points.

Juveniles with developmental disorders may not be able to make the connection between their behavior and the associated rewards earned if waiting to "cash in" their points is required. Juvenile justice professionals may need to provide interim reinforcers for cognitively impaired youth, such as giving them points each shift versus at the end of the day. If tangible reinforcers (*e.g.*, treats, privileges) are not available until the end of the week, these juveniles may need a chart or graph to keep track of their behavior and associated consequences (*e.g.*, chart with stars or points). Giving youth poker chips or stickers when they earn points can serve a similar purpose. Because they are typically concrete thinkers, youth with developmental disorders often need something they can see, touch or hold, versus just being told they "made it to level three." This modification does not necessarily need to occur with all offenders who have intellectual impairments. But it can be beneficial for youth who are having difficulty progressing within a token economy program. It also reduces the number of times juveniles need to ask staff, "What level am I on?" or "How many points do I have?" Some juveniles with developmental disorders ask these types of questions of staff repeatedly throughout the day.

146

Juvenile Offenders with Mental Health Disorders: Who Are They and What Do We Do With Them?

Depending on their level of impairment, some youth with developmental disorders have difficulty making the connection between room confinement/isolation and their negative behavior that elicited the consequence. Juvenile justice professionals should clearly state the connection between youths' negative behavior and the sanctions given, especially when the sanction is room time. Once cognitively impaired juveniles are placed in their own room (or a special seclusion room), they typically need periodic reminders as to why they were placed there. This is especially true if these youth are in a room for more than 20-30 minutes. Due to memory problems or distractibility, juveniles with developmental disorders may be oblivious as to why they were removed from their peers and instructed to go into a room. These youth commonly attribute room confinement/isolation as due solely to "staff being mean." If this is youths' belief, room confinement/isolation is not likely to have much of an influence on the juveniles' negative behavior.

In addition, many juveniles with cognitive limitations do not fully understand the abstract concept of time. Some juvenile justice professionals use warnings of continued room confinement when youth persist engaging in negative behavior (*e.g.*, banging on the door, trashing their room, yelling at peers, repeatedly pressing the buzzer in their room). Warnings, threats or promises of abstract negative consequences—such as an additional two hours, four hours or eight hours of room confinement/isolation—may mean little to cognitively impaired youth. This strategy typically has minimal influence on these juveniles discontinuing their negative behavior. *(Please see Chapters 3 and 14 for additional information on effective behavior management.)*

Reminders

Youth with developmental disorders often need reminders, sometimes repeatedly. Therefore, juvenile justice professionals can become increasingly frustrated due to having to instruct youth to complete what seems to be simple tasks, over and over again. Many cognitively impaired juveniles have memory problems and/or are very distractible. Because of this, they often rely on external cues to keep them focused and on-task. Providing reminders to youth in a "matter of fact" tone (so that juveniles do not feel dumb or inadequate for not remembering) can be helpful. Writing things down for youth also can be an efficient way to facilitate their memories. Providing youth with a list of specific responsibilities (which they can check off upon completion) can help decrease the need for constant verbal reminders, which can be time consuming for staff.

Additionally, juvenile justice professionals should ensure that youth clearly understand what is expected of them. Many cognitively impaired juveniles have learned that "parroting back" what they have been told convinces most staff that the youth understand instructions. But repeating what they have heard does not necessarily mean youth truly comprehend the information. Juveniles with developmental disorders may initially require numerous reminders related to several different behaviors (*e.g.*, make your bed, brush your teeth, put your books away, no phone calls until written assignments are complete). However, most of these youth will be better able to self-monitor—without as much staff assistance—after repeated practice with tasks.

Specificity

Because most cognitively impaired youth think in concrete terms, juvenile justice professionals need to be very specific in their communication. Statements such as, "Clean your room," "You need to be more respectful," or "You can make a phone call when you show me you can handle your behavior more appropriately," are typically too vague for youth with cognitive impairment. These juveniles need staff to be unambiguous in their requests. A "clean" room might refer to no underwear on the floor. Or it could refer to having the bed made, placing all

Developmental Disorders: Mental Retardation, Learning Disorders and Fetal Alcohol Syndrome

books in the closet, and ensuring that extra t-shirts are folded and put away. In addition, juvenile justice professionals and youth typically have different views regarding what constitutes "respectful" behavior. The word "appropriate" is also vague and ambiguous. In contrast, the following statements, "Please make your bed and clean the papers off of your floor," "Keep your hands to yourself," and "You can make a phone call at 3:00 p.m. if you speak to me without using profanity," let youth know precisely what is expected of them.

Positive Directions

When providing directives to youth with developmental disorders, juvenile justice professionals should tell youth what *to* do versus what *not* to do. Rather than saying, "Don't lean back in your chair during group," staff can say, "Keep your feet on the floor at all times." Instead of saying, "Stop trading food with Brian," it is better to say, "You can only eat the food on your own plate." Rather than saying, "Stop yelling," staff can instruct youth to "Speak in a conversational tone," When juvenile justice professionals direct youth to stop engaging in behaviors, many juvenile offenders with cognitive impairments do not know what behavior should take its place. By providing positive directives, staff instruct juveniles to discontinue negative behavior, while also helping them develop more prosocial behavior for the future.

One Directive At a Time

Youth with cognitive impairments can be easily overwhelmed with multiple directives. Because they often cannot hold several instructions in their memory, these youth can forget to do some of what is asked of them. Juvenile justice professionals should make sure not to provide too many instructions at one time. For example, telling youth to "Hang up the phone, help Josh set the table, put those books away, and return the pencil you borrowed," may be too much for youths' brains to handle if they have some type of cognitive impairment. Instructing these

youth to "Hang up the phone" is likely to be more effective. Once the youth complete that task, staff can tell them to "Help Josh set the table." Once the table is set, the youth can then be shown which books to put away. Finally, the youth can be instructed to return the pencil they borrowed. Although this strategy appears time-consuming, it often consumes less staff time—because staff do not need to repeatedly prompt, prod, or coerce youth to carry out multiple directives when the juveniles forget what to do.

However, sometimes providing consecutive verbal directives in the aforementioned manner still takes up too much time for juvenile justice professionals who supervise large numbers of youth simultaneously. In these circumstances, staff can quickly jot down directives (*e.g.*, tasks to complete) on a piece of paper. Youth can be instructed to place a checkmark next to each task when it is completed and a given a time limit as to when the tasks need to be done. This practice should take no more than five minutes of staff time. If juveniles only accomplish two of the four tasks, staff members should direct the youths' attention to the list and ask them to complete any remaining duties.

If juveniles are severely cognitively impaired, they may not be able to complete a single task all the way through without staff breaking the task down into smaller components. "Set the table" may need to be separated into smaller tasks. "Put the cups out" can be an initial instruction. Once youth complete that, staff can instruct them to, "Put the forks on the napkins." After that is completed, youth can be told to, "Bring out the salt and pepper shakers." With repeated practice and experience, most juveniles eventually learn what they need to do and will not always need such specific instructions.

Concrete Communication

Many youth with cognitive limitations focus on the *literal* meaning of words when conversing with others. Therefore, juvenile justice profes-

148

Juvenile Offenders with Mental Health Disorders: Who Are They and What Do We Do With Them?

sionals should speak in concrete terms. For example, sarcasm and humor may be common among staff in juvenile justice facilities. Although humor can be an effective interpersonal strategy with many juvenile offenders, those who are intellectually impaired may not understand a joke. These youth also may not understand when staff members are teasing them. They often feel confused, ignorant and isolated from staff and peers who do understand the teasing/joking. Sarcasm can result in similar dynamics. Juveniles with developmental disorders often do not understand sarcasm and can be puzzled or hurt by it.

Short, Simple Sentences/Slow Speech

Many juvenile offenders find it helpful when juvenile justice professionals take the time to reason logically with them or to explain the rationale involved in requests. This situation is not necessarily true with youth who have cognitive limitations. Adults should avoid overwhelming the brains of these youth. Staff should use short, simple sentences to get their point across. The more succinct staff can be, the better. Because these youth can have difficulty processing verbal information—particularly when hearing language spoken aloud—staff should speak slowly and clearly when communicating with them.

Avoidance of Automatic Attributions

There will be times when youth with developmental disorders do not follow instructions or engage in behaviors that are clearly against the rules. This situation can occur even after several staff reminders. Juvenile justice professionals should first clarify whether youth are aware of what is expected of them. If they know the expectations, are the youth *choosing* not to comply? Do they not *understand* what the expectations mean? Or, have the youth *forgotten* what they are supposed to do because of intellectual impairments? It is easy for juvenile justice professionals to assume that youth are being intentionally oppositional—especially if

the youth have demonstrated acceptable behavior in the past. Even if developmentally disordered juveniles have previously complied with expectations, however, this does not necessarily mean that their cognitive difficulties will not impact future behavior. This is particularly true during periods of increased stress. There are times when youth with developmental disorders purposely break rules or defy authority, and they should receive negative consequences for this behavior. But staff should not automatically attribute youths' negative behavior to malicious motivations. Staff should take the time to clarify the reasons for the misbehavior of cognitively impaired juveniles.

Patience

Because they may not process information as quickly as their peers, youth with developmental disorders may take longer to adjust to the environment of juvenile justice facilities. Facility programming can be confusing to them, and they may need several reminders to accomplish even simple tasks. Juvenile justice professionals may feel that they do not have the time to provide the extra support required by some cognitively limited youth and can become increasingly frustrated with them. However, if staff are patient and *initially* provide these juveniles with the level of structure, consistency and routine they need, most mildly impaired youth eventually adjust to facility programs. At the outset, these youth can be overly dependent on external cues, but many of these youth develop internal cues to help them accomplish what needs to be done—decreasing their reliance on staff support. Both staff and youth should take pride in these juveniles' increasing autonomy and independence.

Chronological Age and Physical Size Do Not Necessarily Indicate a Youth's Cognitive Ability

A number of juvenile offenders with developmental disorders are older adolescents who are big and strong in stature. Adults commonly treat

Developmental Disorders: Mental Retardation, Learning Disorders and Fetal Alcohol Syndrome

these youth as more capable than they really are and hold them accountable for tasks that are too challenging for them. Juvenile justice professionals may not remember that a 6'2" young man with Fetal Alcohol Syndrome weighing 240 pounds could function at the level of a 9-year old. Juvenile justice professionals can easily forget that a 17-year-old young woman with Mental Retardation can overlook basic hygiene without reminders from others. Therefore, juvenile justice professionals, as well as teachers, must be conscious of youths' level of intellectual functioning and not get distracted by their physical appearance or chronological age.

Basic Living Skills

Although most incarcerated youth can benefit from programming that emphasizes basic living skills (*e.g.*, hygiene, socially appropriate clothing, chores, responsible decision-making), this point is particularly true for youth with cognitive limitations. The following are helpful when juvenile justice professionals teach youth how to do a new behavior:

- Verbally explain the behavior to youth
- Model the behavior for youth
- Observe youth engaging in the behavior
- Provide specific feedback regarding what youth are doing correctly/incorrectly

External support and cues from staff will probably be needed when youth are first learning to function more independently. As juveniles continue to practice new skills, however, external supports can be faded out. Patience and persistence on the part of staff is critical, and cognitively impaired juveniles should be reinforced for every small step toward acquiring new skills.

Basic Social Skills

Youth with developmental disorders often have problems with social judgment and language processing. Therefore, these youth often get into interpersonal conflicts with staff or peers and/or are rejected by others. These youth may lack basic social skills such as:

- Walking up to and joining a group of peers
- Letting others speak without interrupting them
- Looking at someone when they are talking
- Making requests of staff
- Discontinuing the poking of peers or the slapping of peers hard on the back

Discussing specific social skills with juveniles and then modeling the particular skills is one of the most effective modes of social skills training. Staff should also role-play various social situations with youth and provide feedback on the juveniles' behavior. Some adolescents with developmental disorders have the social skills of young children. Therefore, juvenile justice professionals should not expect too much too soon from these juveniles and should reward each positive step toward prosocial behavior.

Various Modes of Communication

Due to the deficits in language processing among some youth with developmental disorders, it is important to present these juveniles with information in a variety of modalities. Some of these youth may need to hear things, see things and touch things to fully understand them. Juvenile justice professionals need to provide concrete examples of specific behaviors expected from youth, as well as role-play the behaviors so that the likelihood of miscommunication is minimized. Writing short lists and posting pictures of behavioral expectations can be helpful for cognitively impaired youth who do not respond well to verbal cues. Hands-on instructions and hands-on activities can also be particularly effective for these juveniles.

Use of Peers for Mentoring

Some of the more mature youth in juvenile justice facilities enjoy taking lower-functioning youth "under their wing." The pairing of youth who have a developmental disorder with higher-functioning and responsible peers can be a positive and rewarding experience for all juveniles involved. This outcome is particularly likely when the youth with cognitive limitations achieve some success during the partnership. Higher-functioning juveniles can help cognitively impaired youth with written assignments and basic chores; they also can engage them in leisure activities (*e.g.*, playing cards, listening to music). However, rotating the peers that are used as mentors or "buddies" is important so that these particular youth do not become burned out. In addition, staff should monitor these types of situations to ensure that cognitively impaired youth are not being exploited or misled.

Communication with School Personnel

Juvenile offenders with learning disorders can improve their educational skills dramatically with individualized tutoring and coaching. These youth can learn how to use their academic strengths to compensate for the areas in which their academic skills are weaker. Because many juvenile justice facilities offer small classrooms, computer access, various modes of teaching and individualized instruction, juvenile offenders have opportunities to increase their academic skills (sometimes dramatically) throughout their incarceration.

All juvenile justice facilities must be aware of federal and/or state laws related to the evaluation, education and programming of youth with developmental disorders. There are often specific mandates related to the types of educational services that must be provided to these youth. Because of these requirements, many juvenile justice facilities have access to professionals who are specifically trained to work with youth suffering from cognitive limitations (*e.g.*, special education teachers, school psychologists).

Youth with developmental disorders are typically entitled to an Individualized Education Program (IEP). An IEP is a written plan, typically developed by a team of individuals (*e.g.*, teacher, parent/caretaker, school administrator,

the youth, school psychologist) after they collaboratively identify youths' educational and behavioral needs. Once juveniles' needs are identified, the team makes decisions about what specific actions should be taken to meet those needs. All school personnel, and most juvenile justice professionals, have access to youths' IEPs. These written reports usually offer a great deal of important information about youths' abilities and limitations. These plans can be helpful when juvenile justice professionals develop treatment plans and/or create effective management strategies for youth with developmental disorders. When cognitively limited youth have difficulty in a living unit, juvenile justice professionals can often obtain practical tips or suggestions from school personnel. Correctional educators may be aware of specific intervention strategies that work effectively with particular cognitively limited youth.

Modeling Respect for a Youth

Juvenile offenders often look to juvenile justice professionals for models of socially appropriate behavior. They frequently look to see how staff members are reacting to, and treating, lower-functioning youth. If juvenile justice professionals become irritated with, roll their eyes at, or tease juvenile with developmental disorders, such behavior gives permission to the rest of the youth to act in this manner. Even when they get frustrated with juveniles who are cognitively limited, juvenile justice professionals should always be conscious of how their own behavior appears to the youth around them. Staff should make sure to model patience, understanding and respect.

Focus on Success

Many youth with developmental disorders, whether mild or severe, suffer from feelings of low self-esteem. They often feel stupid and become frustrated when they cannot accomplish things as quickly as those around them; many of these youth are aware that they take longer to grasp certain concepts. Due to their fear of failure, some youth with developmental disorders have given up on academics and may be apprehensive about trying new and unfamiliar tasks or activities in a classroom. In addition, many of these youth are rejected by same-age peers and have few friends. Reinforcement is essential when cognitively limited juveniles engage in positive behaviors. This reinforcement is especially important when these youth engage in behaviors that are outside of their typical repertoire. The more success these juveniles experience, the more likely they will engage in the newly developed behaviors in the future. Helping youth with developmental disorders gain confidence about their skills often results in positive ramifications in all areas of their lives.

> Cognitively impaired juveniles may display poor judgment in social situations with staff and peers, which typically results in interpersonal conflicts and possible assaults by other youth.

Referral for Mental Health/ Medical Evaluation

Juvenile justice professionals frequently supervise youth with developmental disorders who have never been evaluated by medical or mental health professionals. Even if youth have been evaluated in the past, those records are often not forwarded to the juvenile justice facility where the youth reside. Juvenile justice professionals commonly describe offenders with developmental disorders as not "getting" the program, not "being all there," or being extremely "slow." They may also notice that typical sanctions have minimal influence on these youths' negative behavior. Cognitively impaired juveniles may display poor judgment in social situations with staff and peers, which typically results in interpersonal conflicts and

possible assaults by other youth. These youth may also be alienated and rejected by peers due to their unusual and/or immature behavior. Most juvenile justice professionals have good intuition about juveniles who are functioning at a lower cognitive level. Staff usually perceive that "something is not right" with these youth— even if they cannot be specific as to what is wrong. Referring youth suspected of having cognitive impairment to a mental health/ medical professional is essential (even when staff cannot be specific as to the youths' underlying difficulties). The juveniles can then be evaluated and their current level of cognitive functioning determined. Once a referral is made, juvenile justice staff and school personnel should provide clinicians with examples of specific, observable behavior in which the youth engage (positive and negative). They should also mention which management strategies have and have not been effective with these particular youth. Information from a mental health/medical evaluation should be communicated to the staff members responsible for supervising and managing the juveniles'—as well as integrated into the programming and treatment of the youth.

Psychotropic Medication

Many juvenile offenders with Mental Retardation also suffer from an additional mental health disorder. Psychotropic medication may be prescribed to help treat the symptoms of these other disorders. For example, psychostimulants are often prescribed for inattention and impulsivity. Antidepressants, such as the SSRIs, are often prescribed for symptoms of depression and/or anxiety. Mood stabilizing medications and antipsychotic medications may be prescribed for aggressive behavior and/or stabilization of mood. Medication should only be used when absolutely necessary. The primary goals of the medication are to:

- Stabilize the youths' behavior
- Keep youth from harming themselves or others

152

Juvenile Offenders with Mental Health Disorders: Who Are They and What Do We Do With Them?

- Help the youth function more effectively in activities of daily living

Medication should never be used to control or sedate youth with Mental Retardation. Medication should be part of a larger treatment plan and should not take the place of appropriate behavioral interventions. Medication is unlikely to be helpful if the reason the youth are depressed, anxious or aggressive is related to expectations being too high for the juveniles.

Realistic Expectations

Depending on the severity level of juveniles' cognitive impairment, behavioral expectations may need to be modified for some youth. Many juvenile justice programs are based on the philosophy that all youth should be treated equally. Therefore, program modifications should be discussed among members of a staff team, as well as with appropriate supervisory staff. The goal is to help youth with developmental disorders experience some success, no matter how small, so that they will be motivated to make additional positive changes.

For example, some juveniles with cognitive limitations have difficulty sustaining progress with regard to token economy systems (*e.g.*, point system, level system). This situation can be frustrating for youth, particularly if they are putting forward a great deal of effort to fulfill the expectations of a living unit or program. Sometimes, these juveniles are only able to partially complete required behaviors, so they are ineligible to receive the rewards/points associated with the full completion of the behaviors. Eventually, these youth may become discouraged and discontinue putting forth any effort at all. Some juveniles with developmental disorders remain on the lowest level of token economy programs for significant periods of time. This circumstance typically results in these juveniles not having access to many of the incentives their peers have earned by accumulating points or moving upward in the system. When this occurs, cognitively limited youth seem to be penalized for being incapable of

completing certain behaviors. Juvenile justice professionals should ensure that youth with developmental disorders *earn* their rewards, but expectations should be congruent with the youths' capabilities.

Accountability

Having a developmental disorder is not an excuse for juveniles to engage in unacceptable behavior. If juvenile justice facilities have rules such as "no kicking" or "no profanity," those rules are meant to apply to all youth. When they do not comply with unit or facility rules, juveniles (with or without cognitive impairment) need to be held accountable. This practice helps young offenders better understand what is expected of them behaviorally. Juvenile justice professionals should respond to the negative behavior of developmentally disordered youth as quickly as possible. This swift response helps these youth make the connection between their negative behavior and the consequences received. Although all juveniles should be held accountable for rule-breaking behavior, the exact nature of consequences (*e.g.*, points deducted, time in their room) should differ depending on:

- The presence/severity of youths' cognitive impairment
- Youths' ability to comprehend the rules/behavioral expectations
- The specific circumstances surrounding the negative behavior

Community and Transition Services

Federal and state government agencies typically offer a variety of programs and services for youth with developmental disorders (*e.g.*, Department of Developmental Disabilities, Special Education). Therefore, appropriate staff should investigate youths' eligibility for these services before cognitively impaired youth are released from juvenile justice facilities. If youth are eligible for community resources such as educational assistance, funding, residential placements and so forth, these links should be estab-

Developmental Disorders: Mental Retardation, Learning Disorders and Fetal Alcohol Syndrome

lished well in advance of youths' scheduled release date. Allowing an adequate amount of time for planning increases the likelihood that special services can begin as soon as the juveniles return to the community.

Linking juveniles who have developmental disorders to educational services prior to release is also critical. Some of these youth will return to their previous schools, while others will need to transfer to new schools. Youth who receive high school diplomas or GEDs during incarceration may need to be linked with college courses or some type of vocational services in the community.

———————

Juvenile justice professionals may look at this list of recommended management strategies and immediately dismiss it. Most facility staff are inundated with a variety of tasks that must be completed simultaneously. They are often responsible for supervising large numbers of youth, and the thought of using some of these suggestions may seem overwhelming and unrealistic. Some of these recommendations do require additional staff time. Explaining things slowly and making sure that youth truly understand what it being said can take a few minutes. Providing juveniles with reminders or modifying specific consequences for particular youth can be more time-intensive than saying something once or providing the same consequences for all juveniles. However, juvenile justice professionals are typically already spending additional time working with youth who have developmental disorders. Unfortunately, this extra time is usually provided *after* negative incidents occur. The more time juvenile justice professionals can provide to cognitively impaired youth preventively (on the front end), the less likely additional time will be spent responding to negative behavior. Verbal conflicts, power struggles, tantrums, physical forces, restraint incidents and the like, can be decreased when youth clearly understand rules and behavioral expectations. This is particularly true when behavioral expectations are commensurate with youths' level of cognitive functioning. In addition, such practices can reduce frustration for both staff and juveniles, leading to more positive interactions and safer, smoother-running units in general.

Case Example

Charles, 15, is accused of being an accomplice in a gas station robbery. He was with three other boys who held up a gas station attendant, asking for all of the money in the cash register. Charles was picking out a comic book when the crime took place. He said he was unaware that the other boys were going to engage in any criminal behavior. Once they took the money from the cashier, all four boys ran out of the store. Charles tripped and fell; he was the only one of the group who was caught and arrested. Charles did not have much information to give to the police when they questioned him. In fact, the police found Charles to be more like a young child than a teenager, even though he was close to six feet tall. The rotating blue and red lights on the police car continually distracted Charles. He repeatedly asked if he could go for another ride in the police car, as well as turn on the siren.

Once he arrived at the juvenile detention facility, Charles became confused and disoriented. He did not understand why he had been brought there and why he could not sleep at his own house that night. Charles physically interrupted the staff whenever he had a minor question or concern. He would repeatedly poke staff on the arm or back if they did not immediately respond to him. When in his room, Charles would continually push his buzzer to try to get the staff to engage with him. The other youth at the facility teased Charles because he looked and moved somewhat differently from his peers. Staff knew there was something "not right" about Charles, but they were not sure what it was.

Juvenile Offenders with Mental Health Disorders: Who Are They and What Do We Do With Them?

CHAPTER 8

Schizophrenia and Other Psychotic Disorders

"Something is not right with this kid. I'm not sure what it is, but something is not right."

Juvenile Correctional Officer

Terrence, 17, has spent the past two years at one of the most secure training schools in the state and is going to be released within the next six months. Staff recently began to notice a change in Terrence's behavior. Although staff used to describe him as an "odd" youth, they were now describing him as "weird," "crazy" and "totally out of it." Terrence had always kept to himself and was known as a loner within the facility. But lately he has become agitated and angry when forced into group situations. He accuses other residents of stealing his belongings, and he believes that the staff are conspiring to conceal the thievery of his peers. He has difficulty watching television because he believes subliminal messages are being transmitted over the airwaves. He is also fearful that the host of one of his favorite shows is trying to steal his thoughts. Terrence has not told anyone about his experiences with the television for fear that the staff and residents will think he is crazy.

Brian, 16, was brought into a detention center for brutally killing his neighbor's dog. He stated that the dog was constantly looking at him, following him and harassing him. Brian is convinced that the dog was possessed by the devil and was trying to kill him. At one point, Brian thought the dog could read his mind and was trying to get him to follow Satan. Brian exhibited no other unusual behavior, except a recent decline in his schoolwork after he started spending time with several boys at school who were well-known drug users. Brian reported experimenting with methamphetamine in fairly high doses the previous weeks before he was arrested. He had never abused animals before the current incident.

The number juvenile offenders with Schizophrenia and other psychotic disorders is less than the number of juvenile offenders with Attention-Deficit/Hyperactivity Disorder, Anxiety Disorders, or Mood Disorders (Timmons-Mitchell, *et al.*, 1997). However, due to the nature and degree of impairment often associated with Schizophrenia and other psychotic disorders, it is critical that juvenile justice staff:

- Be able to identify these youth
- Refer these youth to appropriate mental health/medical professionals
- Manage these youth effectively within a facility

Failure to do the above can result in negative consequences for psychotic offenders, other residents and facility staff. A single psychotic youth can significantly impact an entire living unit (and sometimes an entire facility) if not identified and managed properly.

Juvenile offenders with psychotic disorders can be some of the most confusing and frightening youth with whom juvenile justice professionals work. This is usually because staff do not understand these youths' behavior, which tends to be unusual and sometimes bizarre. Juvenile justice professionals play an essential role in managing these youth within juvenile justice facilities. Staff interactions with psychotic juveniles and the specific management strategies staff use can affect whether these youths' mental health symptoms are exacerbated or diminished.

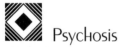 Psychosis

The term *psychosis* refers to impairment in reality testing. Individuals who are psychotic tend to have difficulty differentiating what is real from what is not real. Psychotic individuals may experience and exhibit hallucinations, delusions, disorganized speech, disorganized thinking, and/or disorganized behavior.

Hallucinations

Hallucinations are false sensory perceptions that are not associated with real external stimuli. Although youth can experience hallucinations involving any of the five senses (*i.e.*, auditory, visual, gustatory, olfactory, tactile), the type of hallucination most commonly reported among juveniles is auditory: hearing voices that other people cannot hear. Psychotic youth may report that these voices are coming from inside or outside of their heads. Regardless, they do not perceive these voices as their own thoughts but as someone else talking to them or about them. Some juveniles report recognizing the voices heard (*e.g.*, a brother, uncle, God, the devil), while others report that they do not. Some psychotic youth can decipher exactly what the voices are saying; for others, the voices are more muffled and vague.

In addition, the voices may tell juveniles to behave in certain ways, such as kill themselves or kill staff members. Sometimes, the voices are commenting on the youth or the youths' behavior (*e.g.*, telling them they are stupid or ugly, ridiculing them for something they did). Although less common, some psychotic juveniles see things that others cannot see (*e.g.*, seeing people or animals when the youth are alone in their room). Other youth may feel spiders or insects crawling on their skin. Or they may feel that they have some type of object or creature moving inside of their bodies. Some juveniles may even smell things that no one else can smell.

Delusions

Delusions are personal beliefs that individuals rigidly hold onto, despite obvious proof that these beliefs are false and/or irrational. Examples of delusional beliefs held by psychotic juveniles include thinking that other people are:

- Plotting against them
- Talking negatively about them
- Trying to steal or control their thoughts
- Trying to read the youths' minds

Persecutory delusions are common among youthful offenders suffering from psychosis. Some juveniles believe that the staff are trying to poison them or that all law enforcement and juvenile justice professionals are in a conspiracy against the youth. Some psychotic female juvenile offenders are convinced that they are pregnant, even when they have never been sexually active and multiple pregnancy tests are negative. Some psychotic youth believe parts of their body are diseased, decayed or rotting away, even though all medical tests are normal. In addition, some psychotic juveniles have grandiose delusions, believing they have been "chosen" in some way (*e.g.*, by someone famous, God) or have a special/magical gift or talent. Religious themes are not uncommon among individuals suffering from delusional thinking.

Disorganized Thinking/Speech

Disorganized thinking and speech are common among youth suffering from psychotic disorders. These youth may:

- Speak in sentences that do not make sense or are only loosely related

- Use words that do not make sense

- Talk in rhymes or with a singsong tune

- Repeatedly parrot back what others have said

Some psychotic juveniles are talkative but what comes out of their mouth is often strange and confusing. Juvenile justice professionals often feel as if they are not listening closely enough because they do not understand what psychotic juveniles are trying to convey. However, the reality is that the psychotic youth may not be making much sense. These juveniles may put words or sentences together that are not logical, such as "I didn't call my mom yet because the mirror in the bathroom is getting steamed up." Or psychotic youth may put words and sentences together that are not really related, such as "He wouldn't give me the basketball when I asked, my girlfriend is going

to call me on Sunday, we will probably get to stay up late tonight." Some juveniles with psychotic disorders use words the youth have made up themselves. These word are typically meaningless to listeners, such as "I slid across the floor really fast when I went to the manicon." Or the youths' words may make no sense at all, such as "Pass up king and then the dog no games play." Youth suffering from psychotic disorders may repeat certain words over and over, or they may completely stop talking in the middle of a sentence for no apparent reason. Some psychotic youth take a very long time to answer questions and/or may have little to no speech at all. Even when asked to elaborate, these juveniles may only provide one- or two-word answers or sentences.

Disorganized Behavior

Psychotic youth with disorganized behavior may exhibit:

- Restless or agitated behavior

- A messy appearance

- Bizarre movements or posturing

- Pacing

- Rocking

These juveniles may not shower or brush their teeth for days. And they may repeatedly engage in unusual and stereotypical movements involving specific parts of their body. Psychotic youth with disorganized behavior often appear odd or strange to juvenile justice professionals. They may sit on their beds or in a corner of their rooms and rock back and forth for hours. Within juvenile justice facilities, some psychotic youth like to crawl into tight spaces in their rooms—such as under a bed, in between a toilet and a wall, or a toilet and any type of cabinet. These juveniles can appear extremely tense and nervous. They may wring their hands and walk back and forth in the small space of a dorm room or in one particular segment of a living unit. Some psychotic youth may be unable to remain still and feel like they have to keep moving constantly. However, others remain

Schizophrenia and Other Psychotic Disorders

still, without any movement, for extended periods of time.

———

Juveniles from different ethnic, racial and socioeconomic backgrounds, as well as youth with lower levels of intellectual functioning, may report experiences that can be *misinterpreted* as psychotic symptomatology. For example, a number of young children and cognitively impaired adolescents talk about interacting with imaginary friends. These youth may also report seeing or hearing the voice of superheroes seen on television. In some cultures, seeing visions of deceased relatives or religious figures may be normal and completely acceptable. Determining whether juveniles are delusional or whether their beliefs are related to developmental or cultural issues can sometimes be difficult. For example, some juvenile offenders are adamant that someone is trying to kill them or that law enforcement is arresting them more often than their peers. Depending on the youths' lifestyle or the community in which they live, these youths' beliefs may be fairly accurate and not a reflection of "paranoid" thinking. Staff should always consider developmental and cultural issues while working with juveniles who could potentially be suffering from psychotic disorders.

 SchizophRENiA

Juveniles with Schizophrenia experience psychotic symptoms, as well as impairment in several areas of functioning (*i.e.*, their thinking, emotions and behavior). Schizophrenic youth often have difficulty distinguishing experiences that are real from those that are not real. Their thinking may not be logical, and they often behave strangely in social situations.

Schizophrenia among youth under the age of 13 is rare, with the most common age of onset being late adolescence or early adulthood (American Academy of Child and Adolescent Psychiatry [AACAP], 2001). Males tend to manifest the disorder at somewhat younger ages in comparison to females. And, youth who have relatives with Schizophrenia are at significantly greater risk of developing the disorder themselves.

Symptoms and Associated Features

Hallucinations, delusions, disorganized speech and disorganized behavior are common among juveniles with Schizophrenia. Not surprisingly, these youth tend to have difficulty carrying out their everyday responsibilities. For example, they may have problems with:

- Interpersonal relationships
- Hygiene
- Academic achievement
- Work/vocational programs
- Basic self-care tasks

Youth with Schizophrenia typically exhibit both positive and negative symptoms of the disorder. *Positive* symptoms of Schizophrenia refer to the symptoms that tend to be outwardly evident and bizarre, such as:

- Perceptual experiences that others do not have (*e.g.*, hearing voices that other people cannot hear)
- Rigid and fixed beliefs that are not true (*e.g.*, believing they have magical powers, believing someone is trying to control their mind)
- Problems with thinking or speech (*e.g.*, speaking in a manner that does not make sense to others, making up words)

The *negative* symptoms of Schizophrenia refer to symptoms where there is a shortage of something, such as:

- Not having energy
- Minimal to no speech
- Little emotional tone or feelings
- Indifference to the feelings of others
- No facial expression
- Lack of eye contact

- Loss of interest in people or activities that used to be of interest
- Minimal or no movement
- Inability to concentrate
- Lack of goal-directed behavior

To be diagnosed with Schizophrenia, youth must have several symptoms of the disorder for at least six months. These symptoms cannot be due primarily to another mental health disorder, a medical condition, or the use of drugs and alcohol.

In addition to the symptoms already mentioned, several features associated with Schizophrenia can make the disorder even more disabling (American Psychiatric Association, 2000). Some juveniles with Schizophrenia display emotional reactions that are inappropriate to particular situations. They may laugh or smile when nothing appears to be funny. Or they may cry or become distressed without any apparent provocation. Because some psychotic juveniles have sleep difficulties at night, they may prefer to sleep throughout the day.

Also, they may have considerable anxiety and excessive worries. These worries can often reach delusional proportions, with some youth believing that others are trying to poison them or harm them in some other way. Or, youth may worry excessively about their health, believing that something terrible is happening inside of their bodies and/or that they are dying from some type of illness. Attention, concentration and memory problems are also common, particularly if these youth are hearing voices or responding to some other type of internal stimuli.

Many juveniles with Schizophrenia are unaware that their thinking, speech or behaviors are odd or unusual. They can become defensive when confronted about their delusional beliefs, which frequently results in their holding onto their beliefs even more rigidly. This situation is particularly true if juveniles are paranoid about those around them and/or think that certain individuals are conspiring against

them. Psychotic juveniles' lack of insight about their mental health disorder can significantly interfere with their ability to comply with treatment because they may not think anything is wrong with them. Some of these youth believe that their main problem has to do with those around them. They may believe that other people are "crazy," do not understand things the way they should, or that they just do not "get it."

Most individuals with Schizophrenia are no more dangerous than anyone else. Juveniles with Schizophrenia who are at highest risk for assaultive or violent behavior are those who (APA, 2000):

- Are male
- Are excessive drug or alcohol users
- Are noncompliant with regard to taking psychotropic medication
- Have a history of assaultive or violent behavior

Phases of Schizophrenia

There are several phases of Schizophrenia, and schizophrenic youth could be experiencing any one of the following phases while residing in juvenile justice facilities. The *prodromal* phase is the time period right before youth begin experiencing psychotic symptoms; this is often the point when youth become involved with the juvenile justice system. During the prodromal phase, youths' behavior begins to deteriorate from how they were previously functioning, regardless of whether they typically functioned at a high or low level. For some juveniles with Schizophrenia, the change is subtle and may occur over months or years. For others, the change in behavior is drastic and obvious, occurring over several weeks or even days. During the prodromal period, many schizophrenic youth begin exhibiting strange or odd behaviors. They may develop unusual concerns or preoccupations, and their grades may begin to decline (AACAP, 2001). Some of these youth may even drop out of school altogether. If juveniles in the prodromal phase have a job,

Schizophrenia and Other Psychotic Disorders

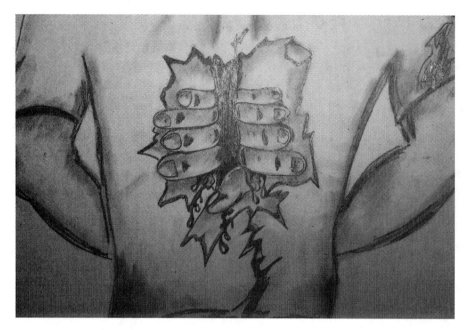

The *acute* phase of Schizophrenia follows the prodromal phase. During this stage of the illness, there is an even more noticeable change in juveniles' behavior. This change is typically associated with a considerable decline in the youths' functioning. Adolescents in the acute phase of Schizophrenia may exhibit full-blown hallucinations, delusions, disorganized speech, and disorganized behavior (AACAP, 2001). If youth are not identified as having a mental health disorder during the prodromal

their work performance typically suffers. They may decide to quit their jobs or may be fired due to their unexplained change in behavior.

During the prodromal phase, juveniles may spend less time with family or friends, preferring to be by themselves. They may also be less concerned about their physical appearance and what others think about them. Depression and irritability are not uncommon. During this time, youth may begin to experiment with drugs and alcohol, or existing substance use may increase. These juveniles may also become verbally or physically aggressive, as well as engage in disruptive and oppositional behavior. This behavior can result in contact with law enforcement and, eventually, juvenile court. During the prodromal phase of Schizophrenia, those who interact with the youth—family, friends, juvenile justice professionals and even some mental health professionals—may assume that the juveniles are "just going through a phase" typical of adolescence. Or, the youth may be misdiagnosed as having Oppositional Defiant Disorder, Conduct Disorder or a mood disorder. (*Please see Chapter 3 for additional information about Oppositional Defiant Disorder/Conduct Disorder and Chapter 4 for information on mood disorders.*)

phase, they are typically identified during the acute phase of the disorder—because their behavior is clearly "different" and often bizarre.

If incarcerated, schizophrenic youth in the acute phase of Schizophrenia come to the attention of line staff, teachers and supervisors fairly quickly. Juvenile justice professionals typically notice that something is "wrong" with youth in this stage of the disorder, although they may not be able to articulate exactly what that is. The behavior of some juvenile offenders with Schizophrenia can be so unusual and strange that the youth may need to be transferred out of a juvenile justice setting. The acute phase of Schizophrenia can last anywhere from one to six months. But if the youths' illness does not respond well to treatment, this phase can last even longer (Werry & Taylor, 1994). The "positive" symptoms of Schizophrenia (*i.e.*, hallucinations, delusions, disorganized speech and behavior) typically diminish with appropriate mental health treatment (*i.e.*, antipsychotic medication), while the "negative" symptoms of the disorder may continue throughout the course of the illness (APA, 2000).

The *recuperative/recovery* phase follows the acute phase of Schizophrenia and typically lasts several months. During this phase of the disor-

160

Juvenile Offenders with Mental Health Disorders: Who Are They and What Do We Do With Them?

der, youths' hallucinations and delusions diminish or may even be completely absent. Their thinking and speech usually become more logical and their behavior much less bizarre. However, even though many symptoms are improved from the last phase of the disorder, juveniles continue to experience considerable difficulty in their ability to function. This difficulty usually occurs because the negative symptoms of Schizophrenia persist (*e.g.*, isolation, lack of energy and motivation, depressed mood, lack of interest in things they used to enjoy). For some youth with Schizophrenia, some of the positive symptoms may continue as well.

During the *residual* phase of Schizophrenia, youth may go for several months or years without having any major psychotic symptoms. Their thinking and behavior may be much improved in comparison to when they were psychotic. However, most juveniles with Schizophrenia continue to suffer some degree of impairment due to the continuation of negative symptoms.

Course of the Disorder

The course of Schizophrenia is variable. For example, some youth with Schizophrenia have been described as odd or strange since early childhood, and they may never have had many friends. Their motor skills and/or cognitive skills can be slow to develop. Therefore, these youth may have been teased in school because they appeared "different" from other students—even at a young age. Rather than interacting with others, some juveniles with Schizophrenia prefer to engage in solitary activities, including fantasy-related games and books or activities that rely heavily on their imagination. Youth whose illness follows this course typically begin exhibiting increasingly unusual behavior as they enter adolescence, culminating in the youth eventually experiencing true psychotic symptoms.

In contrast, some youth with Schizophrenia can appear quite "normal" during their childhood years, with little to no unusual behavior. At some point (usually late adolescence or early adulthood), their thinking and behavior begin to change, eventually leading to full-blown psychotic symptoms. However, for juveniles with Schizophrenia to function absolutely fine one day and then be psychotic (*e.g.*, hearing voices, acting or speaking in a bizarre manner) the next is rare. There is almost always a period beforehand (which can last for days, weeks, months or years) in which youths' functioning deteriorates in comparison to how they were functioning for most of their lives until that point.

A small minority of youth with Schizophrenia go through the phases of the disorder one time only. However, most will experience more than one cycle (Werry, McClellan, & Chard, 1991). Most juveniles with Schizophrenia never return to exactly the way they were before they experienced psychotic symptoms. The majority will have some form of impairment in social, academic, and/or vocational functioning. Individuals with Schizophrenia are also at higher risk for committing suicide, particularly after the acute phase of the disorder resolves (APA, 2000).

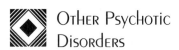 Other Psychotic Disorders

Although Schizophrenia is the mental health disorder most individuals associate with psychotic behavior, many psychotic juvenile offenders do not suffer from Schizophrenia. Their psychotic behavior can be due to a substance use disorder, a mood disorder such as Major Depression or Bipolar Disorder, or a medical condition. When psychotic juvenile offenders enter juvenile justice facilities directly from the community, determining the cause of their symptoms can be difficult. Juvenile justice facilities might admit paranoid youth who report hearing voices and who believe the FBI has implanted computer chips in their heads. If these youth remain quiet during the intake process, their unusual thoughts may not be identified until they are placed in a living unit and begin interacting with peers. Juveniles exhibiting these symptoms could possibly be in an acute phase of Schizophrenia, they could be reacting to prolonged use of high levels of drugs (*e.g.*, methamphetamine), or their behavior could be related to another problem. Even if the cause of symptoms is unknown, the moment juveniles are identified as experiencing psychotic symptoms, juvenile justice professionals should:

- Ensure the youths' safety
- Refer them for appropriate mental health evaluation and treatment

Substance-Induced Psychotic Disorders

Some juvenile offenders—particularly those who are placed in juvenile justice facilities directly from the community—may experience hallucinations and/or delusions as a direct result of their alcohol or drug use. Youth who are *intoxicated* with alcohol, marijuana, methamphetamine/amphetamine, inhalants, cocaine, prescription sleeping medication, hallucinogens, heroin, phencyclidine (PCP), as well as other substances, may experience psychotic symptoms in association with their substance use. Psychotic disorders can also occur in relation to *withdrawal* from alcohol, sleeping medications, anti-anxiety medications and other substances (APA, 2000). Psychotic symptoms in relation to substance use typically occur with high doses of drugs or alcohol. The symptoms may appear after prolonged use of the substance, or they can occur after a short period of time if large enough doses are ingested.

Some drugs alter youths' perception (such as seeing colors and lights, hearing sounds, or seeing inanimate objects move). However, youth typically recognize that these altered perceptions are not real and are the result of their drug experience. This recognition is different from psychosis. If youth are psychotic, they do not connect their unusual thoughts or

behavior to their drug use, and they behave as if their beliefs truly reflect reality. One of the most common psychotic symptoms associated with substance use are auditory hallucinations (*e.g.*, hearing voices). However, some youth report visual hallucinations, such as seeing" bugs" or creatures in their room or on their skin. It is not uncommon for juvenile offenders who use large doses of methamphetamine or cocaine to become very paranoid. They may become extremely irritable, and even combative, if they feel threatened. Some over-the-counter medications, as well as medications legitimately prescribed to youth, have also been known to cause psychotic symptoms.

If hallucinations or delusions are primarily due to the physiological effects of drugs or alcohol, the psychotic symptoms typically decrease and eventually disappear:

- Once the offending substance is removed, and
- the body rids itself of the toxic substance.

However, psychotic symptoms associated with cocaine, PCP and amphetamine/methamphetamine can last for several days or weeks or even longer. This situation can occur even when the substance is removed, and youth are treated with antipsychotic medication (APA, 2000). Some juvenile offenders with an underlying mental health disorder such as Schizophrenia or Bipolar Disorder may experience their first psychotic episode after using substances; their drug use can trigger or exacerbate a full-blown mental health disorder. For this group of juveniles, psychotic and other associated mental health symptoms remain after a substance has been cleared out of their body.

Psychotic Disorders Due to A General Medical Condition

Some juvenile offenders may experience psychotic symptoms as a direct result of an underlying medical condition. A variety of medical conditions can cause hallucinations or delusions including, but not limited to (APA, 2000):

Juvenile Offenders with Mental Health Disorders: Who Are They and What Do We Do With Them?

- Endocrine disorders (*e.g.*, thyroid, parathyroid, adrenal glands)
- Neurological disorders (multiple sclerosis, epilepsy, migraine, nerve injuries of the eyes or ears, infections of the central nervous system
- Conditions associated with metabolism
- Electrolyte imbalances
- Human immunodeficiency virus (HIV)
- Liver and kidney diseases

When they are a direct physiological result of medical conditions, psychotic symptoms usually resolve with appropriate treatment of the underlying medical disorder. However, this outcome is not a guarantee.

Hallucinations associated with medical conditions can occur among any of the five senses: auditory, visual, olfactory, tactile and gustatory. Whereas olfactory hallucinations (*i.e.*, smelling things that other people do not smell) are not common among individuals with Schizophrenia, they have been associated with temporal lobe epilepsy (*e.g.*, smelling burning rubber or other unpleasant odors). Delusions may be fairly simple or very elaborate and can resemble those of individuals with Schizophrenia. Juveniles whose delusions are related to medical conditions may hold strange beliefs related to possessing magical gifts or powers, people following or wanting to hurt them, or unusual beliefs related to religious themes. If their underlying medical condition is not identified, these youth can be incorrectly diagnosed and treated as if they were suffering from Schizophrenia.

Mood Disorders with Psychotic Features

Some youth who experience hallucinations or delusions actually have a mood disorder, such as Major Depression or Bipolar Disorder. Although a significant number of juvenile offenders have a mood disorder, not all of these youth suffer from psychotic symptoms. (*Please see Chapter 4 for additional information about mood disorders.*) Juveniles with severe cases of Major Depression

or Bipolar Disorder may hear voices that other people do not hear. Or they may have unusual beliefs about themselves or those around them (Ulloa, *et al.*, 2000). The content of the voices or the beliefs are usually "mood-congruent," meaning they are consistent with the way the youth are feeling. For example, depressed juveniles may hear voices telling them they:

- Are ugly
- Will never amount to anything
- Are worthless
- Do not deserve to be alive
- Should take steps to end their lives

The delusional beliefs of depressed youth are also usually related to depressive and negative themes, such as thinking:

- They are defective
- Their body is decaying
- They are deserving of punishment due to an inadequacy or failure

Although not as common, hallucinations and delusions completely unrelated to their mood disorder can occur as well. Youth may believe that others can read their mind or can control their thoughts or behavior. Some juvenile offenders with a severe case of Major Depression may feel an inordinate amount of guilt and turmoil over events in which they have little to no involvement. Feelings of guilt and remorse can be helpful when rehabilitating young offenders who have committed crimes, particularly crimes against others. However, depressed psychotic youth can experience tremendous shame over incidents in which they have no responsibility, and they may hold the delusion rigidly.

Youth with severe cases of Bipolar Disorder can become psychotic in either the depressed or manic phase of the disorder. These juveniles also may experience mood-congruent hallucinations and delusions. During an episode of mania, juveniles may hear the voice of God or a prominent figure (from the past or present) telling them that they have been "chosen" for a special mission. These youth may also believe that they have supernatural or magical powers. Some youth with Bipolar Disorder have persecutory delusions and believe people are out to get them because of their special gifts or talents. However, psychotic juveniles with Bipolar Disorder may also experience hallucinations and delusions that are not related to their feelings of grandiosity or inflated self-esteem—such as believing that others can steal their thoughts or can implant evil thoughts into their mind against their will.

AN iNACCURATE diAGNOSis CAN RESULT iN iNAPPROPRIATE TREATMENT ANd POSSibly EVEN HARMFUL iNTERVENTIONS.

Complexities Associated With Psychotic Symptoms

If youth become psychotic while in residence at juvenile justice facilities, determining the nature and cause of the juveniles' symptoms can be difficult. This difficulty can be even more likely if youth arrive at facilities directly from the community—where drug and alcohol use can further cloud the diagnostic picture. Youth with psychotic mood disorders look similar to those with Schizophrenia and are often misdiagnosed as such (Werry, McClellan, & Chard, 1991).

In addition, lack of awareness of juveniles' previous and current drug use and/or their medical history can result in an incorrect diagnosis of Schizophrenia or Bipolar Disorder. An inaccurate diagnosis can result in inappropriate treatment and possibly even harmful interventions. Medical and mental health professionals should conduct comprehensive evaluations of youth exhibiting psychotic symptomatology. Such evaluations should include, but not be limited to, a thorough history of the youth and their psychiatric symptoms, as well

as any relevant laboratory tests. Reassessment is typically necessary after several days or weeks to further determine if a correct mental health diagnosis was given. Even without treatment, youth with a substance-induced psychotic disorder are likely to appear improved after a few days of no substance use. The symptoms of youth with Schizophrenia or a severe mood disorder are not likely to resolve as quickly.

Psychotic Disorders Not Otherwise Specified

There is a particular group of juveniles who do not seem to fit any of the above-mentioned categories of psychotic disorders, even though they experience occasional psychotic symptoms (*i.e.*, hallucinations or delusions). The diagnosis of Psychotic Disorder NOS is usually given to youth if there is not enough information to make a more specific diagnosis or if there is contradictory information about youths' symptoms. Psychotic Disorder NOS can also be given if it is unclear whether youths' psychotic symptoms are due to mental illness, a medical condition, or substance abuse.

Some juveniles who have received this diagnosis do not show any other symptoms besides auditory hallucinations. Consequently, these youth do not meet the criteria for a specific psychotic disorder. In addition to occasional or transient auditory hallucinations, these youth may also suffer from Posttraumatic Stress Disorder, Conduct Disorder, a personality disorder or a developmental disorder (*e.g.*, Autism, Asperger's Disorder).

When they are alone in their rooms and/or under high levels of emotional stress, they may hear voices that other people do not hear. Although they may experience hallucinations, these youth typically do not experience the delusions, unusual thinking and bizarre behavior seen in truly psychotic individuals—such as those with Schizophrenia or Bipolar Disorder with Psychotic Features (Garralda, 1984). Some of these juvenile offenders have experienced auditory hallucinations for significant periods of time. Youth within this category often report knowing that the voices are not real and may describe them as annoying or irritating. They may find the voices frightening, even though they say they are aware that it is "all in my head."

Many of the juveniles in this subgroup have discovered strategies for distracting themselves when they hear voices, particularly when the youth feel emotionally aroused or stressed. Some offenders report that they listen to music, attempt to talk with staff or peers, or try to go to sleep as ways to divert their attention. The experience of having hallucinations—even without delusions or a thought disorder—can place juveniles at higher risk for poor outcomes in comparison to similar youth who do not experience hallucinations (Del Baccaro, Burke, & McCauley, 1988).

There is another subset of youth that make the diagnosis of psychotic disorders challenging. The youth in this category suffer from intermittent psychotic symptoms such as hallucinations or delusions. And these juveniles experience difficulty in their everyday functioning. However, it is typically problems with aggression and emotional outbursts that cause the most disruption in the lives of these particular youth. These juveniles are typically impulsive and exhibit a variety of behavioral problems. The youth also frequently display extreme emotional reactions that are out of proportion to events that trigger them—sometimes on an almost daily basis. These youth have been described as having difficulty distinguishing fantasy from reality, especially during periods of stress or while falling asleep. In addition, juveniles in this subgroup generally want to interact wither peers but are often rejected due to impaired interpersonal skills.

Although these youth have difficulty processing information (e.g., problems with attention and concentration), they do not exhibit the disturbed or bizarre thought processes of youth with a formal thought disorder (i.e., Schizophrenia). These juveniles usually have significant histories of mental health treat-

ment, including psychiatric hospitalization, and most have been treated with psychotropic medication typically used to treat Schizophrenia, Bipolar Disorder, Major Depression or Attention-Deficit/Hyperactivity Disorder. Some have referred to these youth as "multidimensionally impaired" (Kumra, et al, 1998). It is currently unclear whether these youth have a disorder similar to Schizophrenia or if they are a subset of severely impaired youth who have symptoms from a combination of several psychiatric disorders—but who do not fit neatly into any of them. More research is needed to better understand and accurately diagnose this complex and difficult-to-manage population of youth.

 ## Intervention Strategies for Youth with Psychotic Disorders

Before they can intervene effectively with juveniles who have a psychotic disorder, juvenile justice professionals must be able to identify these youth. The following are suggested guidelines for staff when they are *talking* with juveniles who may be experiencing psychotic symptoms (*i.e.*, auditory hallucinations, visual hallucinations, delusional thinking):

- Remain calm and stay with the youth.

- Find a quiet environment with few distractions to talk with the youth one-on-one.

- Be aware that many youth who hallucinate fear being viewed as "crazy." Psychotic juvenile offenders may try to conceal hallucinations by denying that they are hearing voices or by using intimidating stares, angry responses, or one-word answers.

- Help juveniles describe their current or recent hallucination. Assess for thoughts or hearing voices related to self-harm and/or harm to others.

- If youth appear frightened, remind them of where they are and continuously reassure them that they are safe. Keep youth focused on the here and now.

- Answer juveniles honestly if they ask whether staff are also experiencing the youths' hallucination. Staff should firmly let a youth know that they are not hearing the voices a youth is hearing or seeing the objects that the youth is seeing.

- Do not support the delusions of psychotic juveniles. Staff should convey to youth that they believe *the youth* believes the unusual thought. But staff should add that they personally do not believe it. For example, staff can convey that they believe *the juveniles* believe Satan is trying to corrupt the youth. However, staff should be clear that they do not believe Satan is trying to corrupt the youth. Juvenile justice professionals should avoid arguing with psychotic juveniles about the validity of the youths' hallucinations or delusions.

- Try to determine whether hallucinations or delusions are the result of drug/alcohol use or high levels of stress and anxiety.

- Be aware that some psychotic youth may be suspicious of the motives of those around them. Some juveniles may be overly concerned about everyone's actions, the food they are fed, or the medication they are given.

All youth who are known to have a psychotic disorder, report psychotic symptoms, or whom staff are concerned might be experiencing psychotic symptoms should be referred immediately to a mental health/medical professional for evaluation. Mental health/medical professionals affiliated with juvenile justice facilities should be adequately trained to identify psychotic symptoms among a juvenile population. They should be knowledgeable about the various types of mental health and medical disorders associated with psychotic symptoms, as well as effective management strategies to use with these youth. Depending on a particular facility's mental

health/medical resources—as well as the severity of youths' mental health symptoms—some psychotic juveniles can be evaluated and managed in a correctional environment. Others will need to be transferred to a mental health or medical facility.

If they are suffering from a psychotic disorder such as Schizophrenia, or a mood disorder with psychotic features (*e.g.*, Major Depression with Psychotic features, Bipolar Disorder with Psychotic Features), youth will probably require psychotropic medication. Neuroleptics, also known as antipsychotics, have been shown to be effective in the treatment of individuals with psychotic disorders.

If juveniles' symptoms are primarily related to a mood disorder, however, antidepressant medication or a mood-stabilizing medication may also be prescribed. Traditional antipsychotic medications (*i.e.*, Haldol®, Thorazine®, Mellaril®) can have a significant affect on the "positive" symptoms of Schizophrenia (*e.g.*, hallucinations, delusions, unusual thoughts and behavior), but they tend to have less affect on the "negative" symptoms (*e.g.*, disinterest, low energy, dysphoric mood). Atypical antipsychotic medications (*i.e.*, Resperidal®, Zyprexa®, Clozaril®) are also effective in decreasing the positive symptoms of Schizophrenia. However, they may be more effective in reducing negative symptoms in comparison to traditional antipsychotic medications. The sedative effects of neuroleptic medication may become apparent quite quickly, but the antipsychotic effects can take up to several weeks to become evident. Juveniles who are prescribed antipsychotic medication should be monitored closely, as this type of medicine can cause significant and serious side effects. (*Please see Chapter 14 for additional information about psychotropic medication.*)

Some juvenile offenders with psychotic symptoms are evaluated by mental health/ medical professionals within juvenile justice facilities and continue to reside in that environment. In contrast, some facilities may attempt to transfer psychotic youth out of a

Juvenile Offenders with Mental Health Disorders: Who Are They and What Do We Do With Them?

facility but may be unable to locate mental health/medical facilities willing to admit the juveniles. A small number of correctional facilities have been successful in transferring psychotic youth to medical or psychiatric hospitals for an evaluation. However, many of these youth eventually return to the juvenile justice facilities once the juveniles' behavior has stabilized. Regardless of the situation, juvenile justice facilities are housing a number of psychotic youth, and juvenile justice staff are typically expected to supervise and manage them.

If psychotic youth are going to be housed in a juvenile justice facility, staff should consider the following issues:

- Where will the youth be safe? Do they need to be housed in a special unit or in a room with specific safety precautions? Where do the youth feel most comfortable?

- Do the youth need to be monitored on an intensive basis (*e.g.*, 1:1 staffing, every five minutes, every 10 minutes, every 15 minutes)?

- How and when will medication issues be discussed with the youth? Medication is usually a critical piece in the management of youth with psychotic disorders.

- How much, and under what circumstances, can the youth interact with staff and other residents?

- Who has a good relationship with the youth? If the youth become frightened, suspicious or aggressive, they may respond more positively to staff whom they normally trust.

Decisions made in relation to the above issues should be based on the unique characteristics and needs of each individual youth.

Some juvenile offenders with psychotic disorders can be adequately managed within juvenile justice facilities if the youth receive appropriate medication and if staff are trained in effective ways of interacting with this population of youth. Because the behavior of psychotic juveniles can be bizarre and sometimes anxiety-provoking for juvenile justice professionals, staff may want to house these youth alone in their room for extended periods of time. Staff should avoid any temptation to take such actions. All youth with a psychotic disorder should have an individualized treatment plan that is designed and implemented by a diverse group of individuals (*e.g.*, psychiatrist, psychologist, juvenile justice professionals, youth, family, physician, nurse, teacher).

The following guidelines can be helpful for staff when managing youth with psychotic disorders in juvenile justice facilities:

- Keep the juveniles involved in as many scheduled activities as the youth can tolerate, keeping in mind the safety of the psychotic youth, as well as that of the other residents. Levels of involvement will vary, depending on the severity of the youths' psychotic symptoms.

- Do not expect psychotic youth to be able to meet the same expectations as non-psychotic residents. Token economy programs (*i.e.*, point and level systems) may need to be modified for the functioning level of youth with a psychotic disorder.

- If psychotic youth have to be isolated for safety reasons, provide them with rewarding tasks to engage in while they are in their room.

- Speak slowly to the youth, using simple sentences.

- Give precise directions to psychotic juveniles. Respectfully tell the youth what they should do instead of giving them a variety of choices. For example, "Please go take your shower now" versus, "Do you want to shower now or wait until after breakfast?" Choices can be very confusing for these youth.

Schizophrenia and Other Psychotic Disorders

- Check in with the juveniles on a regular basis to make sure that they are comfortable and not frightened. Convey an attitude of unconditional acceptance to increase their ability to trust others.

- Avoid sarcasm or humor. Do not joke or tease the youth about their hallucinations or delusions.

- Avoid laughing, whispering or talking quietly where the juveniles can see staff but not hear them. This can make psychotic juveniles suspicious and upset.

- Help psychotic youth, if appropriate, to interact with peers. Psychotic juveniles may be frightened or confused around other residents.

- Do not become overly involved with the content of youths' delusions. Instead, focus on the underlying theme (*e.g.*, persecution, grandiosity, inadequacy, fear).

- Be aware of aggressive tendencies in psychotic juvenile offenders with paranoid delusions. Paranoid youth may misinterpret interpersonal situations as more hostile than they really are and/or react aggressively to perceived threats or provocation (Lewis, Pincus, Lovely, Spitzer & Moy, 1987). Maintain some physical distance and keep hands in full view when talking with paranoid youth. This practice can decrease juveniles' feelings of being threatened.

- Avoid touching psychotic youth without warning.

- Help youth express their emotions in a socially acceptable manner.

- Support juveniles in taking their psychotropic medication. Paranoia or adolescent issues of control may affect psychotic youths' willingness to take antipsychotic medication. Be creative versus demanding if juveniles refuse.

Case Example

Jacob, 16, has always been described as a good kid, a nice kid. He is a handsome young man, and many of the girls at school have a crush on him. He has always been funny, witty and smart, enjoying both the academic and social aspects of school. It came as a complete surprise to Jacob's parents when his grades began to slip. He started spending less time with his friends and more time alone in his room, listening to music. He stopped having dinner with the family, stating that he was not hungry. When he did spend time with a friend, it was with a new neighbor who smoked marijuana on a daily basis. Jacob's parents were concerned that he was starting to smoke marijuana as well. They talked with a school counselor who said that Jacob was just going through a phase, something typical during adolescence.

Jacob began to smoke cigarettes and became belligerent when his parents talked with him about it. He became increasingly irritable and eventually threatened his mother with a kitchen knife when she would not let him use the telephone. She called the police, and Jacob was arrested and taken to a local juvenile detention facility. Juvenile justice professionals noticed that Jacob appeared to be talking to himself in his room and often said things that did not make sense. Because of this behavior, Jacob's attorney referred him for a psychological evaluation to try to have him declared incompetent to stand trial. Jacob was transferred to a local psychiatric hospital to be evaluated by mental health professionals.

Jacob was admitted to a psychiatric hospital for two weeks, which would allow time for a comprehensive evaluation and observation. The psychologist initially found Jacob to be similar to other youth who presented with substance use and/or behavioral problems. Near the end of the

168

Juvenile Offenders with Mental Health Disorders: Who Are They and What Do We Do With Them?

initial interview, however, Jacob began to giggle and laugh for no apparent reason. He seemed to be looking over his shoulder, as if listening to someone commenting to him from behind. When the psychologist asked if he was hearing voices, Jacob flatly denied it.

When Jacob met with the psychologist the following few days, he continued the inappropriate laughter during the testing sessions. In addition, the length of time between his responses seemed to grow longer. After the examiner asked him basic test questions, Jacob often took 45-60 seconds before he would even begin to answer them. Sometimes, he would wait two to three minutes before answering questions. However, he always answered them, and his answers were usually correct.

The psychologist contacted Jacob's parents to gather additional background information. They stated that they had adopted Jacob within three days of his birth and raised him as an only child in a loving, middle-class home. He had had an uneventful childhood and had seemed to be a well-adjusted and happy young man until earlier that year. They described their frustration with his behavior change, irritability, decline in school grades, and possible drug use. Although everyone told them it was a "phase" that Jacob would grow out of, they felt like something was definitely wrong. When the psychologist pressed them for details about why they were so concerned about Jacob, they relayed several stories of unusual behavior. For example, for the past three weeks, Jacob had been re-arranging the furniture in his room from 11:45 p.m. until midnight every Monday, Wednesday and Friday. In addition, his parents often came home from work to find all of the light bulbs taken out of the lamps in the living room and den. When the psychologist asked Jacob about these behaviors, he calmly stated that "they" came

to visit him at night. As long as he moved his bed into a different location, "they" could not find him. He also stated that he could hear voices coming out of the lamps, so he removed the light bulbs to make them stop. At that point, it was clear that Jacob was definitely experiencing some psychotic symptoms.

The psychologist arranged to have Jacob remain in the hospital for an additional two weeks for further evaluation and possible treatment with medication. Jacob was socially withdrawn in the unit and avoided interacting with the other residents. Even though all of the girls at the psychiatric facility had crushes on him, Jacob seemed to live in his own world. He spent much of his time in his room by himself, laughing and giggling. When forced to spend time in the dayroom with the other residents, he rarely spoke and sat expressionless for hours at a time. When staff attempted to interact with him, he became irritable and angry.

Jacob's hygiene deteriorated at the hospital, and he began to get physically ill from not eating enough food. He was certain that the hospital staff were poisoning him. He refused to meet with the psychologist until arrangements were made for him to see a dentist. He was convinced that his teeth were decayed and beginning to fall out. In reality, he had a beautiful smile.

During this time, Jacob's parents contacted the agency that had arranged for Jacob's adoption. They discovered that a state agency removed Jacob from his mother after she gave birth to him because she was being hospitalized for Schizophrenia at the age of 20.

A joint decision was made between the mental health and juvenile justice agencies to have Jacob remain at the psychiatric hospital. A psychiatrist prescribed antipsychotic medication, but Jacob's behavior continued to deteriorate. After several weeks of taking the medication, Jacob reported that the voices began to decrease. But his social withdrawal continued. His irritability was replaced with a brooding, depressed mood, and his hygiene worsened. The doctors tried to find the best medication for Jacob, but everything they tried caused him to feel sluggish and to want to sleep much of the day. Jacob's parents were devastated when they found out that he had been diagnosed with Schizophrenia because they knew they would probably never have their son back the way he had been. All three of their lives were changed forever.

With proper treatment (*e.g.* psychotropic medication, psychoeducation), Jacob may grow up to be a productive member of society. However, if he does not take his medication regularly, he will likely experience a return of psychotic symptoms. Positive outcomes for Jacob are even less likely if he uses drugs and alcohol.

Juvenile Offenders with Mental Health Disorders: Who Are They and What Do We Do With Them?

CHAPTER 9

Substance Use Disorders: Substance Abuse and Substance Dependence

"I smoke weed when I get up. I smoke weed whenever I eat. I smoke weed all day. I always smoke weed before I go to bed. But, I don't have a problem. It's not like I am doing crack."

James, 16

Martin, 14, has been smoking marijuana and drinking alcohol on a daily basis since the age of 12. His older brothers introduced him to marijuana when he was nine. He never thought anything was wrong with smoking marijuana because it was a common activity in his household, his neighborhood, and even among his friends at school. Martin often goes to school stoned, and he skips class several times a week. He is failing almost all of his academic classes. Martin fights with his mother constantly because he refuses to do chores around the house. He chooses to take long naps or lie on the couch watching television instead. Martin was arrested on a charge related to fighting.

Substance use is widespread among youth involved with the juvenile justice system. In fact, juvenile offenders are at least five times more likely to use alcohol and other drugs when compared to youth in the general population (Deschenes & Greenwood, 1994). A national survey of incarcerated juveniles in long-term, state-operated institutions found that 81 percent of the youth had used drugs at some point in their life. Seventy-nine percent of the juveniles had tried marijuana, 43 percent cocaine, 38 percent amphetamines, and 27 percent LSD. Three out of five of the incarcerated youth reported that they used at least one drug on a regular basis (Snyder & Sickmund, 1995). In addition, the survey found that close to half of the youth in custody reported being intoxicated (drugs or alcohol) at the time they committed their crime (for which they were being held at the juvenile justice facility). This finding was true for offenders who were incarcerated for a variety of crimes, including murder, drug charges, burglary or assault. Only a small minority of these youth said they were solely under the influence of alcohol. Most of the juveniles reported being under the influence of some type of drug or a combination of drugs and alcohol. Moreover, a national program relying on anonymous urine alcohol/drug tests instead of youths' self-report of drug use, found that approximately one-third of juveniles arrested or detained tested positive for at least one illegal drug (National Institute of Justice, 1994).

 ## Common Substances Used By Juvenile Offenders

Some of the most common substances used by juvenile offenders include:

- Alcohol
- Marijuana
- Cocaine/Crack
- Amphetamines/Methamphetamine
- Hallucinogens (e.g., psilocybin mushrooms, LSD)
- Barbiturates
- PCP
- Heroin
- Inhalants (e.g., paint, airplane glue, gasoline, paint thinner, spray paint, fingernail polish remover)
- Ecstasy

Some aspects of juvenile drug use have changed in the last few years, with today's juveniles using several substances that were not as common in the past. For example, some juvenile offenders do not always smoke small cigarette-size "joints" when they smoke marijuana. They may smoke "blunts," which are thickly rolled, cigar-like marijuana sticks. Some juvenile offenders dip regular cigarettes, joints or blunts into formaldehyde or embalming fluid (sometimes known as "wet" or "sherm") for a more intense, hallucinogenic type of high.

"Rave" parties (all-night dance events) have become increasingly common in the past several years. Many youth who attend rave dance parties take Ecstasy, an amphetamine/hallucinogenic drug that helps youth maintain their energy and provides a sense of well-being for an extended period of time. Some juveniles take Ecstasy each and every time they go dancing, which for some youth can be every Friday and Saturday night for a year or more. Some Ecstasy users go dancing and use the drug on weeknights as well.

Both "wet/sherm" and Ecstasy can be incredibly dangerous substances. Smoking cigarettes or marijuana joints dipped in formaldehyde can result in extreme agitation, aggression and violent behavior, as well as damage to juveniles' brains. Ecstasy increases youths' heart rate, blood pressure and body temperature. Using Ecstasy can also result in death.

"Huffing"(purposely inhaling or sniffing various chemicals in order to get high) is also not uncommon among juvenile offenders. Most youth have easy access to chemical substances that they can inhale. Sometimes youth even have access these chemicals (e.g., toxic cleaning supplies) during incarceration. Huffing can kill brain cells. Juvenile justice professionals who work with youth who abuse inhalants typically witness a downward spiral in these juveniles' cognitive ability over time. Youths' thinking usually becomes much slower, and they are often unable to grasp and comprehend concepts they were able to understand before their drug use. Inhalants can damage juveniles' liver or kidney or even cause death by stopping the heart.

Unfortunately, many juvenile offenders do not view these three types of drugs (formaldehyde, inhalants, Ecstasy) as dangerous. In fact, some youth who primarily use Ecstasy and inhalants pride themselves on not being "druggies." These youth refer to marijuana, cocaine and heroin as "real drugs" and say they avoid them because of the potential dangers associated with these substances. Many juveniles who dip their marijuana cigarettes or blunts in embalming fluid refer to "sherm" as "marijuana plus." They usually have little knowledge of the damage these chemicals may be doing to their brain and nervous system.

172

Juvenile Offenders with Mental Health Disorders: Who Are They and What Do We Do With Them?

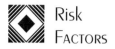 Risk
FACTORS

A variety of factors have been associated with juvenile substance use. Some of these factors are related to youths' family environment, school performance, peers and the community in which youth reside. Some of the most common risk factors for substance use among juveniles include (Hawkins, Lishner, Catalano, & Howard, 1985):

1. Low bonding to family (*e.g.*, lack of closeness or parental involvement in activities with children)

2. Family conflict

3. Poor and inconsistent family management practices (*e.g.*, lack of parental discipline, low parental educational aspirations for their children)

4. Family behavior and attitude toward alcohol and drugs

5. Academic failure

6. Low degree of commitment to school (*e.g.*, truancy, not expecting to attend college)

7. Peer rejection in elementary school

8. Association with drug-using peers

9. Alienation and rebelliousness (*e.g.*, alienated from customary values of society)

10. Extreme economic deprivation (*e.g.*, poverty, poor housing, overcrowding)

11. Neighborhood disorganization (*e.g.*, densely populated cities, low level of attachment to neighborhood)

12. Laws and norms favorable toward obtaining and using drugs and alcohol

13. Availability of drugs and alcohol (*e.g.*, ease of accessibility)

14. Early and persistent behavior problems

15. Physiological factors (*e.g.*, sensation seeking, poor impulse control)

16. Attitudes favorable to drug use

17. Early onset of drug use

Professionals working in the juvenile justice field know that a significant number of young offenders have several, and sometimes many, of these risk factors for substance use. They are also aware that substance use is extremely common among youth involved with the juvenile justice system. Education and prevention efforts are essential to help thwart youths' progression from experimental/recreational substance use to serious substance use disorders. These efforts are particularly critical among juvenile offenders because of their high-risk status. Not all youth who use drugs or alcohol have a substance use *disorder* but many of them do. For example, one study of juvenile offenders found that a high percentage of the youth assessed suffered from a substance use disorder versus occasional use of drugs and alcohol. Forty-six percent of the youth suffered from Alcohol Abuse or Alcohol Dependence, and 64 percent suffered from some type of drug abuse or drug dependence (Davis, Bean, Schumacher, & Stringer, 1991).

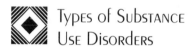 Types of Substance
Use Disorders

Substance Abuse Disorder

Juveniles with substance abuse disorders (*e.g.*, Alcohol Abuse, Cocaine Abuse, Cannibis Abuse) are neither experimenting with drugs and alcohol nor using these substances on an intermittent basis. These youth have a pattern of substance use that causes them considerable suffering and/or significantly interferes with their ability to function in an expected manner (APA, 2000). Juveniles who abuse substances typically experience difficulties meeting expectations at home, school or work. They may repeatedly miss class or receive school suspensions due to their drug and alcohol use. These youth may experience conflict at home because they are not following their parent's/caretaker's requests and/or completing tasks (*e.g.*, chores, curfew) as a result of their substance use. Many juveniles with substance abuse disorders place

Substance Use Disorders: Substance Abuse and Substance Dependence

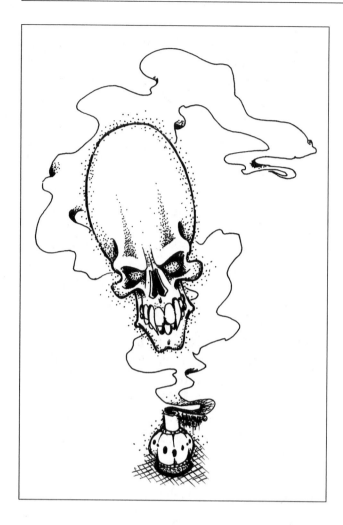

alcohol for a long enough period of time, they may develop a substance dependence disorder.

Substance Dependence Disorder

Individuals who become physiologically *dependent* on alcohol or a particular drug typically develop symptoms of tolerance and/or withdrawal. *Tolerance* refers to youth needing increasingly larger amounts of a substance in order to feel drunk or high. Whereas juveniles may have felt drunk with eight beers, eventually they may need 12 in order to achieve the same effect that eight beers used to provide. *Withdrawal* refers to the appearance of certain physical symptoms when youth stop taking drugs or alcohol. Withdrawal also refers to when youth continue to use drugs or alcohol to avoid experiencing these physical symptoms. The specific withdrawal symptoms experienced by juveniles are particular to the substance ingested and are typically uncomfortable, sometimes painful and potentially lethal (*e.g.*, sweating, heart palpitations, blurred vision, tremors, vomiting, anxiety, seizures).

Most youth involved with juvenile justice have not used drugs or alcohol for long enough time periods to develop the physiological symptoms of tolerance or withdrawal. However, they can still meet diagnostic criteria for substance dependence disorder (*e.g.*, Alcohol Dependence, Cocaine Dependence, Heroin Dependence). These youth use substances in a *compulsive* manner, and their substance use causes them extreme suffering or considerable impairment in their everyday functioning (APA, 2000). On occasions when juveniles with a substance dependence disorder use drugs or alcohol, they have difficulty stopping—even when they have made up their mind to cut down on their substance use. They often use more of the substance, or use it for a longer period of time, than they had planned. Almost all of these juveniles' daily activities revolve around the substance on which they are dependent. These youth spend much of their time trying to buy the substance, getting drunk or high from the substance, and

themselves in situations that are physically dangerous to their health, including driving while high or drunk, repeatedly riding in cars driven by friends who are high or drunk, or getting into physical fights when high or drunk. Youth with substance abuse disorders often have experienced legal problems in relation to their drug and alcohol use. They may have been arrested on a drug charge or for behavior that occurred while they were drunk or high.

Juveniles with substance abuse disorders continue a pattern of drug or alcohol use, despite the negative consequences associated with their substance use. These youth experience difficulties in interpersonal relationships, school, work and so forth due to their involvement with drugs and alcohol. However, these juveniles continue to use the substance(s) anyway. If youth continue to *abuse* drugs or

Juvenile Offenders with Mental Health Disorders: Who Are They and What Do We Do With Them?

recovering from the effects of their substance use.

As one can imagine, these behaviors greatly interfere with the youths' ability to go to school or have meaningful relationships with people other than substance-using friends. These juveniles may drop out of school or may be suspended or expelled. If the youth have a job, they may end up quitting or being fired for behaviors related to their substance use. Juvenile offenders with a substance dependence disorder typically have experienced numerous negative consequences in relation to their use of drugs and/or alcohol. They may have suffered psychologically, physically and/or legally, and they are aware that these costs are directly related to their significant substance use. However, these youth continue their pattern of drug and alcohol use.

 ## Screening For Substance Use Disorders Among Juvenile Offenders

All juveniles should be *screened* for substance use disorders upon entering juvenile justice facilities. Screening is a brief process used to identify those youth who are in need of a more extensive substance abuse assessment/evaluation. The goal of the screening is to uncover signs or symptoms of a serious substance abuse problem, not to provide youth with a specific substance-related diagnosis. Some juvenile justice facilities use a standardized substance abuse screening tool, whereas other facilities have designed their own screening tool.

Key areas that should be addressed when screening for substance use disorders include:

- Current intoxication or withdrawal from alcohol or drugs
- History of substance use:
  - Age youth began using drugs and alcohol
  - Youths' drug(s) of choice
  - Typical pattern of substance use
  - Motivation for using substances

- Negative consequences associated with substance use
- History of substance use treatment (*e.g.*, inpatient, outpatient)
- Family history of substance use disorders
- Youths' perception about their need for substance abuse treatment/level of motivation for treatment

The Center for Substance Abuse Treatment (CSAT) has published guidelines regarding the screening and assessment of juveniles who use drugs and alcohol, including youth in juvenile justice settings. *Screening and Assessing Adolescents For Substance Use Disorders* is a publication that addresses key issues in substance use assessment and summarizes common measurement instruments for assessing youths' drug and alcohol use (Winters, 1999).

Examples of *screening* tools for substance abuse among adolescents are:

- The Drug Use Screening Inventory-Revised (DUSI-R) (Tarter & Hegedus, 1991)
- The Personal Experience Screening Questionnaire (PESQ) (Winters, 1992)

Examples of *assessment* tools for substance use among adolescents include:

- The Adolescent Diagnostic Interview (ADI) (Winters & Henly, 1993)
- The Personal Experiences Inventory (PEI) (Winters & Henly, 1989)

There are no "typical" substance-abusing youth. Juvenile justice professionals should screen all juveniles for substance abuse regardless of their age, gender, socioeconomic status, ethnicity or culture. Staff should ask youth for clarification if the name of a drug or type of drug a juvenile is talking about is not clearly recognizable. The way youth use particular substances (*e.g.*, smoking, snorting, injecting) should also be clarified.

Most substance abuse screenings rely on juveniles' self-report of their drug and alcohol

Substance Use Disorders: Substance Abuse and Substance Dependence

use. In general, self-report about substance use tends to be fairly reliable among adolescents (Oetting & Beauvais, 1990). However, some juvenile offenders may be motivated to overstate or understate the extent of their drug and alcohol use. Some juveniles may minimize or deny recent substance use if ingesting drugs or alcohol is a violation of their probation/parole order. Other juveniles may not want to be referred or mandated to attend substance abuse treatment. However, some juveniles may view significant substance use as status enhancing and may actually over-report their true usage. This over-reporting is even more likely if peers are in close proximity while youth are being screened.

Juvenile offenders with a substance use disorder may not have used any drugs or alcohol for several days or weeks before a screening is conducted. This situation occurs most often when youth are transferred from one residential setting to another. For example, juveniles held at short-term detention facilities prior to placement at a long-term training school do not have recent access to drugs and alcohol. These juveniles' report of no recent drug and alcohol use may not be an accurate representation of the youths' typical substance use habit, which means important treatment issues can be overlooked. Therefore, evaluating juveniles' history of substance-related problems and treatment, in addition to current symptoms and behavior, is important.

If concerns arise from juveniles' substance abuse screening, youth should be referred to professionals specializing in substance use disorders for a comprehensive substance abuse assessment/evaluation. A comprehensive drug and alcohol assessment helps staff to better understand:

- The nature of youths' substance use

- The severity of youths' substance use

- Any problems related to youths' substance use (e.g., academic achievement, family relationships, medical issues)

Collateral sources (e.g., family members, teachers, juvenile justice facility line staff, probation officers) and well-designed, standardized assessment instruments can be helpful in collecting this information. Collateral sources can often provide details surrounding youths' pattern of substance use and associated problems that the juveniles may be unaware of or unwilling to report themselves.

A comprehensive substance use assessment typically results in a written report that identifies:

- The nature and severity of youths' drug and alcohol use

- A diagnosis of a substance use disorder (if present)

- Any recommendations for treatment

 DRUG RECOGNITION/ DRUG TESTING

Drug recognition and drug testing are additional forms of screening and assessment that can be used with youth who are involved with the juvenile justice system. These methods are not meant to replace the screening and assessment strategies previously mentioned but can serve as adjuncts, corroborating self-reported information from youth. They also can be used throughout the course of juvenile justice supervision (e.g., probation, parole) and/or substance abuse treatment to detect relapse and/or help youth remain motivated.

Drug Recognition Techniques

Drug recognition techniques typically rely on standardized processes of detecting signs and symptoms of drug and alcohol use. These techniques do not rely on youths' self-report and are used to supplement information gathered from a screening interview. Drug recognition techniques are useful for identifying youth who are under the influence of drugs or alcohol or who have recently ingested these substances.

The following characteristics are common signs and symptoms of substance use. The presence of these factors does not necessarily indicate alcohol or drug use, but if present, indicate the need for further evaluation of juveniles:

- Dilated or constricted pupils
- Red, watery eyes
- Elevated or lowered vital signs (*e.g.*, heart rate, pulse)
- Muscle stiffness
- Impaired memory
- Slurred or very rapid speech
- Coordination difficulties/slow reactions
- Impulsive or erratic behavior
- Poor hygiene
- Runny nose/sores in or around nose
- Confusion
- Odor of alcohol or chemicals (*e.g.*, paint, gasoline)
- Needle marks on arm
- Profuse sweating
- Drifting off or falling asleep at inappropriate times

If staff detect signs or symptoms of substance use, additional information should be collected regarding youths' behavior. Investigating whether juveniles' current symptoms differ significantly from their normal behavior is important. In addition, high levels of stress and fear and the emergence of mental health symptoms can all play a role in youths' unusual behavior and should be ruled out. Excluding all nondrug-related causes of juveniles' actions is essential. If it is determined that youth have recently used drugs or alcohol, care should be taken to establish which specific substance(s) were ingested/used and how long ago.

Drug recognition techniques provide immediate information to staff about youths' possible drug and alcohol use. This type of screening is inexpensive and minimally intrusive for juveniles. It can be used separately or in conjunction with drug/chemical testing for substance use.

Drug Testing

Drug testing (also known as chemical testing, laboratory testing, or toxicology screening) is the analysis of various body materials or bodily fluids to determine recent drug or alcohol use. Chemical testing is one of the most accurate strategies for determining current or recent substance use (McLellan & Dembo, 1995). Drug testing can be used for initial screening and assessment purposes, as well as while monitoring the treatment compliance of juvenile offenders with a substance abuse disorder. Chemical testing techniques can often, although not always, increase

---

DRUG RECOGNITION TECHNIQUES PROVIDE IMMEDIATE INFORMATION TO STAFF ABOUT YOUTHS' POSSIBLE DRUG AND ALCOHOL USE.

---

the truthfulness of juveniles' self-report regarding their recent drug and alcohol use. However, drug testing can be an intrusive process because it involves analyzing parts of juveniles' bodies/physiological functions. It also tends to be more expensive than most of the other substance use screening strategies, making it less practical for many juvenile justice settings.

Some of the most common chemical tests for drugs and alcohol are:

- Urine analysis
- Breath analysis
- Saliva analysis
- Blood analysis
- Hair analysis

When used, drug testing should only be part of a comprehensive assessment of juveniles' substance use behavior and not be the only screening measurement. Chemical testing strategies can provide information on the specific substance(s) youth may have recently

Substance Use Disorders: Substance Abuse and Substance Dependence

used. But they provide no information on the consequences of youths' substance use or their motivations for using drugs and alcohol. In addition, some substances are eliminated from the body fairly quickly (*i.e.*, alcohol) and are difficult to detect. However, other substances (*i.e.*, chronic use of marijuana) may be detected after several days, weeks or even months after youth have stopped using the drugs. The accuracy of test results will depend on:

- How long ago the juveniles used the substance(s)

- Which substance(s) the juveniles used

- The particular method of drug testing being used

Drug testing might be considered in the following situations with juveniles who are suspected of having a substance use disorder:

- Admission to juvenile justice facilities directly from the community

- After youth return to juvenile justice facilities from community visits

- At any point during incarceration if there is reasonable suspicion of substance use

- During the course of community supervision if probation/parole staff notice:

  —Sudden, dramatic and unexpected changes in mood and/or behavior

  —Increased aggression/violent behavior

  —Ongoing failure to comply with rules/expectations

  —Youth are living on streets and/or in shelters

  —Frequent relapses with substance use

Urine analyses (UAs) are one of the most commonly used methods of chemically testing juvenile offenders for alcohol and other substance use, particularly when they are on probation or parole. Some juvenile offenders are aware of strategies that can modify the accuracy of urine drug tests. By engaging in certain behaviors, youth can decrease the

probability that specific substances will be detected in their urine. For example, drinking extremely large quantities of water or ingesting the herb Goldenseal can alter drug test results. Some youth have tried drinking vinegar or small amounts of bleach to alter the accuracy of urine tests.

Drug testing all youth suspected of substance abuse is unlikely due to:

- The large number of juvenile offenders who use drugs and alcohol

- The limited resources of most juvenile justice agencies

All juvenile justice agencies using drug tests should have clearly written policies and procedures for conducting these types of analyses. These policies and procedures should clearly address critical issues such as:

- Obtaining proper consent

- Identifying specific consequences resulting from positive findings

 MANAGING JUVENILE OFFENDERS WHO HAVE SUBSTANCE USE DISORDERS

Drug and alcohol *treatment* is typically conducted by professionals specializing in the assessment and treatment of individuals with substance use disorders. Substance abuse treatment is beyond the scope of this chapter. However, the following are some guidelines for juvenile justice professionals when *managing* juvenile offenders who have a substance use disorder. These suggestions are applicable whether or not juveniles are currently receiving, have received, or are scheduled to receive formal substance abuse treatment.

If Youth Appear To Be Intoxicated or Withdrawing From Drugs or Alcohol:

SEEK IMMEDIATE MEDICAL ATTENTION Intoxication and withdrawal from drugs or alcohol can be extremely dangerous and potentially lethal. If youth arrive at juvenile justice facilities intoxicated or in withdrawal from drugs or alcohol, they should be immediately evaluated and monitored by medical professionals.

OBTAIN A HISTORY OF DRUG AND ALCOHOL USE

Determining what substance(s) youth have recently ingested is critical. Information also should be gathered about youths' history of behavior when intoxicated, as well as any withdrawal complications. Any information on past aggression, suicidal behavior, psychotic behavior and the like while the youth have been intoxicated is also helpful. Some juveniles who have previously experienced withdrawal symptoms may be able to inform staff about what intervention strategies have been helpful or harmful in the past. Historical information should be gathered from as many sources as possible (*e.g.*, youth, medical records, staff, parents, treatment providers).

DO NOT LET THE YOUTH JUST "SLEEP IT OFF"

Juvenile offenders who are intoxicated or withdrawing from alcohol or drugs often want to go into their room and sleep for several hours or even days. This desire to sleep is particularly strong if youth are physically uncomfortable or in pain. Such an intervention is not appropriate unless under the direction of a medical professional who has evaluated the youth. Even in these cases, the juveniles should still be medically monitored on a frequent basis.

General Substance Abuse Strategies

REFER YOUTH FOR SUBSTANCE ABUSE TREATMENT SERVICES

Some juvenile justice facilities have separate living units/cottages specifically designated for substance abuse treatment, similar to inpatient/residential treatment programs in the community. Other facilities offer treatment on generic units/cottages through treatment groups or individualized treatment-related coursework related to substance abuse. At a minimum, most juvenile justice facilities offer "educational" groups on substance abuse issues. Most drug and alcohol treatment groups are cognitive-behavioral in nature. Therefore, treatment staff should ensure that materials related to substance abuse are modified for youths' particular developmental or cognitive level. Some facilities offer substance-abusing youth the opportunity to attend Alcoholics Anonymous (AA) or Narcotics Anonymous (NA) meetings. These types of groups tend to be most effective for youth when they are modified for an adolescent population. Even when formal substance use treatment is not available onsite, the combination of abstinence from chemicals, substance abuse information, and AA/NA groups can be powerful for some offenders.

DO NOT ALLOW YOUTH TO GLORIFY DRUG USE

Drugs and alcohol are a significant part of the lives of juvenile offenders with substance use disorders. Because of this, these youth are typically accustomed to spending large amounts of time talking about substances with their peers and relaying incidents associated with being drunk or high. Many of these juveniles glorify their drug use and continue to idealize their drug-using experiences during incarceration. Staff should have substance-abusing youth focus on the negative and dangerous consequences of their alcohol and drug use. This focus provides a more realistic picture of how the juveniles' substance use affects their lives— as well as those around them. In addition, facility staff should not discuss their own current alcohol use (*e.g.*, being hung over from a party the night before) with youth.

PAIR SUBSTANCE-ABUSING JUVENILES WITH NONSUBSTANCE USING PEERS

Most juveniles who abuse substances spend much of their time with other youth who abuse substances. Many of these juveniles think

Substance Use Disorders: Substance Abuse and Substance Dependence

substance use is a part of being "cool." Having substance-abusing youth spend time with youth who are "hip" or "cool" but who do *not* use drugs or alcohol can be helpful. Clean and sober youth may be able to introduce substance-abusing juveniles to new activities and ways of thinking about issues and lifestyle choices. The impact may even be greater if the nonsubstance-using youth used to be heavy users of drugs or alcohol, but they are currently clean and sober. Many juvenile offenders with a substance use disorder cannot even imagine what their life or lifestyle would be like without drugs and alcohol.

EMPHASIZE THEIR SUCCESS IN REMAINING CLEAN AND SOBER

For many juvenile offenders with substance use disorders, incarceration may be the most consistent period of time when the youth have not consumed drugs and alcohol. Juvenile justice professionals should point out to these youth the length of time they have functioned without any drugs or alcohol in their body—particularly if the youth have been locked up for a significant period of time (*e.g.*, weeks, months, years). While in the community, many of these juveniles never thought they could have "survived" such a lengthy period of time completely clean and sober.

HELP JUVENILES DEVELOP NEW INTERESTS AND ACTIVITIES

Many juvenile offenders with substance use disorders have few interests and activities that they enjoy while sober. Juvenile justice professionals can help these youth explore new activities and skills to which they have not have been exposed—or to which they have never experienced without being drunk or high. Some new behaviors may initially seem uncomfortable for these juveniles. But staff should continue to support the youth and reinforce every effort made to engage in positive and pro-social activities, without the use of substances.

BE ALERT TO VISITORS

A significant number of substance-abusing youth involved with juvenile justice have parents, siblings or extended family members who also have a substance use disorder. Some family members of incarcerated juveniles may bring small amounts of drugs to facilities during visiting hours. Some drugs can be exchanged and transported fairly inconspicuously (*e.g.*, pills, LSD on a stamp). Therefore, staff need to be vigilant about ensuring that no drugs are exchanged during visits and brought back into a facility.

SECURE COMMUNITY TREATMENT SERVICES

Some juvenile offenders are in need of formal substance abuse treatment, but this type of treatment may not be provided during the youths' incarceration. Other juveniles receive formal treatment within juvenile justice facilities but may need additional treatment upon release. In either case, juvenile justice facility and community supervision staff should work together to secure treatment services in the community *before* the youth are released.

DO NOT GIVE UP ON THE YOUTH

Substance use disorders are multifaceted and complex. Even after substance-abusing youth have abstained from using drugs and alcohol for a significant period of time, some of these youth relapse and ingest substances again. Relapse should be anticipated, prevented if possible, and addressed if it occurs. Reinforcing youth for the period of time they were able to remain clean and sober is essential. There should be a significant focus on motivating juveniles to return to a substance-free lifestyle, rather than solely providing sanctions for returning to previous substance-using behavior.

Case Example

Michael, 16, has been arrested for the first time and is terrified. Michael and his best friend were arrested for stealing a pack of

180

Juvenile Offenders with Mental Health Disorders: Who Are They and What Do We Do With Them?

cigarettes from a small market in a strip mall. Michael hates being at the detention facility. He is afraid that one of the boys on the living unit is going to beat him, rape him or even kill him. He views himself as superior to his peers at the detention center and keeps trying to convince the staff that he does not belong in the facility.

Michael loves to dance and often attends all-night "rave" parties at which he dances for six or more hours at a time. Initially, he only went dancing on the weekends, but over the past five months, he has begun to go dancing on weeknights as well. Michael tells his mother he is spending the night at his best friend's house. Michael and his friends always take "E," also known as Ecstasy, whenever they go dancing. He says it gives him "tons of energy" and makes him feel "love" toward everyone with whom he dances. He says the lights of the dance clubs and the sound of the music are much more intense when he takes Ecstasy. Michael says he can feel the music pumping "through every cell of his entire body."

Michael purposely does not associate with the students at school who use marijuana, cocaine and amphetamines. He refers to them as "potheads" and "speed freaks," and he swears he would never put "that kind of crap" in his body. He felt very strongly about this commitment, even though on two separate occasions he passed out while he was taking Ecstasy. Both times, he was unconscious for several minutes and does not remember much about the episodes. His friends reported that Michael was complaining about feeling sick and then just dropped to the ground as if he had fainted. When Michael awoke, he was still feeling slightly ill, but he did not appear to have any significant physical symptoms.

Due to his late night dancing, sometimes staying up for 24-hours-at-a-time, Michael began to have problems staying awake in school. He lost his part-time job as a busboy because he would fall asleep during his shift. He also became irritable with family members and began getting into frequent fights with his older sister. Michael's family was shocked when they heard about his arrest.

CHAPTER 10

Co-Occurring Mental Health and Substance Use Disorders

"Most of us who are addicts aren't mentally ill. It just helps us with our depression. We do every drug we can get our hands on."

Rita, 17

Shawna, 16, drinks alcohol every weekend and occasionally uses large amounts of cocaine. She rarely drinks by herself, but she binge drinks on the weekends at parties. She typically passes out and/or throws up by the end of the night. Shawna uses cocaine whenever she meets someone at a party who has some, even if it means exchanging sexual favors for it. She loves the weekend and always looks forward to being drunk or high. During the week, Shawna keeps to herself at school. She has difficulty concentrating in class and spends much of her time drawing disturbing pictures in her notebook, writing gloomy poetry or daydreaming about the weekend. She has difficulty sleeping at night, so she stays up late drawing pictures while listening to music related to death or destruction. About once a month, Shawna cuts her forearms with razor blades as a way to release built-up tension. She feels ugly and stupid, and she believes that she will never have a boyfriend. Shawna states that alcohol and cocaine give her the confidence she needs to talk to her peers, as well as flirt with boys. She was arrested on a shoplifting charge.

The term *co-occurring disorders* describes two independent medical disorders that occur at the same time. Within the mental health and substance abuse fields, however, the term typically describes the simultaneous presence of a mental health disorder (*e.g.*, Major Depression, Attention-Deficit/Hyperactivity Disorder, Posttraumatic Stress Disorder) *and* a substance use disorder (*e.g.*, Alcohol Abuse, Cannabis Abuse, Cocaine Abuse, Heroin Dependence). Although some youth involved with the juvenile justice system have a mental health disorder *or* a substance use disorder, many juvenile offenders have *both* types of disorders. One study found that 39 percent of juvenile offenders with a substance abuse disorder also had a co-occurring mental health disorder—not including Conduct Disorder or Oppositional

182

Juvenile Offenders with Mental Health Disorders: Who Are They and What Do We Do With Them?

Defiant Disorder (Milin, Halikas, Meller, & Morse, 1991).

The notion that some mentally ill juveniles also have a substance use disorder is not new. Throughout the years, a variety of terms have been used to describe this complicated subset of youth with co-existing disorders including, but not limited to:

- "Dually diagnosed"
- "Double jeopardy"
- "Mentally Ill Chemically Affected/ Abusers" (MICA)

Regardless of the label used, each of these terms refers to youth who have *both* a major mental health disorder and a substance use disorder. The term "co-occurring disorders" will be used in this manner throughout the rest of this chapter.

Identifying juvenile offenders with co-occurring disorders can be challenging because they are such a diverse group of adolescents. There is no *typical* juvenile with co-occurring disorders because each youth's clinical presentation is related to his or her particular combination of mental health and substance abuse symptoms. In addition, juveniles may present themselves differently at different times due to:

- The level of stress they are experiencing
- The degree of access they have to alcohol or drugs
- The potentially changeable nature of both of these types of disorders

Assessing, treating and managing youth with co-occurring mental health and substance use disorders is different than that for youth who have only one of these types of disorders.

Some juveniles with co-occurring disorders are particularly uncomfortable receiving a mental health or substance use diagnosis. For example, a number of youthful offenders with co-occurring disorders readily admit that they have a substance abuse problem. But they are unwilling to acknowledge that they also suffer from a mental health disorder. This situation typically occurs when youth perceive having a problem with drugs as "cooler" than being viewed as "crazy" or mentally unstable. In fact, substance use can often be a status enhancer for youth involved with the juvenile justice system, whereas mental illness tends to tarnish youths' reputation. However, there is a subset of juvenile offenders with co-occurring disorders who are willing to acknowledge their mental health diagnosis. They may even be willing to talk to mental health professionals about their psychiatric symptoms and to take psychotropic medication for their mood or behavior. But these same youth may not be ready to talk to professionals about their drug and alcohol use. In fact, they may be completely unwilling to discuss issues related to decreasing or entirely discontinuing their substance use. It is critical for juvenile offenders with co-occurring disorders to understand the nature of *both* their mental health and substance use disorders; the relationship between these disorders; and the affect these disorders have on their lives.

 Relationship Between Mental Health and Substance Use Disorders

Mental health and substance use disorders can interact with each other in a variety of ways (Peters & Bartoi, 1997):

SET OFF

Substance use can *set off,* or trigger, the emergence of a mental health disorder if youth are biologically/genetically predisposed to mental illness. For example, juveniles whose mothers suffer from Bipolar Disorder may never experience symptoms of mania until the youth begin using PCP.

PRODUCE

Substance use can *produce* psychiatric symptoms. For example, alcohol is a depressant. If juveniles ingest large-enough amounts of alcohol and/or ingest alcohol for a long enough period of time, these youth could develop

Identifying juvenile offenders with co-occurring disorders can be challenging because they are such a diverse group of adolescents. There is no *typical* juvenile with co-occurring disorders because each youth's clinical presentation is related to his or her particular combination of mental health and substance abuse symptoms.

depressive symptoms. If juveniles' heavy alcohol use continues for a significant time period, they could eventually meet diagnostic criteria for Major Depression.

WORSEN
Symptoms of mental illness may *worsen* when youth use alcohol and other drugs. For example, youth with suicidal ideation may take action to try to kill themselves while they are drunk or high. Juveniles may have thought about suicide in the past, but they may have been too scared to make an actual attempt. Alcohol and drugs can intensify feelings of depression, lower inhibitions or raise youths' feelings of courage. Additionally, youth with Schizophrenia can experience a significant worsening of psychotic symptoms when using hallucinogenic drugs.

IMITATE
Substance use can look very *similar* to the symptoms of a mental health disorder. For example, youth who have no history of mental health symptoms may develop significant paranoid delusions about their family and friends after heavy use of methamphetamine.

COVER UP
Symptoms of a mental health disorder may be *covered up,* or hidden, by juveniles' drug and alcohol use. Heavy use of alcohol, marijuana or other drugs may conceal symptoms of a mental

health disorder or alter the way symptoms are expressed. Symptoms of a mental health disorder may not be identified until youth are abstinent for a significant period of time.

UNRELATED
Juveniles may have both a mental health disorder and a substance use disorder, but the two disorders may *not be related* to one another. However, a common factor may underlie them both. For example, youths' genetic makeup may result in an increased vulnerability for the development of mental illness and/or substance abuse.

Some experts believe that juveniles with mental health disorders are *self-medicating* with alcohol and drugs. Others propose that drug and alcohol use is a major risk factor in the development of psychiatric symptoms. It is also possible that both disorders are caused by the same underlying factor(s). At this time, the *exact* relationship between mental illness and substance use is uncertain. However, one thing is clear: juveniles with co-occurring mental health and substance use disorders are at significant risk for multiple problems.

There are a variety of possible negative outcomes for youth who have both mental health and substance use disorders. The following have all been associated with substance abusing individuals who also have mental health symptoms (Kaminer, Tarter, Bukstein, & Kabene, 1992; Peters & Hills, 1993):

- Faster progression from initial substance use to drug dependence
- High rates of hospitalization
- Interpersonal difficulties
- Poor medication compliance
- Decreased probability of successfully completing treatment

Juveniles with co-occurring disorders are also at higher risk for a completed suicide (Brent *et al.*, 1993).

Some juvenile offenders with co-occurring mental health and substance use disorders may

184

Juvenile Offenders with Mental Health Disorders: Who Are They and What Do We Do With Them?

be placed in restrictive settings or receive high levels of juvenile justice supervision due to factors other than their criminal behavior. Questions about previous/current substance use, previous/current mental health symptoms, and previous/current substance abuse or mental health treatment are often included in juvenile justice risk assessments instruments. Even if youths' criminal history or current criminal behavior is not severe, juveniles with co-occurring disorders may receive a juvenile justice "risk" score in the moderate or severe range—due to the other problems in their lives. The appropriate identification and management of juvenile offenders with co-occurring disorders can help these youth to be more effective and successful in their daily lives. And it also can result in juvenile justice placements that best fit youths' particular needs.

 ## Screening and Assessment of Co-Occurring Disorders Among Juvenile Offenders

All youth should be screened for substance abuse and mental health disorders, as well as suicidal risk, when they enter juvenile justice facilities. However, youth can be re-screened at any point during juvenile justice supervision. Re-screening should occur if staff notice negative changes in youths' behavior and/or during times of transition (*e.g.*, sentencing, release to community supervision). If mental health and/ or substance abuse symptoms are detected during screening, youth should be further evaluated to assess the nature of these symptoms and the possible presence of a full disorder(s).

Any further assessment of youth with co-occurring disorders should include an examination of the interactive effects of their symptoms, including:

INFLUENCES OF SUBSTANCE USE ON MENTAL HEALTH SYMPTOMS

- Do the juveniles' mental health symptoms occur only when the youth are using

substances? Do drugs or alcohol make pre-existing mental health symptoms worse? Do mental health symptoms decrease during periods of abstinence?

INFLUENCES OF MENTAL HEALTH SYMPTOMS ON SUBSTANCE USE

- Do the youth increase their substance use when they are experiencing mental health symptoms? Do the juveniles use specific drugs in order to decrease particular mental health symptoms? Do the youth decrease their substance use when they are experiencing mental health symptoms? Do the youth use drugs and alcohol only when they are experiencing mental health symptoms?

TREATMENT ISSUES

- How has previous mental health treatment, if any, affected the youths' substance use behavior? How has previous substance abuse treatment, if any, affected the youths' mental health symptoms? How motivated are the youth to receive mental health treatment? How motivated are the youth to receive substance abuse treatment?

Most juvenile justice staff have not been trained to identify youth with co-occurring disorders. Some staff members may be able to recognize mental health symptoms but are reluctant to ask about substance abuse. Other staff may be better at recognizing substance abuse symptoms but have never been trained in mental health issues. Even when staff have some knowledge about both mental health and substance abuse disorders, most are not trained in the various ways the symptoms of these two disorders can interact (*e.g.*, imitate, worsen, set off). Once educated about co-occurring disorders among adolescent offenders, juvenile justice professionals are likely to become more adept at identifying these youths, as well as referring them to appropriate health care professionals.

No specific assessment tool has been developed especially for youth with co-occurring disorders. Most mental health and substance abuse assessment instruments were developed for use with youth who have a mental health or substance abuse disorder. There are a few instruments available that inquire about both mental health and substance abuse symptoms, and a few of these tools have been used to screen and assess juvenile offenders with co-occurring disorders. Unfortunately, even with such tools, determining whether youths' problems are primarily related to a mental health disorder or substance use is difficult (*e.g.,* Is the youths' heavy alcohol use a response to feelings of anxiety? Is the youths' depression a result of their heavy substance use?). In addition, most available mental health and substance abuse assessment tools have not been validated for youth with co-occurring disorders—particularly youth with co-occurring disorders who are involved with the juvenile justice system. (*Please see Chapters 9 and 13 for additional information about Screening and Assessment and Substance Use Disorders.*)

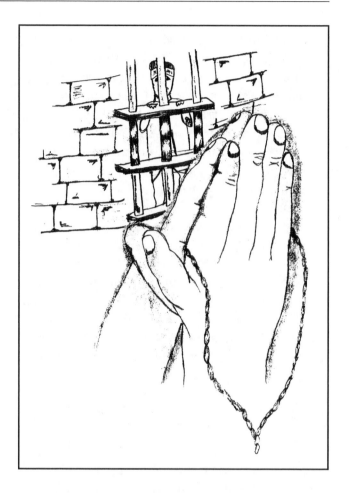

At this time, one of the best approaches for assessing co-occurring disorders among juvenile offenders is to conduct a comprehensive evaluation of youths' mental health and substance abuse symptoms—using a combination of reliable and valid mental health and substance abuse assessment tools. Assessment results related to each independent disorder should be integrated, along with an assessment of how youths' mental health and substance abuse symptoms impact one another. Information related to youths' family, intellectual functioning, health, juvenile justice status, criminal behavior and social history should be integrated as well. Data should be gathered from as many collateral sources as possible (*e.g.,* arresting officer, family/caretaker, school personnel, juvenile justice staff, treatment providers).

The relationship between various mental health disorders and substance use disorders is complex. The disorders may co-exist independently, or there may be an interactive relationship between them (*e.g.,* self-medication, substance use is masking mental health symptoms). In addition, drug recognition testing with these juveniles can sometimes be difficult because some of the signs and symptoms of substance use are similar to those of mental illness. Therefore, the screening and assessment of co-occurring disorders must be considered an ongoing, continual process covering the multiple domains that affect juveniles' functioning.

Currently, there is little to no empirical information about whether or not youth with certain mental health disorders prefer to use particular types of substances. For example, some juvenile offenders with Attention-Deficit/Hyperactivity Disorder report that using methamphetamine and cocaine helps them to focus. However, other juvenile offenders with Attention-Deficit/Hyperactivity Disorder report that they prefer the effects of alcohol and marijuana

186

Juvenile Offenders with Mental Health Disorders: Who Are They and What Do We Do With Them?

because these substances help to slow the youth down.

When screening and assessing youth with co-occurring disorders, clinicians may have difficulty obtaining accurate reports of juveniles' mental health and substance use behaviors. For example:

- Youth with severe mental health disorders may not be accurate reporters of their current mental health or substance use symptoms.

- Youth with severe mental health disorders may not be accurate reporters of their mental health or substance use histories.

- Youth with severe mental health disorders may be confused about how their substance use and mental health symptoms are related.

- Juvenile offenders who use substances daily may be unable to report whether mental health symptoms are present during periods in which the youth are clean and sober.

- Juveniles' mental health and substance use symptoms may be so strongly inter-related that it may be unclear whether specific symptoms are related solely to substance use or to a mental health disorder.

- Previous medical records and juvenile justice files may list several different mental health and substance use diagnoses, provided by several different professionals.

- Previous evaluators may have neglected to inquire about mental health or substance use symptoms, only focusing on one area and not the other.

- Previous evaluators may not have had expertise in the manifestation of mental health or substance use disorders among adolescents (versus adults), so they misidentified or did not identify important issues.

- Youth may purposefully provide inaccurate information. *(Please see Chapter 13 for additional information related to self-report information.)*

Other issues complicate the screening and assessment of youth with co-occurring disorders. Youth who have a mental illness may be particularly vulnerable to the effects of substance use. Therefore, these youth may develop significant problems with drugs and alcohol even when using lower dosages of substances than their peers (Peters & Bartoi, 1997). Because they are not using excessive amounts of the drug, their substance abuse disorder may be overlooked—even though the amount they are using is causing significant problems in their lives. In addition, the consequences of substance use for juveniles with mental illness can appear differently than for youth who do not have a mental health disorder. For instance, substance use among mentally ill juveniles can result in paranoia, aggression, hyperactivity, depression, anxiety/agitation and noncompliance with psychotropic medication. The period of risk for onset of substance abuse and major mental illnesses (*e.g.,* Schizophrenia, Bipolar Disorder) is the same—further confusing diagnostic issues.

CLARIFICATION OF DIAGNOSIS

Some juvenile offenders exhibit behaviors that appear to be indicative of a mental health disorder but that are really due to intoxication or withdrawal from drugs or alcohol. Therefore, waiting through a substance-free period is often necessary to determine whether youths' symptoms are primarily related to a substance use or a psychiatric disorder. Even when juvenile offenders appear to have co-occurring substance use and mental health disorders, the youths' presenting symptoms can be entirely substance-induced. These youth may look and act as if they were mentally ill. However, their unusual or distressing symptoms are the direct physiological consequence of medication, illegal drug use or toxin exposure (APA, 2000). For example, the hallucinatory experiences of youth using

Co-Occuring Mental Health and Substance Use Disorders

PCP, LSD or psilocybin mushrooms can mimic a psychotic mental health disorder. "Crashing" after using high doses of amphetamine or cocaine can result in severe feelings of depression, including suicidal ideation, for days after cessation of substance use. If youth are suffering exclusively from a substance-induced disorder, their problematic symptoms will probably diminish with each day that they abstain from the causal agent. If significant mental health symptoms continue even after youth have been abstinent from drugs and alcohol (time periods will vary depending on the type of substance used), the symptoms are not likely due primarily to the effects of substances.

For youth residing in the community prior to incarceration, adequately assessing the causes of unusual or problematic symptoms can be difficult (and sometimes impossible) if the youth were regularly using drugs and alcohol. Due to the delayed withdrawal syndrome associated with some substances, waiting several weeks or months of a substance-free period may be necessary to make a definitive diagnosis of a mental health disorder. However, delaying the identification of mental health symptoms for a few weeks or more will likely postpone mental health treatment, which may be needed. Therefore, when working with juveniles exhibiting both mental health and substance abuse symptoms, it is recommended that clinicians:

- Evaluate youth according to agency protocols
- Provide a *provisional* mental health and/or substance use diagnosis
- Treat any symptoms, if necessary
- Reassess juveniles after about a week or so of no substance use

 TREATMENT ISSUES RELATED TO JUVENILES WITH CO-OCCURRING DISORDERS

Treatment interventions and management strategies for juvenile offenders with co-occurring disorders largely depend on youths' par-

ticular combination of mental health and substance abuse symptoms. The management strategies outlined in each of the individual chapters of this book provide helpful guidelines that can be used with youth who are experiencing a variety of mental health and substance use disorders. However, managing juveniles with co-occurring disorders is more complex and challenging than managing youth who primarily have either a mental health or a substance use disorder. Screening, assessing, diagnosing and treating this multifaceted group of adolescents requires an increased amount of collaboration between service systems (*e.g.*, mental health, substance abuse, juvenile justice) and service providers. A collective sense of responsibility regarding youth with co-occurring disorders is necessary to:

- Adequately share important information between various systems/service providers
- Bring together the variety of appropriate resources needed to intervene effectively these youth

Which Disorder Should Be Treated First?

One of the most prominent issues in the history of the treatment of youth with co-occurring disorders is associated with the decision as to which disorder should be treated first. One school of thought has been that treating a primary disorder of mental illness first may be enough to resolve youths' substance use disorder. The assumption has been that youth use drugs and alcohol primarily in response to their mental health symptoms. This philosophy underlies the view that youth with co-occurring disorders often "self-medicate" their mental illness. However, another school of thought has been that treating a primary disorder of substance abuse first will result in diminished mental health symptoms. This view suggests that youths' depression, attention problems and the like are primarily a result of their drug and

188

Juvenile Offenders with Mental Health Disorders: Who Are They and What Do We Do With Them?

alcohol use. Both of these strategies are simplistic and ineffective with the majority of juvenile offenders with co-occurring disorders. Many youth with co-occurring disorders do not achieve successful outcomes within *mental health* treatment programs if their drug and alcohol use is not adequately addressed. In addition, many youth who have co-occurring disorders do not achieve successful outcomes in *substance abuse* treatment programs if their mental health disorder(s) is not adequately addressed.

When juveniles have both a mental health and substance use disorder, the decision regarding which disorder to treat first can actually hinder the youths' ability to receive appropriate treatment. For example, some mental health treatment programs will not accept mentally ill juveniles if staff believe that the youth have a primary problem with drugs and alcohol. Some substance abuse treatment programs will not accept substance abusing youth until their mental health disorder has stabilized. When clinicians work with juveniles who have co-occurring disorders, both disorders should be viewed as important, and the youth should receive treatment for both of them.

There are three models related to the timing of treatment for individuals with co-occurring disorders (Ries, 1995):

SEQUENTIAL MODEL OF TREATMENT

- In this model, treatment is provided sequentially. Juveniles typically receive treatment from one system (mental health or substance abuse) and when that treatment is complete, they receive treatment from the other system. Historically, this model has been a common approach to mental health and substance abuse treatment for youth with co-occurring disorders. The system that initially treats the youth is usually determined by:
  - Which disorder seems more severe at the particular time treatment is sought

  - Whichever system youth happen to come into contact with first
  - Which particular agencies contract with the juvenile justice system
  - Which treatment services are available in a particular juvenile justice facility
  - Which treatment services are most accessible in youths' community

After youth with co-occurring disorders initially receive mental health or substance abuse treatment, they are then referred to receive treatment from the other system. Under this model, the coordination of services can be confusing, and the sharing of information between involved parties can be difficult. Providing treatment in a sequential manner may be appropriate for juvenile offenders with co-occurring disorders who have:

- intermittent episodes of mental health or substance abuse problems (*e.g.*, episodic depression, occasional drinking binges), or
- more significant problems with one disorder versus the other.

PARALLEL MODEL OF TREATMENT

- In this model, treatment is provided in a parallel manner. Youth receive treatment from the mental health system and the substance abuse system simultaneously. For example, juveniles might attend a substance abuse treatment group twice a week and also meet with a mental health professional once or twice a week. Youth may receive quality treatment within both systems, but there is often minimal coordination and integration between the two settings/systems. Youth, their family, and juvenile justice professionals are often responsible for the coordination of services and the sharing of information. Juveniles may receive conflicting messages from treatment providers (e.g., substance abuse agencies may require

Co-Occuring Mental Health and Substance Use Disorders

youth to remain abstinent from all mind-altering substances, including the psychotropic medication they receive from mental health professionals). The parallel model of treatment is most beneficial when there is significant communication and collaboration among all individuals providing treatment services to juveniles.

INTEGRATED MODEL OF TREATMENT

- In this model, treatment is provided in an integrated manner. Youth receive treatment for both their mental health and substance use disorders at the same time, in the same setting, possibly even from the same clinician(s). Treatment staff are typically cross-trained in both mental health and substance abuse issues. An integrated treatment program provides comprehensive treatment, combining elements of both mental health and substance abuse. These types of programs usually have a strong case management component, which helps ensure that juveniles receive consistent messages and that clinical information is shared among all individuals involved in the treatment. The integrated treatment model is likely the best treatment format for juvenile offenders who have persistent co-occurring disorders (Drake, Mercer-McFadden, Mueser, McHugo, & Bond, 1998).

Collaboration is critical when supervising juvenile offenders with co-occurring mental health and substance use disorders. Professionals from the mental health, substance abuse and juvenile justice systems must work together to identify youths' problem areas, as well as develop treatment plans. Collaboration and integration between these three systems should begin during the screening phase and continue through any necessary assessments, treatments and aftercare services. Sharing important information about the juveniles' symptoms, behav-

iors and treatment needs is necessary if these youth are to receive an accurate diagnosis and an appropriately individualized treatment plan. In addition, as youth with co-occurring disorders move through the juvenile justice system, important information from previous evaluations (mental health and substance abuse) should be communicated to individuals responsible for supervising the youth.

Psychotropic Medication

Many juvenile offenders with co-occurring disorders are prescribed psychotropic medication for a mental health disorder. Some of these youth take a combination of several medications at the same time. Regardless of the model of treatment services with which youth are involved (sequential, parallel, integrated), additional monitoring needs to occur when juveniles with co-occurring disorders are prescribed psychotropic medication. This area is of particular concern when youth are released back into the community from juvenile justice facilities. Important issues to keep in mind include:

- The use of alcohol and street drugs while taking psychotropic medication can significantly interfere with juveniles' prescribed medications, which can result in an increase in mental health symptoms.

- Even when youth with co-occurring disorders agree to remain substance-free, there is a considerable likelihood that they will engage in alcohol or drug use. Substance use relapse is not uncommon among juvenile offenders, even after youth complete substance abuse treatment. Combining alcohol and street drugs with psychotropic medication prescribed for youths' mental health disorder can result in physiologically harmful, and potentially lethal, consequences.

- Most clinicians are cautious about prescribing psychotropic medications with high addictive potential to juveniles with alcohol and drug use disorders. However, if clinicians decide to prescribe one of these types of medications, even on a short-term basis, youth should be closely monitored.

- Some substance abuse treatment providers, agencies or support groups may not approve of youth with co-occurring disorders taking psychotropic medication. This situation can be confusing for juveniles and can result in medication compliance issues.

Enhancing Motivation

There are a variety of reasons why youth may not be motivated to engage in treatment for their co-occurring mental health and substance use disorders. Some juveniles with co-occurring disorders do not see their mental health symptoms and/or substance use as problematic. Or some youth may be willing to admit they have difficulties in one area but not in the other. In addition, many juvenile offenders with co-occurring disorders have already experienced either the mental health or substance abuse treatment systems. Some of these youth have long histories with both systems. Although their experiences vary, most juvenile offenders with co-occurring disorders do not describe previous mental health and substance abuse interventions in encouraging terms. Previous treatment outcomes were often short-lived or never realized. Motivational enhancement strategies such as "Motivational Interviewing" can be helpful when treatment providers work with this often challenging and multifaceted population of juveniles (Miller and Rollnick, 1991). *(Please see Chapter 14 for additional information about Motivational Interviewing.)*

Case Example

Enrique, 16, was brought to a detention facility after being arrested for trespassing. Enrique and his two friends had climbed onto the roofs of several houses in the neighborhood and were yelling obscenities into their neighbors' chimneys. Getting into trouble for these types of activities is not uncommon for Enrique. He has been arrested numerous times on charges related to trespassing, malicious mischief and disturbing the peace. Enrique's mother feels helpless and unable to control her son's behavior. She has always described him as a "handful" and says "he was hyperactive from the day I brought him home from the hospital."

Enrique was diagnosed with Attention-Deficit/Hyperactivity Disorder and prescribed Ritalin from the ages of 6 to 12. Enrique refused to take his Ritalin or any prescribed medication once he turned 13 because he did not want to be seen as a "wimp" at school. As he entered his teenage years, Enrique began experimenting with marijuana and eventually became a daily user. His grades began to slip, and he started to skip class. At the age of 15, Enrique was exposed to methamphetamine at a party. He liked the way he felt when he took it and began using it several times a month or more. When Enrique and his friends "get hyped up on meth," they usually run around the neighborhood causing trouble. Enrique's father is a practicing alcoholic and does not see a problem with the boys' "just having some fun."

CHAPTER 11

Suicidal Behavior Among Juvenile Offenders

"So many of these kids threaten suicide for attention, it's hard to know who to believe."

Juvenile Correction Officer

Stefan, 15, had been becoming increasingly depressed and agitated during his stay at the juvenile detention facility. Stefan had been arrested on numerous occasions, but he never remained in the detention facility for more than a few days at a time. Given the serious nature of his current charge, Stefan was afraid that the judge was going to commit him to the state juvenile justice system.

He was particularly afraid of being sentenced to the training school where the "big boys" go. He had heard stories from his peers that being threatened, intimidated, beaten and raped at the training school was common—especially for someone who had never been there before. Stefan decided he would rather die than live in that "hell." He tried to hang himself with a sheet in his room after everyone went to bed.

Suicide is the third leading cause of death among individuals between the ages of 15-24 (Centers for Disease Control, 1997) and is a national health care problem. Currently, no national data are available on the extent of suicidal behavior among incarcerated youth. However, national studies of adult prisoners found that the annual rate of suicide in prisons was double the rate of suicide for the general population (Hayes, 1995; Hayes & Rowan, 1988). The rate within jails was nine times higher! Even without national research data on juvenile offenders, most juvenile justice professionals would agree that suicidal behavior is a

significant issue within juvenile justice facilities. There are two types of staff members working directly with youth in juvenile justice facilities: those who have encountered suicidal youth and those who will.

One study looking at suicidal behavior in a juvenile detention population found a high degree of suicidal behavior in the histories of these youth. More than one-third (34 percent) of the juveniles had thought about killing themselves at some point in their lives, and 14 percent had thought about killing themselves within the past week. Almost one-fifth (19 percent) of the juveniles had made at least one suicide attempt, and 10 percent of the youth reported making two or more suicide attempts (Rhode, Seeley, & Mace, 1997).

Another study found that 21 percent of juvenile offenders had had contact with an inpatient hospital, 21 percent had made suicidal threats, and 13.5 percent had engaged in actual suicidal behaviors by trying to hang, drown, poison or strangle themselves (Davis, Bean, Schumacher & Stringer, 1991). Other studies also have found high rates of previous suicidal behavior among youth involved with the juvenile justice system (Alessi, McManus, Brickman, & Grapentine, 1984; Dembo, et al., 1990).

The Office of Juvenile Justice and Delinquency Prevention (OJJDP) published a report on various conditions of confinement within juvenile justice facilities (Parent, Leiter, Kennedy, Livens, Wentworth, & Wilcox, 1994). Lower rates of suicidal behavior were found within facilities that trained their staff in suicide prevention, as well as within facilities that conducted suicide screening at admission. Rates of suicidal behavior increased for youth who were housed in isolation. When different types of juvenile justice facilities were compared, juvenile *detention* centers had the highest number of youth suicidal behaviors. Reception centers had the next highest rate, followed by training schools and then ranches. The higher number of suicidal behaviors among detention and reception centers may reflect the fact that youth residing in these types of facilities are often admitted directly off the street (immediately upon arrest). Being arrested and brought to a juvenile detention/reception facility can be stressful for youth—particularly if they have never spent time in one of these types of facilities before. Juveniles residing in detention facilities are often:

- Fearful about what is going to happen to them

- Unclear about how long they will remain in the facility

- Confused about the social norms in a juvenile correctional environment

- Intoxicated and/or high on drugs

In contrast, when youth transfer from short-term detention facilities to longer-term residential facilities (*e.g.*, training schools, camps, ranches), the situation is usually different. Youth typically:

- Have a fairly good idea of how much time they are going to spend at a facility

- Have abstained from drugs and alcohol during the time they were in detention

- Have some familiarity with juvenile justice settings, even if only through the brief time they spent in a detention center

Although juveniles typically engage in fewer suicidal behaviors in long-term residential facilities versus short-term detention centers, youth in training schools—and other long-term juvenile justice programs— can still be at high risk for suicide.

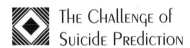 The Challenge of Suicide Prediction

Accurately predicting which youth will and will not commit suicide is a difficult and complex task. Although suicide among adolescents is a significant problem, it is still a fairly infrequent act, which makes it difficult to study and predict. In addition, much of the research done on youth suicide has been weak methodologically, which makes drawing firm conclusions from the results difficult. To better understand what leads up to suicidal behavior, some studies investigate suicide "completers" (juveniles whose suicidal behavior has resulted in death) by reviewing these youths' medical records and talking with significant people in the youths' life. However, it is not clear whether juveniles who *complete* suicide are the same as juveniles who *attempt* suicide. Additionally, the reliability of retrospective information from medical records/third parties is also an issue. In fact, retrospective information may not even be accurate when juvenile suicide attempters are asked what led up to their own suicidal behavior. Youths' memory of their thoughts, feelings and behaviors prior to a suicide attempt may or may not reflect what was truly going on at that time.

One of the main reasons retrospective investigations are conducted on suicide attempters and suicide completers is to determine which risk factors are prevalent among this population of youth. Risk factors can help determine which juveniles are at *high risk* for suicide, but they cannot predict whether an individual youth will or will not become suicidal (Hughes, 1995). Many youth in the general population possess risk factors for suicide, but most of them will never try to kill themselves.

Risk Factors for Suicide

A variety of risk factors consistently have been found to be associated with suicidal behavior among adolescents. When working with youth who have any of the risk factors below, juvenile justice professionals should be alert to the possibility of suicidal behavior.

PREVIOUS SUICIDAL BEHAVIOR

Adolescents who have made some type of suicide attempt in the past are at higher risk to make another suicide attempt in the future. Whether juveniles' previous suicide attempt involved overdosing on pills, cutting their wrists, running in front of a car or attempting to hang themselves does not matter. Any type of previous suicide attempt places youth at higher risk for another suicide attempt. In general, females tend to have higher rates of suicide attempts, whereas males tend to have higher rates of completed suicides (those that actually result in death).

When asked whether they have ever thought about suicide, many juvenile offenders reply, "Everybody thinks about killing themselves." Some adolescents, particularly those involved with the juvenile justice system, think about

what it would be like to be dead. At times, some of these youth even wish they were dead. However, vague thoughts about death and dying are very different from detailed thoughts about killing oneself (*i.e.,* incarcerated youth who plan to hang themselves with their bed sheet during the overnight shift when there are fewer staff members on duty). Thinking about suicide is also very different from youth taking specific actions to purposely end their lives, such as: swallowing a bottle of pills, cutting their wrist or strangling themselves with their tee shirt. Suicidal thoughts with a specific plan, as well as previous suicide attempts, are both very strong predictors of future suicide attempts (Berman & Jobes, 1994; Shafii, Carrigan, Whittinghill, & Derrick, 1985).

Actual suicide attempts are not common and are not a normal part of adolescence. Juveniles may state that their previous suicidal behavior was done solely to obtain attention from significant people in their lives (*e.g.,* family members, juvenile justice professionals, peers, romantic partner). Even so, the behavior is still an important risk factor for future suicidal behaviors. There is no way to know the true motivation of youth during a previous suicide attempt. Furthermore, juvenile offenders can use a variety of behaviors to get attention from others. Youth who choose suicidal behavior as a method to gain attention should always be assessed by a mental health professional. All forms of suicidal behavior can be indicative of a mental health disorder and increase youths' risk of a completed suicide. Therefore, all suicide attempts in juveniles' histories should be explored and evaluated.

SUBSTANCE ABUSE

A significant percentage of youth who have made suicide attempts, including youth who have died as a result of these attempts, have problems with drug and alcohol abuse. In fact, many juveniles are intoxicated at the time they attempt to kill themselves (Berman & Jobes, 1994; Brent *et al.*, 1987). Alcohol is a depressant,

Juvenile Offenders with Mental Health Disorders: Who Are They and What Do We Do With Them?

and barbiturates and tranquilizers can also have a depressant effect. If youth are already feeling hopeless and sad, their depressed feelings can be intensified when drinking alcohol or using depressant types of drugs. In addition, alcohol and other drugs can reduce juveniles' inhibitions. If youth were contemplating suicide while sober, they may be more willing to take action to end their lives while intoxicated or high, due to feeling less inhibited.

MENTAL HEALTH DISORDERS

The majority of youth who make a suicide attempt suffer from at least one mental health disorder (Brent, Perper, Goldstein, *et al.,* 1988). The most common disorders found among youth at risk for suicide are mood disorders (*e.g.,* Major Depression, Bipolar Disorder), personality disorders (*e.g.,* Borderline Personality Disorder), and Conduct Disorder. Juveniles suffering from Major Depression are likely to have a negative and pessimistic view of themselves and their current situation, as well as their future. When depressed adolescents feel hopeless and perceive their current negative situation as never changing, they may view suicide as the only viable solution to their problems. Juveniles who suffer from a mood disorder, Conduct Disorder *and* a co-occurring Substance Abuse Disorder may be at particularly high risk for suicide (Shaffer, *et al.,* 1996). This particular combination of serious disorders is not uncommon among incarcerated youth, placing many of these juveniles at high risk for suicidal behavior.

AGGRESSIVE AND VIOLENT BEHAVIOR

The juvenile justice system is filled with aggressive and violent youth, and juveniles at high risk for hurting others are also at high risk for hurting themselves. In fact, many suicidal youth experience homicidal ideation the week before they kill themselves (Brent *et al.,* 1993). A considerable number of suicidal youth within juvenile justice facilities have long histories of aggression. Some of these youth may have even been assaultive toward staff or peers during incarceration. Most juvenile justice professionals do not view violent and aggressive youth as significant suicide risks. Instead, these professionals are more likely to consider sad and withdrawn youth to be most in need of emotional support and close monitoring for suicidal behavior. This assumption is dangerous and potentially lethal. The risk for a suicide attempt can be just as high for aggressive, assaultive and violent youth as it is for withdrawn youth expressing tears. Aggressive, violent youth may also be in need of emotional support and close monitoring for suicidal behavior.

FAMILY FACTORS

Parental psychopathology, including mood disorders, substance abuse and antisocial behavior, are common among juveniles who have made suicide attempts (Brent & Perper, 1995). Youths' increased risk of suicide may be associated with a genetic, biological vulnerability to mental health disorders. Suicide runs in families regardless of the type of psychiatric diagnosis youths' parents may have. Or youths' increased risk may be associated with environmental factors related to being raised by a parent with a mental health disorder (*e.g.,* family disorganization, poor parental supervision). High rates of conflict, parental absence, negative communication patterns, rigidity, and a lack of support within the family have also been linked to adolescent suicide.

In addition, being exposed to suicidal behavior (attempted or completed suicide) by parents, siblings or relatives places juveniles at higher risk of committing suicide themselves. Even having a parent or relative think about or threaten suicide can increase youths' suicide risk (Shafii, Carrigan, Whittinghill, and Derrick, 1985). Why exposure to suicidal behavior among family members increases juveniles' own risk of killing themselves is unclear. If a suicidal family member suffers from a mood disorder, youth may inherit a biological predisposition to also suffer from a mood disorder. In addition, being exposed to suicidal behavior in their family may suggest to youth that suicidal behavior is an acceptable way to deal with problems and difficult situations. Either way, exposure to suicide among family members increases the likelihood that juveniles will view suicide as an option for themselves if they are distressed.

POOR SOCIAL SKILLS/FEW FRIENDS

Having poor social skills or few friends can place youth at higher risk for making a suicide attempt. Juveniles who have died from suicide attempts have been described as "loners," "bizarre," "withdrawn," "lonely," "supersensitive," "angry" and "impulsive" (Ladely & Puskar, 1994). If they are isolated and tend to withdraw from others, youth may not have many people in their lives to whom they can turn during difficult times. Some juveniles who do have a support system have never developed the skills to reach out and inform significant others about their distress and need for assistance. In addition, parents, teachers, peers and juvenile justice professionals may not be as motivated to comfort, assist, or provide emotional support to youth who are angry and impulsive—or who act unusual and strange. Each of these factors can result in suicidal youth feeling increasingly isolated and alone.

STRESSFUL EVENTS

Stressful life events also have been associated with suicidal behavior among juveniles, and interpersonal conflict is one of the most significant stressors related to youth suicide (Marttunen, 1994). Interpersonal conflict among juveniles often includes:

- Arguing with parents or other significant adults

- Breaking up with a girlfriend/boyfriend

- Experiencing change in relationships with peers

Other stressful events linked to adolescent suicidal behavior include (Ladely & Puskar, 1994):

- School suspension

- Recent sexual assault

- Recent change in school

- Suicidal behavior by someone known to youth

- Significant harassment of gay and lesbian youth by peers

Most professionals working closely with juvenile offenders are aware that many of these youth have experienced significant stressors during their lifetime—with some youth experiencing severe and traumatic events. Many juvenile offenders have been physically or sexually abused, and their homes may be filled with domestic violence and parental substance abuse. A significant number of these youth live in dangerous communities where physical assaults, prostitution and shootings are common. In addition, many juvenile offenders have been suspended or expelled from school, and some of them have dropped out completely.

Incarceration can be stressful and frightening for some juveniles. Separation from friends, family and other significant supports in youths' lives can be difficult for adolescents. Not knowing what is going to occur legally or how much time they will spend in a juvenile justice facility also can be anxiety-provoking. However, being told what *is* going to happen can be just as stressful—particularly if juveniles are told that they must remain in a facility for a significant period of time or that they have received new legal charges.

Peers in a living unit can also create stress, especially when they are physically large and aggressive. Juvenile offenders typically share very small living quarters with a number of youth with whom they may not get along. Many youth fear for their physical safety during incarceration and may be too afraid to sleep at night. In addition, some juvenile offenders experience the presence of juvenile justice staff members as stressful. Most of these youth are not accustomed to a structured and authoritarian atmosphere, and some staff members can be

196

Juvenile Offenders with Mental Health Disorders: Who Are They and What Do We Do With Them?

confrontational and demanding. Constantly being told what to do, how to do it, and when to do it can be very difficult for some of these juveniles. *(Please see Chapter 1 for additional information about the stress of incarceration.)*

Not all incarcerated youth find juvenile justice facilities stressful. There is a small subset of youth who do not mind being incarcerated and on some level feel "at home" in an institutional environment. Some of these youth have been to a particular juvenile justice facility several times and have developed relationships with certain staff members. Other youth are happy to have three hot meals, a shower and a bed. A number of youth feel safer in juvenile justice facilities than the neighborhoods in which they reside. Moreover, it is not unusual for some of the juveniles' relatives and friends to reside at the same facility as the youth.

Even if a juvenile correctional environment itself is not stressful for youth, just being removed from the community can have stress-producing repercussions. For example, some juveniles have had their cars or belongings stolen or sold by family members while the youth were incarcerated. Girlfriends/boyfriends of youthful offenders have ended their romantic relationship with incarcerated youth (or become romantically/sexually involved with someone new) due to prolonged physical separation.

While locked up, some juveniles have heard by telephone that their parent overdosed on drugs or was assaulted/killed by a stepparent. Other youth have been informed that their best friend was severely beaten by a rival gang member or shot by an unknown assailant. Feelings of guilt, shame, helplessness and frustration can arise in juveniles who are incarcerated during a period when significant others are harmed. These youth often have thoughts such as, "I should've been there," "I could've done something," or "This wouldn't have happened if I wasn't locked up." These types of thoughts and the associated guilt can remain with juveniles for weeks, months or even years.

Stressful life events do not necessarily need

to be as serious as the incidents just mentioned. In fact, what is perceived as a stressful event to youth may not seem like cause for major concern to those around them. Juveniles and the staff who work with them frequently have different views regarding the significance of certain events. In fact, two different youth can perceive the significance of an incident very differently.

Youths' *perception* of an event is critical when assessing stressors and juveniles' risk of suicide. For example, juvenile offenders have made suicide attempts after hearing that their girlfriend/boyfriend began dating someone else. Other young offenders have become suicidal when they were told that they must remain in a juvenile detention facility for one or two nights versus being immediately released. Adults know that adolescents have numerous girlfriends/boyfriends throughout their teen years and that broken-hearted youth are likely to have a new romantic interest within weeks. And juvenile justice professionals often do not regard youth having to remain in detention for one or two nights as a major event—particularly in comparison to the many youth who remain in detention for weeks or months at a time.

Regardless, adolescent offenders may think that their current situation is the absolute worst thing which has ever happened to them. They may view the situation as a "crisis" that is going to ruin their entire lives. Some juvenile offenders have stated, "If I can't be with my girlfriend/boyfriend, I don't want to live," or "I can't stay overnight in this facility. I would rather be dead than have to spend the night here." At the moment they make these types of statements, juveniles may actually feel that strongly about their situation. At the time, some of these youth believe that being dead is better than enduring the suffering they are experiencing or the suffering they anticipate experiencing.

Juvenile justice professionals should be careful not to place their own value judgments on what is or is not stressful for youth. For example, James, a 16-year-old juvenile incarcerated at a juvenile detention center, repeatedly complained about his lack of privacy at the facility. He told the staff that his roommate was "bugging" him and that he could not stand sharing such a small room with someone else. James became increasingly agitated and withdrawn over the following two weeks and continued to complain about his roommate situation, saying he "couldn't take it anymore." Juvenile justice staff viewed James' complaint as typical and did not perceive his situation as serious or in need of any action. In fact, they told him he was "acting like a baby" and that he "needed to pull it together." James asked to stay behind when the rest of the unit went to the gymnasium to play basketball and attempted to hang himself in his room. Fortunately, a staff member happened to check in on him and intervened before James suffered any serious injury. The staff perceived James's roommate situation as understandably annoying and not unusual given a correctional environment. But for James, the situation was too stressful to bear.

These risk factors repeatedly have been shown to be associated with increased risk for youth suicide. Anyone who works with juvenile offenders can think of at least one youth who has one or two of the risk factors listed above. Most juvenile justice professionals can think of multiple youth who have three, four or even five risk factors for suicidal behavior. For example, it is not unusual to find juvenile offenders who:

- Have little to no contact with their father
- Argue continually with their mother and siblings
- Have been diagnosed with Conduct Disorder
- Abuse alcohol and/or marijuana
- Are angry and assaultive
- Lack adaptive social skills
- Have a history of academic problems
- Have numerous school suspensions

These youth may also be depressed, and they commonly experience interpersonal conflict with juvenile justice staff during incarceration.

Given what is known about risk factors associated with youth suicide, we can safely say that many (if not most) juvenile offenders—particularly incarcerated youth—are at high risk for suicidal behavior. However, that does not necessarily imply that all juvenile offenders will try to kill themselves. In fact, despite having several risk factors, most youth involved with juvenile justice do *not* engage in suicidal behavior. This situation makes identifying those youth who will make an actual suicide attempt even more complex. It is important for juvenile justice professionals to be aware of youths' risk factors, document these risk factors, and consider them when making decisions about juveniles' risk for suicide.

A critical aspect of suicide prevention among juvenile offenders is to undertake extra precautions with those youth who are the *highest* risk for suicide within this very high-risk population. Juvenile justice professionals should be most concerned with youth who are an *imminent* suicide risk: those youth who are *currently* suicidal. Special safety measures should be taken for juveniles who are planning to kill themselves, threatening to kill themselves, and/or engaging in suicidal behavior. However, staff also should continue keeping a close eye on the other youth in their care, in case one of them becomes imminently suicidal.

Although many juvenile offenders have several significant risk factors for suicidal behavior, putting all of them on "suicide precautions"/"suicide watch" (increased level of observation and monitoring) is not practical. Doing so also is unnecessary because not all youth with suicide risk factors require intensive supervision and programming restrictions. The vast majority of juvenile offenders do not make a suicide attempt. However, because a small minority of these youth does try to end their lives, staff need to be aware that at any time, any one of

Juvenile Offenders with Mental Health Disorders: Who Are They and What Do We Do With Them?

the youth under their care could try to kill themselves. Only worrying about sad and withdrawn juveniles who are crying in the corner of a living unit is dangerous (and potentially lethal). Being concerned solely with young offenders who publicly announce that they are going to kill themselves is also a mistake. Juvenile justice professionals need to be just as concerned about depressed youth who do not talk about their suicidal thoughts—as well as angry and aggressive youth who repeatedly get into fights. These youth may be just as likely to make a serious suicide attempt as youth who appear more obviously distressed.

 ## Common Misconceptions About Suicide

There are many misconceptions about youth suicide, including:

MISCONCEPTION:
- Juvenile justice professionals should avoid talking directly about the topic of suicide with juvenile offenders. If youth were already thinking about killing themselves, talking about it might upset them and cause them to actually do it. If youth were not already thinking about suicide, talking about it might put the idea in their heads.

REALITY:
- An important part of reducing youths' risk of harming themselves is to discuss the issue of suicide directly and openly with them. Most juveniles feel relieved after talking about their suicidal thoughts and feelings with someone they trust.

MISCONCEPTION:
- Suicidal adolescents always want to die.

REALITY:
- Many suicidal adolescents experience unbearable psychological pain and/or want to escape from an intolerably

stressful situation. Some suicidal youth have been dealing with a difficult problem(s) for a long time and do not want to think about or deal with it anymore. Some juveniles may be focused on wanting others to feel guilty or sad if the youth die. Other juveniles are aware that engaging in suicidal behavior may help them secure certain resources within a facility. Even if they are motivated to escape emotional pain or a stressful situation, many juveniles do not fully grasp the notion of the finality of death.

MISCONCEPTION:
- Juveniles who are serious about killing themselves always have a detailed plan as to how they will commit suicide.

REALITY:
- Many youth who make serious suicide attempts develop specific plans regarding how they are going to end their lives. However, some juveniles make impulsive suicide attempts with little forethought as to how they are going to do it. Juveniles' decision to kill themselves may be made only moments before they engage in suicidal behavior.

MISCONCEPTION:
- Improvement in a youth's mood is a good way to determine when a suicidal crisis is over.

REALITY:
- Some depressed youth will make a suicide attempt once they start feeling better and actually have the energy to carry out their suicide plan. In addition, if youth are ambivalent about killing themselves, they may experience relief and an improvement in mood once they make a final decision to go through with it.

MISCONCEPTION:
- Suicidal behavior among adolescents is typically caused by one issue or event.

REALITY:

- A suicide attempt may appear to be the direct result of a certain incident or issue. However, suicidal behavior among juveniles is complex and typically related to the interaction of a variety of factors in youths' lives. There may be one incident that serves as the "last straw," but suicidal youth usually have various stressors in their histories or associated with their current situation.

MISCONCEPTION:

- Suicidal behavior among youth typically happens without warning.

REALITY:

- Most suicidal youth provide warnings and clues about being suicidal. Many juveniles tell at least one person that they are thinking about killing themselves (*e.g.*, peer, family member, teacher, mental health professional, juvenile justice professional). Some youth express their suicidal thoughts in poetry or artwork.

MISCONCEPTION:

- If juvenile offenders really want to kill themselves, there is nothing anyone can do about it.

REALITY:

- Most suicides in juvenile justice facilities are prevented. There is a great deal juvenile justice professionals can do to prevent youth from ending their lives.

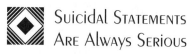 Suicidal Statements
Are Always Serious

Juvenile justice professionals must take seriously all suicidal statements made by juveniles. Even if staff members perceive youth as being "manipulative" and/or "trying to get attention," juveniles' statements related to killing themselves should be taken seriously. Figuring out why particular youth are threatening suicide or

engaging in suicidal behavior can be difficult. Juvenile justice professionals should avoid making determinations about youths' motivation for suicidal behavior and instead focus on the actual suicidal behavior itself. The notion that juveniles are trying to avoid having to do their chores is less important than the fact that they tried to strangle themselves with their t-shirt. It is not unusual for incarcerated youth to be sent to their room for brief periods of time as a sanction for negative behavior. These juveniles may shout out to staff, "If you send me to my room, I'm going to kill myself." Staff may conclude, perhaps correctly, that the youth are attempting to avoid being sent to their room. However, these juveniles may still try to kill themselves once inside their room.

Adolescent offenders are typically not very good at judging which behaviors will result in death and which behaviors will not. Youth who want to "scare" staff may tie something around their neck, attach it to something on the wall or ceiling in their room, and start to hang themselves. These juveniles may expect a staff member to check on them before anything dangerous happens. Many young offenders are unaware that this type of behavior can result in brain damage and/or death in as quickly as a matter of minutes. Along the same lines, most juveniles do not know how many pills or what type of pills it takes to scare significant others versus truly overdose. And most youth are not aware of exactly what type of cut they should make or how deeply they should cut their wrists, in order to die versus solely gain the attention of those around them. Youth who do not purposely intend to kill themselves still can end up dead accidentally.

In addition, many youth within the juvenile justice system are impulsive and do not appreciate the long-term negative consequences of suicidal behavior. Impulsive juvenile offenders who are extremely angry with staff—or who feel rejected/emotionally hurt by a staff member—may make a suicide attempt to "pay staff back." Impulsive youth often do not

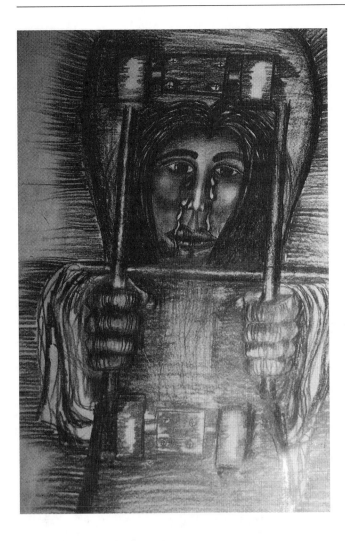

realize the finality of death. In the moment, these juveniles are not thinking about how their lives would completely end if they died. They often do not consider that they would never see their friends, family or girlfriend/ boyfriend again. Instead, these youth can become totally preoccupied with how they can most effectively impact the staff, making them "pay" for what they have done to the youth.

This combination of impulsivity and an intense focus on retaliation can significantly interfere with youths' realization that their suicidal behavior will be most harmful to themselves. These youth can make a serious, and potentially deadly, suicide attempt in a matter of minutes. Therefore, *all statements of suicidal behavior should be taken seriously.* Regardless of youths' intention or motive, their behavior could result in death.

When juvenile offenders engage in suicidal behavior, they are trying to meet some need. This need could be related to ending unbearable psychological distress, escaping an intolerable situation, trying to influence juvenile justice professionals' behavior, and so forth. Distinguishing between juveniles who are "serious" about suicide versus those who are "manipulative" or "attention-seeking" is difficult and can be dangerous. Juveniles have a variety of ways to elicit attention and/or influence staff behavior other than making suicidal statements or engaging in a suicide attempt. Youth who choose this type of behavior to meet their needs always should be evaluated by a mental health professional. Once youth are evaluated, a specific treatment plan should be developed that takes into account the particular issues and unmet needs (*e.g.*, ending emotional pain, wanting increased contact with staff) that are relevant to individual youth.

 ## The Continuum of Suicidal Behavior

Suicide is a *behavior.* Similar to many other behaviors, it can be viewed as occurring on a continuum. The continuum of suicidal behavior ranges from mildly serious to extremely serious.

Suicidal Ideation	Suicidal Ideation With Plan	Suicide Attempt	Completed Suicide
Mildly Serious	Moderately Serious	Extremely Serious	

Suicidal Ideation

Before youth make a suicide attempt, they typically have some type of thought about wanting to be dead and/or wanting to kill themselves. These thoughts may occur weeks, months or years before the youth take any action to harm themselves. For some juveniles, these thoughts may occur only a few moments before the youth make a suicide attempt. Although many youth involved with juvenile justice do not think about suicide, a significant number of them do. And some of these youth think about killing themselves while incarcerated. Examples of suicidal ideation include:

- "I wish I were dead"
- "I just want to go to sleep and never wake up"
- "I want to kill myself"
- "I want to die"

Suicidal juvenile offenders may ask staff or peers numerous questions about death or what happens after someone dies. Thoughts about death and dying may also be evident in youths' writings and/or drawings.

Suicidal Ideation with a Plan

Although a considerable number of juvenile offenders have vague or passing thoughts about suicide, having a well thought out plan as to how they would kill themselves is much less common. Juveniles who have thought about the details as to how they would end their lives are likely to be a higher risk for a suicide attempt—versus youth with only vague thoughts about death and dying. Examples of suicidal ideation with a plan include:

- "I'm thinking about hanging myself with a t-shirt in my room."
- "I'm going to save up all of my psychiatric medication and take it all at once."
- "I'm going to cut my wrist with a fork that I will steal from the cafeteria."

Finding out how much detail is included in youths' suicide plan is important. This information helps determine juveniles' level of risk for suicide and can influence how staff monitor the youths' behavior in a juvenile justice facility. Juvenile justice professionals should be concerned about any youth with suicidal ideation, particularly when their thoughts are accompanied with a specific plan. Staff concern should increase as the details of youths' suicide plan become clearer. Juveniles with a detailed suicide plan are likely to be a higher suicide risk

than youth with vague ideas related to killing themselves. Examples of a detailed suicide plan include:

- "I'm going to hang myself with my sheet during the overnight shift when I know the staff only checks us every twenty minutes."
- "I have been saving up my antidepressant medication for the last two weeks and am planning on taking all of it this weekend when I know the doctor will not be here."

Keep in mind that these are guidelines—given the difficulty in predicting suicide among youth, there is no guaranteed way to know which juveniles will or will not make a suicide attempt.

Suicide Attempt

Most individuals refer to a suicide attempt as any behavior youth engage in with the intent of trying to end their lives/kill themselves. Death may seem like the only option to youth who are hopeless and depressed, and who want to escape excruciating psychological pain or a very stressful situation. However, some youth engage in what appears to be suicidal behavior (*i.e.*, self-inflicted behavior that could result in death), even though ending their lives is not their intent at all.

As mentioned earlier, juvenile offenders may attempt to hang themselves or overdose on their psychiatric medication as a way to influence staff behavior. However, youths' ability to distinguish a toxic from a nontoxic dose of medication, or determining how long they can survive with something around their neck tends to be poor. Death can result in either of these situations, regardless of youths' intent. Therefore, regardless of youths' underlying motivation, these types of behavior should be considered suicide attempts. In juvenile justice facilities, suicide attempts could include, but are not limited to:

- Hanging themselves with a sheet, t-shirt or shoelaces

Juvenile Offenders with Mental Health Disorders: Who Are They and What Do We Do With Them?

- Cutting their wrists
- Taking large amounts of pills/medication
- Drinking shampoo/soap
- Submerging their head in a toilet in an attempt to drown themselves
- Diving off the upper bunk of a bed onto a cement floor
- Choking themselves with a sheet, blanket, t-shirt, underwear or bra
- Trying to suffocate themselves by placing plastic trashcan liners over their heads

---

WhEN dOCUMENTiNG suicidAl bEhAvior, sTAFF shOUld rECOrd youThs' ACTIONs ANd Avoid mAkiNG dETERMiNATIONs AbOUT ThEir MOTIVATION (E.G., youTh iNTENdEd TO diE, youTh wERE TRyiNG TO GET ATTENTION, youTh WANTEd TO Avoid COMplETiNG A TAsk).

- Swallowing cleaning supplies

There are numerous methods youth can use within juvenile justice facilities if they want to kill themselves. Tear-resistant blankets have been purchased by several facilities. But some youth have found a way to rip these blankets and tie them around their neck in an attempt to die. There are also a variety of ways that juveniles can gather a potentially lethal quantity of medication, which they can use to overdose. Some youth save the psychiatric medication prescribed for them by not swallowing their pills ("cheeking") for several days or weeks. Other juveniles are able to obtain psychiatric medication from their peers who are willing to help them commit suicide. Some juveniles request daily doses of nonprescription aspirin/pain reliever in order to save them and take them all at once. Even when they are placed in a room where there is no access to sharp materials, youth always can try to choke themselves

with their clothing, bang their head against the wall, or dive head first off of their bed onto a cement floor. Most juvenile justice facilities have taken precautions and safeguards to remove sprinkler heads from the ceilings of the rooms where youth are housed. Many have also removed any protruding objects in youths' cells and/or suicide-resistant rooms so that youth are unable to access anything from which to tie a sheet, blanket or t-shirt to hang themselves. If a facility has not taken these precautions, they should do so immediately.

Completed Suicide

A completed suicide occurs when juveniles' suicide attempt results in death. A significant number of juvenile justice professionals have intervened with youth who have made a suicide attempt. However, only a small group have been involved with youth whose suicide attempt actually resulted in death. A completed suicide can be a devastating and profoundly emotional experience for staff, the other youth in a facility—and for a juvenile justice facility as a whole.

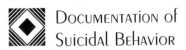 DOCUMENTATION of Suicidal BEhAvior

Documentation within the juvenile justice system is critical. Documentation related to juveniles' suicidal behavior should be similar to the documentation of any other type of juvenile behavior (*e.g.*, aggressive behavior, escape behavior, sexual behavior). When documenting suicidal behavior, staff should record youths' *actions* and avoid making determinations about their *motivation* (*e.g.*, youth intended to die, youth were trying to get attention, youth wanted to avoid completing a task). The suicide-related terms mentioned above (*i.e.*, suicidal ideation, suicidal ideation with a plan, suicide attempt, completed suicide) or similar terms should be used to describe youths' actions. These objective behavioral descriptions facilitate communication because all staff reading the records know what is being conveyed. Documentation should be specific, such as:

- "Brian is expressing suicidal ideation."
- "Cassandra has suicidal ideation with a plan to kill herself by cutting her wrist with glass from her eyeglasses."
- "Shawn was found climbing on top of his sink with a sheet around his neck."

Behavioral observations related to youths' depression, irritability or aggression should also be documented. Documentation related to suicidal behavior should focus on what is *factual* and *observable*, not what the staff *think* or *feel* is occurring with suicidal juveniles. Comments about youth being manipulative or engaging in suicidal behavior for attention should not be documented because there are no means to determine whether this information is accurate.

In addition, documenting words such as "attention," "manipulation," and suicide "gesture" can result in some juvenile justice professionals not taking seriously the behavior of suicidal youth. Documentation is one of the most important ways to inform staff on all shifts about which juveniles need to be monitored closely and why. It also provides critical information to clinicians who evaluate and help develop intervention strategies for suicidal youth. *(Please see Chapter 4 for additional information about Major Depression.)*

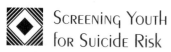 Screening Youth for Suicide Risk

Many youth within the juvenile justice system possess several of the known risk factors for suicide and often experience multiple stressors, legal and otherwise. Therefore, all staff working directly with juvenile offenders should be able to screen youths' risk for suicide. *This is not to imply that juvenile justice professionals should be responsible for making determinations regarding which youth should receive intensive monitoring and/or be placed in suicide-resistant rooms.* But juvenile justice professionals (particularly line staff within juvenile justice facilities) are often the primary individuals who refer suicidal

juveniles to mental health/medical professionals for an evaluation, as well as intensive monitoring and special housing decisions.

All youth exhibiting suicidal behavior (statements or actions) should be referred to a mental health/medical professional for a more in-depth suicide assessment. To make appropriate referrals, juvenile justice staff need to be able to identify which youth are at high risk for killing themselves. Further, staff need to be especially able to identify and refer juvenile offenders who are an *imminent* suicide risk: those youth who are currently suicidal and in need of immediate intervention.

Unfortunately, there is no surefire way for juvenile justice professionals to know *exactly* which youth will or will not make a suicide attempt. However, focusing on the following four areas can help staff better identify youths' risk for suicidal behavior in order to help determine which juveniles need to be referred to a mental health/medical professional:

- Observable behaviors
- Youths' history
- Interview with youth
- Institutional hazards/safeguards

Observable Behaviors

Juvenile offenders do not always talk to juvenile justice professionals about their thoughts of suicide; some youth may even deny having such thoughts when directly asked about suicidal ideation. Therefore, relying on cues from youths' behavior for indications of suicide risk is critical for staff.

Staff should pay close attention to the following list of observable behaviors because they may indicate that juveniles are at risk for suicidal behavior. Displaying only one of these behaviors is not enough to indicate suicide risk by itself. However, exhibiting a combination of these behaviors could indicate that youth are at high risk for killing themselves.

- Sad/depressed mood
- Increased irritability

204

Juvenile Offenders with Mental Health Disorders: Who Are They and What Do We Do With Them?

- Diminished interest/pleasure in activities they used to enjoy
- Complaints of fatigue/feeling tired all of the time
- Excessive levels of guilt or shame
- Difficulty concentrating or making decisions
- No emotion or apathy
- Threatening behavior/aggression
- Restless or agitated behavior
- Very slow speech or behavior
- Lack of appetite or overeating
- Sleeping too much or too little

Issues in Youths' History That Could Indicate Suicide Risk

Exploring their history is an important part of gathering information regarding youths' risk for suicide. If their history contains one of the following factors, juveniles are not necessarily an imminent suicide risk. However, the more risk factors youth have in their history, the higher the likelihood that they could engage in serious suicidal behavior.

- Previous suicide attempt
- Knowledge of/exposure to someone else's suicide
- Prior/current psychiatric hospitalization
- Prior/current psychiatric medications
- Multiple traumas
- Impulse and/or mood disorder
- Abuse of drugs and/or alcohol
- Difficulty controlling anger/irritability
- Prior/current psychiatric diagnosis
- Family history of mental illness
- Violent behavior

Interview With Youth

There are a variety of checklists, scales and assessment tools available to assess suicide risk. However, a thorough and carefully conducted interview with juveniles can also provide much of the information needed to determine whether youth are at high risk for suicide. All staff members who work directly with youth in the juvenile justice system should be comfortable asking youth about suicidal thoughts and behavior. Typically, a brief interview (5 to 10 minutes) with youth can provide juvenile justice professionals with enough information to determine whether youth:

- Are an *imminent* suicide risk
- Are in need of a referral to a mental health/medical professional

Being able to conduct a suicide screening in a short period of time is critical because most staff working in juvenile justice facilities are required to monitor and manage numerous offenders simultaneously. Most juvenile justice professionals do not have the luxury of pulling youth aside for an in-depth exploration of the juveniles' motivations, thoughts, beliefs and intentions about suicidal behavior.

If they are concerned that youth may be at high risk for suicide (based on the youths' observable behavior or history), staff should approach the youth and discuss such concerns with them. Staff should express to the juveniles the types of behaviors that have led to their concern (*e.g.*, social withdrawal, not eating, increased irritability, statements about wanting to die). Staff should then ask the youth *directly* if they have been thinking about killing themselves.

If juveniles admit to thinking about suicide, staff should ask the youth if they have thought about how they would go about killing themselves. The goal is to determine whether the youth have only had passing thoughts about suicide—or whether they have thought about it seriously enough to have a plan as to how they would end their lives.

Youth with recent or current thoughts/actions related to suicide should be immediately referred to a mental health/medical professional. If youth report having a plan related to killing themselves, juvenile justice professionals should ask the following questions to help identify the youths' level of risk. This information should be provided to the mental health/medical professional who conducts an evaluation. Unfortunately, some facilities do not have access to a mental health/medical professionals 24-hours-a-day/seven days a week. Collecting additional information about youths' plans can help facility administrators/supervisors develop the best intervention strategy for juveniles—until they can be seen by a mental health/medical professional.

The following acronym can be used to help guide further questioning: **SAL.**

S: SPECIFICITY—How specific is the youths' plan to kill themselves? For example, have the youth decided:

- What method they would use?
- When they would make a suicide attempt?
- Where they would kill themselves?

Staff should gather as much detailed information as possible from youth. As the number of details of youths' plan increases, so does the youths' risk of suicide. In addition, the information gathered should be used to help design an individualized intervention plan for the juveniles.

A: ACCESS—After obtaining details related to youths' suicide plan, juvenile justice professionals need to determine whether juveniles have access to what they need to carry out their plan. Juveniles with a plan to shoot themselves in the head should not have access to a gun while residing in a juvenile justice facility. Youth currently taking psychiatric medication have increased access to pills with which they can overdose. And incarcerated youth who plan to hang themselves most likely have easy access to t-shirts, sheets and blankets. The more access juveniles have to carrying out their plan, the higher their risk of making a suicide attempt.

L: LETHALITY—Lethality refers to how likely it is that youths' plan to kill themselves will actually result in death. For example, taking

three aspirins at one time is not as lethal as taking a 30-day supply of antidepressants at one time. Juveniles' plan to hang themselves in the middle of the "dayroom" during a group activity is not as lethal as a plan to hang themselves in their own room during the overnight shift. The higher the lethality of youths' plan, the more juveniles are at risk for a completed suicide attempt.

After they have obtained the answers to *SAL* from potentially suicidal youth, juvenile justice professionals should try to obtain answers to the following questions, if time allows.

"Have the youth ever made a suicide attempt in the past?"

If yes, follow-up questions should include:

- "When was the last time the youth made a suicide attempt?"
- "What did they do to try to kill themselves?"
- "Was hospitalization required after the suicide attempt?"

"Have they ever thought about suicide and not made an attempt?"

If yes, staff should inquire about:

- "What did the youth do to cope in that situation instead of trying to kill themselves?"

If juvenile justice professionals are comfortable doing so, asking youth if they have any scars or markings from previous suicide attempts can be helpful. Physical scars and markings can sometimes provide additional information about the seriousness of previous suicide attempts.

When inquiring about suicidal thoughts and behavior, juvenile justice professionals should ask questions in a calm, neutral, "matter of fact" tone. All information collected about youths' risk of suicide should be clearly documented and communicated to a supervisor. Youths' answers to the previous questions form the basis of a referral to a mental health/medical professional. These answers also provide critical information to the clinician responsible for evaluating the youth and developing an associated intervention plan.

Interviews with potentially suicidal youth rely heavily on what juveniles choose to disclose. Youth may not feel comfortable sharing the details of their suicidal thoughts, feelings and/or plans with juvenile justice professionals. Or youth may not want to admit to suicidal thoughts or behavior because staff will take action to thwart the youth—which will interfere with their plan to die. Therefore, staff must pay close attention to all four areas of suicide assessment and not rely solely on juveniles' self-report when making decisions about which youth to refer to a mental health/medical professional. That said, most youth (particularly those in emotional pain) will be honest when asked about suicidal thoughts and behavior—especially if the staff members asking the questions are calm, nonjudgmental and genuinely caring.

Sometimes youth deny thoughts about suicide, but staff are still concerned due to the youths' observable behavior and/or history. In these situations, staff should refer the juveniles to a supervisor and/or mental health/medical professional. It is always better to err on the side of caution to ensure youths' safety.

Facility Hazards/Protective Factors

There are a variety of factors related to the way a juvenile justice facility is designed that can either increase or decrease the risk of juvenile offenders making a suicide attempt.

Potential facility *hazards* include, but are not limited to:

- Low number of staff per number of youth requiring supervision
- Over-reliance on isolating/secluding juveniles
- Easily reached protrusions/projections in rooms (*e.g.*, sprinklers, bunk beds, light fixtures, towel racks, door handles)

- Access to psychotropic medication/street drugs
- Cottage/unit layout (*e.g.*, all rooms not in full view, no windows on room doors, long hallways)
- Clothing/uniforms with shoe laces, belts or zippers
- Routine monitoring (*i.e.*, staff conduct room checks on a predictable basis)

Potential facility *protective* factors include, but are not limited to:

- Brief meetings/tie-ins at change of shift. (This provides communication from one shift to another so that all staff are aware of which youth need to be monitored or more closely supervised.)
- An adequate staff-to-youth ratio
- Availability of support staff (*e.g.*, chaplains, volunteers, interns)
- Thorough room searches
- Tear-resistant blankets and mattresses (*i.e.*, no mattress cords)
- Ongoing staff training in suicide prevention and intervention
- Clearly written suicide prevention policy
- Special monitoring of youth at high risk for suicide
- Availability of mental health/medical professionals

When identifying which youth need to be referred to a mental health/medical professional due to high risk for suicide, staff should consider all four factors of suicide assessment: observable behavior, youths' history, interview with youth, and hazards/protective factors related to a facility where juveniles are residing. Relying on a combination of these factors instead of only one will be likely to result in more thorough and accurate mental health/medical referrals.

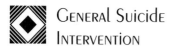

General Suicide Intervention

At the very *minimum,* all juvenile justice facilities should:

- *Screen* every youth for suicide risk upon arrival at a facility, at important transition points throughout the system (*e.g.,* transfer to the adult system, another juvenile justice facility, or a treatment program, placement on probation/parole, release to the community), and whenever indicated by youths' statements or behavior

- Provide *mandatory suicide prevention and intervention training* to all staff before they begin interacting with youth in a juvenile justice facility. Ongoing "refresher" training sessions on suicide should also be mandatory for all staff who work directly with youth and should be provided on a yearly basis.

- Have a *written suicide prevention/ intervention plan* with detailed policies and procedures for responding to the needs of suicidal adolescents. This plan should include some type of monitoring system in which juveniles at high risk for suicide are provided with an increased level of observation (*e.g.,* constant/continuous observation, observation every 10 minutes). When they are monitored every 5, 10 or 15 minutes, youth should be observed at staggered intervals, never exceeding 15 minutes at a time (Hayes, 1999). Some facility plans require suicidal youth to be placed in special rooms. Others allow youth to remain in their own room with increased observation by staff. All juvenile justice professionals should be aware of the details of their facility's suicide prevention/intervention plan.

The following are *additional guidelines* for managing suicidal juvenile offenders. When working with juveniles who are suicidal, juvenile justice professionals should:

- Take all talk or threats of suicide seriously.

- Directly ask youth if they are thinking about suicide.

- Talk with youth about their suicide plan (if they have one) and gather as many details as possible.

- Listen to youth and let them convey what they are upset about. Reflecting back what staff hear youth say helps juveniles feel understood.

- Help youth think about solutions other than suicide. Suicidal juveniles may have difficulty problem-solving on their own.

- Help youth see the light at the end of the tunnel, but be careful not to oversimplify or minimize the juveniles' current problems.

- House youth in a suicide-resistant room when possible.

- House juveniles in the least-restrictive manner possible given their current level of suicide risk. Some suicidal youth are able to function with the general population of residents as long as they are closely monitored.

- Seek consultation from mental health/ medical professionals.

- Have mental health/medical professionals available on-site or by telephone 24-hours-a-day, seven days a week.

- Have actively suicidal youth assessed by a mental health professional at least once a day. In addition to interacting with suicidal youth on a daily basis, mental health professionals should gather information about suicidal youths' current behavior from various staff members (including juvenile justice professionals, teachers and any other professionals with whom the youth have come into contact).

- Set up a protocol for easy communication between staff (*i.e.,* within and between

208

Juvenile Offenders with Mental Health Disorders: Who Are They and What Do We Do With Them?

juvenile justice and mental health professionals) regarding which youth are suicidal and the strategies being used to observe and manage them.

- Trust their judgment/intuition if they think youth are in danger of killing themselves. Even if youth deny suicidal ideation or most staff do not believe youth are suicidal, concerned staff members should take necessary precautions for the youths' safety.
- Err on the side of caution regarding suicidal behavior, regardless of what staff think youths' motivation might be.

Working with youth who have made serious suicide attempts and/or having worked with youth who have died by suicide can be traumatic and painful. Line staff must intervene with youth who have hung themselves, overdosed on medication, swallowed toxic chemicals, or sliced their wrists. Some of these staff members have had to perform life-saving procedures on juveniles such as CPR . Oftentimes, staff must return to work immediately after this type of disturbing incident to supervise the other youth in close proximity.

Not surprisingly, both the staff and other youth are often distressed and confused after a juvenile makes a serious suicide attempt or dies by suicide. It is important for administrators within the juvenile justice system to have specific policies and procedures in relation to debriefing crisis situations such as these immediately after they occur. Suicide debriefing should be provided to all of the youth and staff on the suicidal juvenile's unit. Debriefing should also be provided to any other youth or staff in the facility who had a relationship with the suicidal juvenile. Staff members may experience tremendous amounts of guilt if they were unable to revive a juvenile who has taken his or her own life. Or staff may feel guilty if a juvenile killed himself or herself on a day when they were not present (*e.g.*, believing the death could have been prevented if they were working

that shift). Intervening with suicidal youth, particularly on a repeated basis, can have significant emotional and psychological effects on an individual. Facility staff should be supported after they have an interaction with seriously suicidal youth. And some staff may need more support than others.

When working with juveniles who are suicidal, juvenile justice staff should *not*:

- Leave youth by themselves if they are a high risk for suicide. Staff should remain with the juveniles until assistance arrives and/or the youth are being monitored in a safe place.
- Challenge youth by telling them staff can prevent the juveniles from killing themselves.
- Lecture youth on the value of life.
- Talk sarcastically or jokingly about the juveniles' situation.
- Rely on a "no-suicide contract" as a guarantee that youth will not make a suicide attempt. Signing this type of contract can provide staff with additional information about the level of juveniles' suicide risk. But contracts should not be relied upon as assurance that youth will not kill themselves. Juveniles can sign no-suicide contracts with sincere intentions and then change their mind later.
- Be sworn to secrecy. Juvenile justice professionals should tell youth that they do not plan to discuss the juveniles' situation with everyone. But staff should inform youth that staff will tell those individuals who need to know. Staff should make it clear that their main concern is keeping the youth safe.
- House juveniles in a room with little to no contact with staff.
- Strip youth of their clothes (except shoelaces and belts) or use mechanical restraints unless absolutely necessary for the youths' safety.

- Rely solely on closed-circuit television for monitoring suicidal youth.
- Ignore suicidal threats because staff do not think juveniles are serious.

———

Some juvenile justice facilities automatically place suicidal youth in special isolation/segregation cells. This type of decision should be made in collaboration with mental health/medical personnel. Removing suicidal youth from peers and standard juvenile justice programming can add to youths' feelings of alienation and depression. After juveniles' risk of suicide is assessed, they should be housed in the least-restrictive manner possible given the severity of their suicidal behavior. Removal of juveniles' clothing (other than belts and shoelaces) and the use of mechanical restraints are typically unnecessary for most juvenile offenders expressing suicidal ideation. These management strategies should only be used as a last resort when youth are unable to keep themselves safe without this type of intervention.

Many incarcerated juveniles who express suicidal ideation can participate in much of the standard facility programming—as long as they are provided more intensive levels of supervision and monitoring (*e.g.*, 15-minute checks, 10-minute checks, 5-minute checks, continuous visual observation). If youth are unable to attend school in a classroom with peers due to safety concerns, school-related activities should be provided for these juveniles to complete individually. When placed in a cold and empty room by themselves, suicidal youth have little to focus on—except all of their reasons for being depressed and the various ways that they can attempt to kill themselves. Juvenile justice and mental health professionals can help suicidal youth clarify why they want to die and help the youth cope with their negative circumstances in

a more adaptive and prosocial manner. If juveniles' self-harming behavior is so severe that it necessitates placement in an isolation/segregation room, staff support becomes even more critical *(Please see Chapter 15 for additional information about isolation/seclusion rooms.)*

Case Example

Christina, 16, felt like everything in her life was going wrong, and things were never going to get any better. The girls on her cottage at the juvenile justice facility were getting on her nerves. She was getting into fights with several of her peers and was convinced that most of the staff hated her. Christina was doing poorly in the school at the facility and blamed her declining grades on her favorite teacher being away on vacation for the past three weeks. Christina did not like the other teachers and refused to accept their guidance or support. Christina recently found out that her fiancé, a 24-year old man whom she had been dating for three months, was seen kissing another young woman. When Christina confronted him on the telephone about this issue, he told her that she was over-reacting and that he no longer wanted to be involved with her. She was devastated and felt alone and unwanted. Christina fought with her mother constantly and felt that her mother favored Christina's stepfather over her. Christina was adamant that she would not return to live in her mother's house. Christina's plan to live with her fiancé was no longer feasible. She was afraid that she would be living alone on the streets with no one to take care of her. She concluded that she would be better off dead. Christina planned to take a fork during dinner so she could cut her wrist with it.

210

Juvenile Offenders with Mental Health Disorders: Who Are They and What Do We Do With Them?

CHAPTER 12

Self-Injurious Behavior Among Juvenile Offenders

"Cutting is my way of staying in control and coping.
It helps me. Please don't make me stop."

Sarah, 16

i've been cutting myself for a very long time. i'm 20 now. i started when i was six. when things get to be too intense around me, a lot of stress, i don't know how to feel better, so i cut, and then it releases something inside and i feel able to cope. sometimes the tension and thoughts bound up inside my head, guilt maybe or sadness or whatnot, so i cut to make that a little easier to handle. its really hard to deal with things all the time and the pain inside that is emotional, it hurts so bad. physical pain is easier to deal with. so cutting helps relieve the emotional stuff. i don't do it to be bad. I don't do it to cause trouble. i just rely on it to help me through things i wouldn't be able to get through without it. cutting keeps me calm.

*—Excerpt from a letter sent to the author from
a young woman struggling with self-injury*

Self-injury is becoming a common behavior in juvenile justice facilities. Although known by various names—self-injury, self-mutilation and cutting—this type of behavior reflects youths' deliberate attempt to harm their own body. Although there is no national prevalence data on the incidence of self-injury in juvenile justice, self-harming behavior appears to be on the increase among juvenile offenders. Most self-injurers in corrections engage in superficial cutting and carving, but some young offenders have engaged in more serious and dangerous self-harm behaviors. Regardless of the severity of their self-injury, self-injurers pose a safety and security risk in juvenile justice facilities and can be extremely disruptive to the milieu (environment).

Self-mutilating juvenile offenders can be frightening for staff, as well as the other youth. Both administration and line staff can end up feeling hopeless and frustrated when trying to supervise these juveniles. Although training in suicidal behavior is mandatory in most, if not all, juvenile justice facilities, most staff receive little to no training in the identification and management of *self-injurious* behavior.

 ## What Is Self-Injury?

Self-injury refers to deliberate, nonlife-threatening, socially unacceptable, self-inflicted harm to the body. This behavior tends to begin during the adolescent years and can continue into early adulthood without appropriate intervention. The most common form of self-injury among juvenile offenders is cutting, carving or burning of the skin. Many juvenile offenders have cuts, scratches, burns or bruises on their arms and other parts of their body. Some of these injuries are the result of accidents or physical altercations and would not fit the description of self-injury. Self-injurious behavior is characterized by cuts, burns and the like that are done purposefully and voluntarily to the youth, by the youth. Adults and most other youth typically see the behavior as strange or bizarre.

Tattoos and trendy piercings are becoming more common among today's teenagers, and many juvenile offenders have pierced ears, eyebrows, tongues, belly buttons, and/or other body parts. These behaviors, in and of themselves, do not constitute self-injury. Burning of the skin as part of a cultural and/or ritualistic tradition also does not constitute self-injury. For example, engaging in cutting or burning rituals as part of youths' rite of passage is the norm in some cultures (Favazza & Favazza, 1987). Other adolescents may engage in the cutting or burning of their own skin as part of initiation into, or identification with, a certain group or gang. In addition, some juveniles burn or carve their skin as part of a contest or game to see which youth is the toughest (most "macho") and who can take the most pain. None of these behaviors typically fits the description of self-injury as being used in this chapter.

Youth who self-injure often engage in self-harming behavior as a coping strategy during stressful or emotionally-laden situations. One of the ways that self-injury differs from the above behaviors is that self-mutilation is usually done for the purpose of:

- Regulating youths' emotions
- Getting their emotional needs met in some way

In contrast, the current popularity of adolescent piercings and tattoos is typically related to youth wanting to:

- Look a certain way
- Express their identity
- Fit in with a certain group/culture

For juveniles who already have multiple piercings/tattoos, there can be a fine line between fashion and self-injury. Exploring their motives if youth intend to obtain additional piercings/tattoos can be important. There is a significant difference—between juveniles who are expressing themselves and those who experience a "high" from the pain. Self-injurers often become preoccupied with continuing to obtain additional piercings/tattoos. Self-injurious behavior appears to be more common among today's youth than in the past. But that does not imply that self-injury is a normal part of adolescence. Self-injurious behavior is typically a symptom of a larger underlying problem and should be evaluated whenever it becomes apparent.

Factors Associated with Self-Injurious Behavior

Self-injury occurs among both male and female juvenile offenders but is more prevalent in girls. Although all self-injurers are different and present with their own set of issues, there are some features that are commonly associated with this type of behavior (Walsh & Rosen, 1988):

- Low self-esteem
- Impulsivity
- Repulsed by their bodies/disgusted by the way they look

- Childhood illness or surgery
- Eating Disorders (Anorexia Nervosa, Bulimia, Compulsive Overeating)
- Gender identity issues/confusion over sexuality
- Disgust over their sexual organs and/or menstruation
- Sexual or physical abuse
- Loss of parent (particularly separation without permanent termination, such as foster care, group home, divorce)
- Overly restrictive or neglectful parenting
- Excessive violence at home
- Drug/alcohol abuse
- Inhibition of emotional expression in childhood
- Inability to form stable interpersonal relationships
- Inability or unwillingness to take adequate care of their health and hygiene
- Traumatic experiences during childhood and/or adolescence
- Rigid, "all or none" thinking, including perfectionism

Many self-injuring juveniles go through a series of behaviors before actually harming their bodies. This series of behaviors is sometimes referred to as the *self-harm syndrome* (Kahan & Pattison, 1984). Typically, an event occurs and self-injurious youth have some type of reaction to the event. In most cases, an interpersonal interaction precipitates the act of self-injury. The youth then experience an irresistible urge to cut, carve or burn themselves. The youths' feelings begin to intensify, and their emotions are experienced as overwhelming and out of control. Strong emotions can feel intolerable to youth who self-injure, and they often do not know what to do to escape their mounting anger, anxiety or tension. Because they are increasingly upset, thinking clearly and logically can be difficult for these youth. They may find it hard to take an objective view of their

situation and generate an adaptive coping response. At this point, the youth may go somewhere private and inflict some type of bodily injury onto themselves. After engaging in an act of self-mutilation (e.g., cutting, carving, burning, scratching), the youth typically experience immediate (albeit temporary) relief and a sense of calm. When the sense of calm begins to fade, some self-injurious youth feel embarrassed and ashamed because of the harm they have caused to their body.

 ## Self-Injurious Behavior Versus Suicidal Behavior

Many youth in the juvenile justice system who have engaged in self-injurious behavior have been identified and treated as if they were suicidal. Although some self-injurious youth do become suicidal, these two behaviors are not the same. The intention behind these behaviors is very different. Some suicidal youth want to die. They engage in suicidal behavior in hopes that it will end their lives. Other suicidal youth may not necessarily want to be dead. But their suicidal thoughts and behaviors are a reflection of extreme hopelessness and/or a lack of ability to resolve emotional pain. They want the pain to end and may see suicide as their only option to "escape." Youth engaging in self-injury typically have no intention of killing themselves, and their behavior is not related to wanting to die. Self-injurers also experience a great deal of emotional pain and want the pain to diminish. These juveniles describe cutting and carving as a coping skill—many of them would become suicidal if they did not engage in self-injurious behavior. These youth often view self-injury as *life-sustaining* behavior.

Self-injurious behavior is typically not as lethal as suicidal behavior and tends to cause less physical damage to youths' bodies. Suicidal juveniles often try to hang themselves, cut their veins and arteries, overdose on medication, drink toxic substances, and so forth. Each of these behaviors could cause a great deal of

Self-Injurious Behavior Among Juvenile Offenders

physical damage and/or result in death.

In contrast, most self-injurers within juvenile justice engage in superficial cutting or scratching on their arms or legs. Even if done repeatedly, the damage caused by the typical self-injurer is not life-threatening and tends to result in less damage to the body than serious suicide attempts. The repetitive, chronic nature of self-injury also can help to distinguish this behavior from a suicide attempt.

Suicide attempts are typically responses to some kind of situational and/or emotional crisis. Once the crisis is resolved, youths' suicidal thoughts tend to recede. Most juvenile offenders who have made a suicide attempt have not made an attempt more than a few times.

Self-injurers, however, tend to self-mutilate over and over again. Their cutting, carving or burning is often used as a coping response to overwhelming stress or emotions. Depending on the amount of stress in their lives, youth might self-mutilate on a weekly or even daily basis.

Although they are not the same, suicidal and self-injurious behavior are not necessarily mutually exclusive and can overlap. Some self-injuring juvenile offenders become suicidal and make serious suicide attempts (self-injury is a risk factor for later suicidal behavior). Once the suicidal crisis is resolved and the self-injuring youth no longer want to die (or no longer feel completely hopeless about their situation), however, they are likely to return to self-mutilating behavior to cope with stress.

 ## Forms of Self-Injurious Behavior

Although juvenile justice facilities are designed to be highly safe and secure settings, there are still many ways that self-injurious youth can harm themselves while incarcerated. The following are some items that incarcerated juvenile offenders have been able to access and use for self-mutilation purposes. Youth obtained some of these items— and even used them— while being closely supervised by juvenile justice professionals. This list is certainly not exhaustive. Almost *anything* can be used for self-mutilation purposes if youth are creative.

- Staples
- Thumbtacks
- Paper clips
- Pencils
- Pens
- Erasers
- Safety pins
- Combs
- Brush bristles
- Barrettes
- Earrings/nose rings
- Eye glasses
- Teeth
- Fingernails
- Fork
- Knife
- Broken spoon
- Snap/zipper on uniform/clothing
- Eyelet on tennis shoes
- Belt buckle
- Metal pieces on handle of mattress
- Rocks/gravel from outside
- Hitting fist against cement wall
- Banging head against metal door
- Pulling out eyelashes
- Pulling out strands of hair
- Punching self in stomach
- Broken bits of plastic (e.g., Nintendo, remote control, game pieces)
- Playing cards
- Paint chips
- Corn chips/potato chips
- Pull top from pop can
- Piece of aluminum from pop can

Juvenile Offenders with Mental Health Disorders: Who Are They and What Do We Do With Them?

— Dental floss
— Metal clasp on ace bandage
— Broken tongue depressor
— Toxic chemicals
— Pieces of floor tile
— Peach pits
— Dried apple core
— Dried orange peel
— Chicken bones

Youth who self-injure vary in their method and severity of self-harm behavior. Some self-injurers have a preferred method of self-injury (*e.g.*, they always burn their arms by rubbing them with an eraser, they always cut their forearm with a razor blade), whereas other youth will use anything they can get their hands

---

These youth may need to make deeper and larger cuts, or experience more intense levels of pain, to continue experiencing gratification and relief from their self-harm behavior.

---

on (*e.g.*, staple, pen, playing card, fork, fingernail). The majority of self-injurers engage in superficial scratching, cutting and carving. Forearms are one of the most common targets. However, a number of these youth purposely try to disguise their self-harming behavior. They may cut on areas where others will not see their markings or scars, such as their legs, chest, upper arms, ankles, neck or between their toes. A small subset of self-injuring youth engage in dangerous and severe forms of self-harm behavior. For example, some juveniles have tried to break their own kneecaps with a hammer. Others have aggressively ripped out medical stitches, inserted sharp pencils deep into healing wounds, held Drano pipe cleaner in their mouth for the burning sensation, or inserted a radio antenna into their penis. This type of self-

injurer typically begins with superficial wounding but engages in more severe forms of self-mutilation over time. These youth may need to make deeper and larger cuts, or experience more intense levels of pain, to continue experiencing gratification and relief from their self-harm behavior.

 ## Why Do Youth Self-Injure?

Juvenile offenders engage in self-injurious behavior for a variety of reasons. For some youth, one factor will be predominant; for others, a combination of factors is at play. The following are some of the most common reasons why juveniles cut, carve and burn themselves. For most youth, self-injuring is related to not being able to express their thoughts and emotions in language. Instead, these youth rely on action to express themselves. Strong feelings are often experienced as intolerable, and many of these juveniles will cut, carve or burn themselves to reduce this emotional experience.

TENSION
A number of self-injurious juveniles describe feeling "pent up" and tense much of the time. They describe feeling as if they were going to "explode." These youth often walk around feeling edgy and uptight until they can no longer stand it. Once youth cut or carve themselves and observe blood oozing out of their skin, they typically experience a sense of relief. They are then relaxed. After a period of time, feelings of tension eventually return, and the youth again self-injure to return to a sense of calm.

DEPRESSION
Some youth believe that they are deserving of punishment. They feel bad about themselves and think they are worthless as human beings. Some depressed self-injurers describe feeling exonerated when cutting or burning themselves. Their "badness" seems to flow out of them with

the blood from their cuts or the fluid from their burns.

ANGER

Self-injurers typically have difficulty expressing their anger in a socially appropriate manner, and some self-injuring juvenile offenders report strong feelings of anger toward those around them. Most of these youth, however, would rather hurt themselves than others. They do not want to view themselves as mean or angry people, and would rather take their aggression out on their own bodies rather than someone else. Some juveniles who self-injure report feeling overwhelmed by their anger, which leads to feeling out of control. Engaging in self-injury often calms them, distracts them, and helps them regain a sense of control over their thoughts and emotions.

ANXIETY/DEPERSONALIZATION

A significant number of juvenile offenders who self-injure suffer from Posttraumatic Stress Disorder (PTSD). Posttraumatic Stress Disorder is an anxiety disorder associated with the experience of traumatic events in youths' lives. Many youth involved with juvenile justice have experienced significant traumatic events (*e.g.,* sexual abuse, rape, physical abuse, witnessing the death of a loved one, being shot). For some offenders, their level of anxiety is so severe that the youth experience feelings of depersonalization. When their anxiety reaches a high level, the youth can begin to depersonalize and feel "unreal." The world around them seems fuzzy and difficult to comprehend.

Youth who have experienced depersonalization have described feeling as if they were not in their body. But instead, they feel as if they are looking at their bodies from above, watching themselves go through automatic, robot-like motions. Although they can see peoples' mouths moving and can hear the voices of those speaking to them, these youth cannot make out what the individuals are saying. During an episode of depersonalization, a disconnect

seems to occur between juveniles' experience and their physical body. Not surprisingly, depersonalization can be frightening, with juveniles feeling that they are going crazy.

Many self-injurers cut and carve during periods of heightened anxiety and depersonalization. The pain of the self-injury and/or watching blood flow from their body can jolt them back into feeling more real. It can also help the youth experience a clearer sense of their physical boundaries—where they physically begin and end. The physical sensation associated with self-harming behavior has been described by some of these youth as "grounding." They say it helps them feel "whole" again. *(Please see Chapter 6 for additional information about Posttraumatic Stress Disorder.)*

PAIN

Some youth who self-injure actually enjoy the sensation of pain they experience during an act of self-harm. They may even describe an inner feeling of being "high" while cutting or burning. For some juvenile offenders, the association of pain and nurturance is confused because they came from households in which they experienced severe physical abuse. However, a number of self-injurers describe having a higher pain tolerance than their peers. These youths' bodies are often able to withstand fairly high amounts of tissue damage in comparison to those around them. In fact, many self-mutilators describe feeling little to no pain during the actual act of self-injury. The experience of pain often comes later as wounds begin to heal.

COMMUNICATION WITHIN INTERPERSONAL RELATIONSHIPS

Some juveniles use self-injurious behavior to communicate with individuals to whom they are close. If they feel hurt, criticized or rejected by juvenile justice professionals or friends, some youth cut themselves to show their distress versus communicating with words. Incidents of self-injury also have been associated with anticipated loss (Rosen, Walsh, & Rode,

1990). Self-injurious youth often engage in self-harm behaviors a few weeks before they are going to be released from a juvenile justice facility or treatment program. The same is often true a few weeks before staff members are about to leave for vacation or to leave permanently to work in another setting. Many self-injuring youth have difficulty putting into words their fears or sadness over an upcoming separation. This difficulty can be particularly evident for juveniles who have experienced significant losses earlier in their lives. Most youth know that if they engage in self-injurious behavior, they are likely to be comforted and nurtured. Therefore, many juveniles view self-injury as an effective way to connect with individuals about whom they care.

SEVERE MENTAL ILLNESS

Although rare in juvenile justice, some psychotic individuals (*i.e.*, youth with Schizophrenia) may engage in severe forms of self-injury. This situation is especially true if individuals are suffering from command hallucinations (*e.g.*, voices telling them to hurt themselves) and/or delusions. This type of self-injury is often related to feelings of guilt around religious or sexual issues. Psychotic individuals tend to self-injure to cleanse themselves or punish themselves for perceived wrongdoing or sins—rather than as a coping mechanism to manage strong feelings. Psychotic self-injurers have removed their own eyeballs, cut off one of their breasts, and attempted self-castration. These self-injurers tend to engage in a single, but severe, self-harming incident, which typically leaves them feeling exonerated and pure again. Youth with significant mental retardation may also engage in a variety of self-injurious behaviors, including head banging, lip biting and face slapping.

ATTENTION SEEKING
AND CONTROL OF STAFF

In some juvenile justice facilities, self-injurious behavior can result in rewarding consequences for youth. Although youths' self-harming behavior initially may have been associated with internal motivations, it can then be maintained by reinforcing external events. Or, juveniles who have never engaged in self-harm behavior may observe peers receiving positive consequences after self-injurious incidents. These youth may then engage in the behavior themselves in hopes of receiving similar benefits (*e.g.*, contagion effect).

Attention from adult staff members is one of the strongest reinforcers youth can receive within juvenile justice facilities. Some youth will engage in almost any behavior (positive or negative) to be on the receiving end of staff attention. This situation is particularly true if the attention from staff is one-on-one and free from distractions. In most juvenile justice facilities, staff typically respond to incidents of self-injury with special attention. These youth are typically sent to a medical professional to observe and/or clean any wounds. Line staff, supervisors and mental health professionals are often asked to speak with the youth, and mental health assessments and evaluations may occur. In addition, after youth self-injure, they are often placed on some type of intensive monitoring, with staff members regularly observing and documenting the juveniles' behavior. Depending on the policies and procedures of particular facilities, these responses may be automatically set in motion—regardless of whether the youth superficially scratch their arm or seriously mutilate parts of their body.

Some juvenile offenders spend a great deal of time devising ways to provoke reactions from staff, as well as exert some control over staff behavior. Obtaining a desired reaction and/or exerting control over staff can be very satisfying for incarcerated youth. Cutting, carving, scratching or mutilating their bodies in another manner almost always guarantees a reaction from staff. Being frightened of, confused by or disgusted with self-mutilating behavior is completely natural. Juveniles know this. In addition, youth also may know that self-injury

Self-Injurious Behavior Among Juvenile Offenders

results in transfer to a psychiatric hospital, a special needs unit—or another setting that they perceive as less "correctional" and less restrictive. Or, self-injurious youth may enjoy having the identity of being a "cutter" because it makes them feel special in some way and/or because some of the staff are afraid of them. Most juvenile justice facilities have established policies and procedures in relation to self-injury. Therefore, staff often have no choice but to give self-injuring youth extra attention and to respond in ways that inadvertently reinforce the self-harm behavior (*i.e.*, providing youth with exactly what the youth hoped to achieve).

Not all youth in juvenile justice settings engage in self-injurious behaviors for attention, and staff should not assume that youth do. Many self-injuring youth use their self-harm behavior as a coping mechanism for strong and overwhelming emotions. When these youth have difficulty communicating their thoughts, feelings and needs through language, they rely on action instead. Even if juveniles engage in self-injurious behavior as a strategy to solicit extra attention from staff, self-harming youth should be evaluated by a mental health/medical professional. There are a variety of ways of obtaining staff attention in juvenile justice facilities. Cutting on their skin or relying on other self-harming behaviors as a means to that end is not normal for youth.

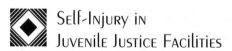 Self-Injury in Juvenile Justice Facilities

Self-injurious behavior is becoming more common in juvenile justice facilities, and there are probably a variety of reasons for this. First, there is a greater incidence of mental health disorders among juvenile offenders in comparison to juveniles in the general population. A significant number of these youth suffer from feelings of depression and anxiety. Many of these youth have experienced trauma during childhood and adolescence, and specifically meet diagnostic criteria for Posttraumatic Stress Disorder—a mental health disorder commonly associated with self-injurious behavior. A large percentage of juvenile offenders have difficulty expressing their emotions in socially appropriate ways. And a considerable number of these youth struggle with overwhelming feelings of anger and depression.

Living in an institutional setting can encourage regressive behavior. Even before entering a juvenile justice facility, many juvenile offenders demonstrate poor coping skills in the community. These youth often rely on alcohol and drugs, running away, sexual activity, self-injurious behavior, or aggression/violence in order to cope with strong emotions, frustrations and disappointments. Many juvenile justice programs focus on helping youth learn more socially adaptive coping strategies. But this effort can be challenging, depending on the setting in which youth reside.

While youth are incarcerated, most decisions are made for them (*e.g.*, where, what and when to eat; where and when to sleep; with whom they will live; what activities they will engage in). Juveniles even have to ask permission to use the restroom and may not be allowed to go at desired times. Restrictive environments (juvenile justice facilities or psychiatric facilities) in which youth are dependent on others for their basic needs can result in juveniles relying on more primitive ways of coping—instead of mature, independent coping strategies (Favazza & Favazza, 1987). Self-injury is one type of primitive coping strategy juvenile offenders still have access to when they cannot rely on aggression, running away, sexual behavior, or drugs/alcohol.

When they are involved with the juvenile justice system, youth are likely to experience negative feeling states. Incarceration can be a positive, life-changing, growth-inducing experience for some young men and women. But it also can be filled with periods of fear, anger, frustration, disappointment, depression, and anxiety. Periods of desperation and demoralization are not unusual if youth are incarcerated

Juvenile Offenders with Mental Health Disorders: Who Are They and What Do We Do With Them?

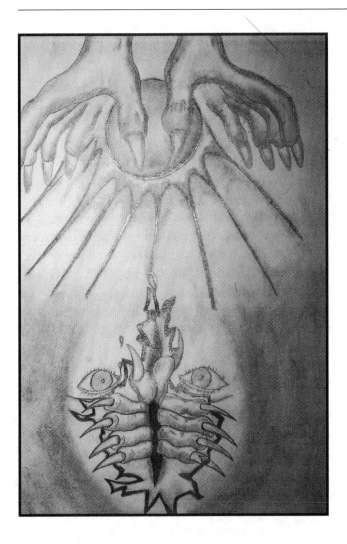

are a very high-risk time for self-harm behavior among juvenile offenders, and this can be especially so for antisocial youth (Favazza & Favazza, 1987). Individuals with antisocial tendencies often require more stimulation and excitement than individuals without antisocial tendencies. Antisocial youth are often thrill seekers and enjoy engaging in high-risk activities. Residing in a small room with minimal stimuli within a juvenile justice facility can be daunting for this type of youth. They sometimes cut or scratch themselves just to feel some kind of stimulation. In fact, some of these juveniles have described banging their fist or head against the wall "just to feel alive."

Another possible reason why self-injury is not uncommon in juvenile justice facilities is that youth may believe (and often rightly so) that this type of behavior will lead to a variety of rewarding results (*e.g.*, staff attention, transfer to another setting, psychiatric medication).

 ## Potential Protective Factors Within Juvenile Justice Facilities

The following factors within juvenile justice facilities can help decrease the incidence of self-injurious behavior among youth in custody:

Support System

Youth who self-injure need support, particularly from adults. Juvenile justice professionals are typically saddled with a variety of responsibilities and multiple youth to supervise simultaneously. Therefore, spending a great deal of time providing individual support to self-injurers is difficult. Mental health professionals, medical professionals, chaplains, volunteers, recreation staff, mentors, interns, and the like, can all serve a critical role in providing emotional support to juveniles who self-injure. Self-injurious youth must have access to adults with whom they can talk *before* the youth engage in self-harm behavior. With necessary supports in place, youth may not need to rely on self-injury as a way to deal with their negative emotions. In

for a significant period of time. Self-injury is most likely to occur during times of negative emotional experiences.

Feelings of boredom also have been associated with self-injury, and many juvenile offenders complain about being bored while incarcerated. Youth often do not think about harming themselves when they are busy with friends in the community or when engaged in school or other programs in juvenile justice facilities.

However, youth may have thoughts of self-injury when they are alone in their room and have little contact with others. In fact, some youth self-injure only during periods of solitary confinement/isolation. And a small subset of juveniles have never cut or scratched themselves until placed in isolation for a significant period of time. Periods of isolation/seclusion addition, they are less likely to injure themselves in order to gain attention from staff if youth are already receiving attention from the adults around them.

Activities

One of the best ways to prevent juvenile offenders from engaging in self-injurious behavior is to keep them occupied: program, program, program. If youth are busy with school, treatment groups, recreation, group activities, writing assignments, and so forth, there is little time for them to think about self-injury—and even less time to engage in it.

Consistent Rules and Schedules

Many youth who self-injure typically do not like change or transitions. These youth need to feel safe and secure in their surroundings. An adjustment in the daily schedule, or a change regarding one or two staff members, can be very unsettling and anxiety-producing for juvenile offenders who self-injure. Consequently, keeping unit schedules and staff teams as consistent as possible is best. Due to the nature of the juvenile justice system, however, change is typically a common occurrence. Therefore, informing self-injuring youth of any upcoming major changes is important. In addition, staff should provide extra support to these youth during times of major transition (*e.g.*, moving to a new unit, being assigned to a new staff member, transferring to a treatment program, being released into the community), as these can be high-risk periods for vulnerable youth such as self-injurers.

Minimal Access to Sharp Objects

Juvenile justice facilities are designed to be safe and secure settings. Therefore, there is typically less access to sharp objects in correctional institutions in comparison to the community. Juvenile justice professionals are trained in conducting searches of youths' rooms to remove any items that can be potentially dangerous to the youth, peers or staff. However, even with

careful and frequent searches of youth and youths' living quarters, some juveniles are still able accumulate items for self-harm. Even seasoned juvenile justice staff members have been outsmarted by creative youth who were able to find something to injure themselves—despite being intensively monitored and having little access to personal items. Clearly, minimizing access to sharp objects is best if youth are unable to keep themselves safe. However, removing access to *every* sharp object is impossible. For example, staff cannot take away youths' teeth and nails, and youth know that.

 GENERAL SELF-INJURY INTERVENTION GUIDELINES

Self-Injury Is A Symptom Of A Broader Psychological Problem

Juvenile offenders who self-injure often suffer from anxiety and/or depression, and many have experienced significant traumatic events. In order to treat youths' self-injurious behavior, additional mental health issues must be addressed as well. Therefore, most self-injurious youth require a mental health evaluation to identify any underlying psychological problems. Depending on the nature of youths' mental health status, psychotropic medication may be a necessary part of a treatment plan.

Self-Injury Is Unacceptable

Within juvenile justice facilities, the safety and security of youth in custody must be maintained at all times. Just as aggression toward others is unacceptable in these facilities, so is aggression toward oneself. Juvenile justice professionals (and mental health/medical professionals, if available) should have a frank discussion with youth about their self-injurious behavior. Staff should convey an understanding that the youths' self-injury may have been effective at reducing the juveniles' negative feelings in the past. However, staff should also convey that self-harm cannot be tolerated in the current environment.

220

Juvenile Offenders with Mental Health Disorders: Who Are They and What Do We Do With Them?

Thought Patterns Preceding Self-Injurious Behavior

Juveniles should learn to identify situations that trigger their self-harm behavior. Most self-injurers harm themselves in response to inter-personal situations. However, youths' accompanying thoughts about a situation are often more relevant than the specifics of the situation itself.

SOME juveNile offendeRs use tHeir self-injuRious beHavioR TO scARe sTAff ANd peeRs, ANd TO foRce THem TO keep THeiR disTANce fRom THe youtH.

For example, youth typically do not cut on themselves because they did not get a second helping of dinner. The reason is usually related to their thoughts about why the staff chose to give a second helping to someone else (*e.g.*, "I never get anything", "That staff hates me," "This place is so unfair," "I never get my needs met"). A negative phone call with their boy-friend/girlfriend is usually not the trigger of youths' self-injury. But the thoughts they have about the phone call and what was said (*e.g.*, "I think they are cheating on me," "They don't love me like I love them," "I am never going to be with them again," "I am not good enough for them," "They don't care about me") are more likely the triggers of their mutilating behavior. Juveniles' negative thoughts often result in their experiencing negative feeling states such as anger, sadness, disappointment or frustra-tion. These youth then engage in self-injury to manage these uncomfortable emotions and/or to modify the dynamics of interpersonal rela-tionships.

Tolerating Negative Feeling States

Juveniles who self-injure often cannot tolerate the experience of anger, anxiety, sadness or frustration. They often feel like their emotions are welling up inside of them and as if they are going to "explode." These youth are usually searching for ways to relieve the pressure they perceive as building up inside them. Self-injurious behavior relieves this pressure and restores youth to a sense of calm. Self-injurers need to be taught that they *can* tolerate nega-tive emotions without exploding. Cognitive-oriented treatment approaches can be helpful in restructuring youths' thoughts about tolerat-ing these negative feelings (Walsh & Rosen, 1988).

New Coping Skills

Everyone experiences anger, disappointment, frustration and anxiety; it is a part of being human. When juvenile justice professionals work with juveniles who self-injure, the goal is not for youth to stop experiencing negative emotions. Instead, the goal is to help the juve-niles learn to *cope* with these emotions in a socially appropriate manner. Juveniles who self-injure need to develop additional *skills*—so that they no longer have to rely on self-harm behav-iors as the main way to soothe themselves and deal with painful emotions.

Adaptive Social Skills

Much of juveniles' self-injurious behavior is related to interpersonal relationships, and these youth often respond to perceived rejection and criticism from others by hurting themselves. Although they crave connection with others, most self-injurious youth have difficulty main-taining stable relationships with adults and peers. These juveniles commonly misperceive communication from others during interper-sonal interactions. In addition, youth may use their self-injury to coerce others to spend time with them, pay attention to them, or nurture them. Ironically, youths' self-injurious behavior usually results in significant others eventually avoiding or rejecting them. Some juvenile offenders use their self-injurious behavior to scare staff and peers, and to force them to keep their distance from the youth. Regardless of youths' interpersonal motives for self-injury, most of these juveniles need to learn to express their relationship needs in words.

Identification of What Is Reinforcing The Behavior

Juvenile justice professionals need to identify the reinforcement patterns associated with youths' self-harm behaviors. By its very nature, self-injury is a difficult behavior to change because it is constantly being *negatively reinforced*. Negative reinforcement occurs when the probability of a behavior is increased by taking away or stopping something negative. When self-injurious youth feel uncomfortable and experience painful emotions, cutting or scratching themselves reduces those negative feelings. Something negative is being taken away (painful feelings), so the self-injurious behavior is being reinforced—negatively reinforced. Youths' painful emotions diminish most, if not every, time the juveniles cut or scratch themselves. Consequently, they are likely to engage in this behavior again the next time they are upset.

In addition, adults and peers who come into contact with self-injurious youth can inadvertently provide *positive reinforcement* for the youths' maladaptive self-harming behavior. Positive reinforcement occurs when the probability of a behavior is increased by providing a positive consequence. Many self-injurious juvenile offenders receive special attention from line staff, supervisors, medical professionals, mental health professionals, and peers after engaging in self-harming behavior. For most youth in juvenile justice facilities, attention, support and nurturance from others is very rewarding. Each time self-injury leads to extra support from others, self-injurious behavior is positively reinforced. Therefore, the behavior is likely to occur the next time the youth are upset and/or want to engage with people. Individuals providing attention to these youth usually believe they are doing what is in the best interest of the juveniles. These individuals usually are not aware that they may

actually be increasing the likelihood that the youth will continue this maladaptive behavior. This does not mean that everyone who comes into contact with self-injurious youth should avoid or ignore the juveniles. Such a response would be unethical and cruel. Adults and peers should respond to youths' self-injurious marks and injuries in a *matter-of-fact* manner, and juvenile justice professionals should take whatever precautions are necessary to keep the youth safe. Any extra attention and support provided to these juveniles should be focused on:

- What triggered the incident of self-injury
- What alternative strategies the juveniles can use in the future when they are upset
- What alternative strategies the juveniles can use in the future when they want to engage others

Attention And Support When Youth Is Not Engaged In Self-Injurious Behavior

Juveniles who self-injure should be reinforced for *not* engaging in harmful behavior. If youth desire attention or nurturance from staff, these should be provided to help prevent further incidents of self-injury. However, extra staff and peer attention should be provided *before* youth do something to harm themselves, as well as when the youth display appropriate coping skills. The goal is for juveniles to learn "I actually get more attention and support when I am *not* hurting myself versus when I do hurt myself." Most juvenile offenders have not received this message. This concept is not only important for self-injurious youth to learn but also for all juveniles in a living unit to learn. Some youth might imitate the self-injurious behavior of their peers to receive perceived rewards. This behavior can easily spread through an entire unit, with several youth mutilating themselves during the same time period. Juvenile justice professionals should emphasize that one of the best ways to receive positive consequences from staff is for youth to engage in socially adaptive behavior.

Emotions Versus Self-Injurious Behavior

Whenever youth self-injure, staff should focus on the underlying feelings that triggered the self-harm incident. Once youth are better able to identify their emotions and express them through words, the less they will need to rely on self-injury as a way to communicate how they feel. Some juvenile justice facilities have policies mandating that youth be secluded/isolated after an episode of self-injury. If youth are placed in seclusion/isolation, they should be given specific assignments to complete during the time they are removed from their peers. These assignments should focus on:

- *What happened* right before the youth made the decision to cut or carve on themselves (*i.e.,* what was the triggering event)
- What the youth were *thinking* in response to this triggering event
- What the youth were *feeling* in response to this triggering event
- How the youth will handle a similar situation more *adaptively* in the future

Staff should limit their interaction with isolated/secluded youth to monitoring their safety and discussing the youths' answers to their incident-related assignment. If juveniles continue to try to engage the staff, staff members should remain focused on helping the youth identify what triggered the self-injury; clarify the youths' thoughts and emotions; and facilitate the youths' problem-solving about what alternative coping responses can be used in place of self-injurious behavior. Identifying youths' thoughts and feelings about interpersonal events is critical to understanding what led up to their self-injury. Juveniles' *reaction* to a triggering event typically requires modification versus the external event itself. Helping juveniles understand their emotional reactions

and problem-solve future situations will make self-injury less likely to occur when similar situations arise.

Respect For The Youth

Feeling frightened or disgusted by youths' self-injurious behavior is a natural reaction for juvenile justice professionals. This reaction is particularly likely if juveniles' wounds are bloody or located on an atypical body part. However, staff should maintain a matter-of-fact attitude and tone when dealing with self-injurious juveniles. Whether they verbalize it or not, many of these youth are ashamed of their behavior and know that it is unusual or weird. If staff appear uncomfortable, frightened or grossed out by youths' injuries or scars, the youth will be less likely to talk to staff about harmful behaviors being done in secret. These youth will also be less willing to engage in discussions about underlying thoughts and feelings with the staff. Conveying an understanding that the youth have used self-injury as a coping skill and/or a way to get their needs met in the past is important. Staff should emphasize that the youth are not crazy or weird. However, conveying that it is unacceptable to use self-injury as a coping mechanism in a juvenile justice facility is just as important. Staff should also communicate that they are committed to keeping the youth safe and helping them learn more acceptable ways of dealing with their emotions and interpersonal relationships.

Not Giving Up

Juveniles who self-injure can be extremely disruptive to a living unit within a juvenile justice facility. These youth can be frustrating for staff to work with, demand a great deal of staff time, and consume a considerable amount of a facility's resources. However, a significant number of self-injurious juveniles do get better and no longer rely on hurting themselves as a way to cope with their emotions. As with other maladaptive coping skills used by many juvenile offenders (*e.g.,* drugs and alcohol, aggression, running away, sexual behavior), decreasing self-injurious behavior is not likely to be quick or easy. If youth have relied on this coping strategy for a significant period of time, eradicating it may take a lengthy period of time. Relapse regarding self-injury will occur, and it should be expected and planned for with help from a clinician. Staff (*e.g.*, juvenile justice, mental health, medical) should help youth identify high-risk situations that may trigger an episode of self-injury and provide the youth with extra support during these times. Consistently reinforcing youths' new coping strategies and positive social skills as they are displayed is key. Likewise, rewarding the juveniles when they do not engage in self-injury during difficult times also is critical. Eventually these new, more adaptive, skills will be naturally reinforced by the positive interactions the youth begin to have with others.

Case Example

(Excerpt from a letter sent to the author)
I have been hurting myself since I was about four years old—that I can remember. It started as hitting my head, or pulling the sides of my face until I had a nose bleed. At some point, thereafter, it turned into cutting and burning. I can assure you that none of this is done for attention as I never told anyone about "my secret." It isn't until quite recently that anyone in my family found out, and I have asked him not to share it with anyone else. He has honored my request but is there for me if I need him. I have yet to discuss it with him. It is still "my secret." There are many theories as to why people hurt themselves. I'm not going to say that since I do it, I know why. I can tell you that most times after I hurt myself, I do sit there and wonder,

"What the hell did I just do? How could I do something like that?" It is not for attention, it is not for fun, it is not to have something to do. It is to keep me alive. That of course being the other myth—that self-injury is a failed suicide attempt. If I had wanted to die, I would be gone by now. It is only because I want to continue to live that I have hurt myself. It pulls me through the day, the night, the situation I am in, and enables me to feel again so that I can carry on. From all the readings I have done, it seems that childhood abuse is the most common "factor" in people that SI (self- injure). I have been told by four separate therapists that my story of my childhood is one of the worst cases of child abuse they have come across. One woman was a therapist for over 20 years. It is not something I am proud of. It is with great embarrassment I say that my father raped me until I moved out of the house at age 20. My mother was quite a sadistic person. Perhaps SI, feeling some kind of pain, was the only thing that made sense. I don't know. Why have I decided to say so much? In the hopes that there will be a better understanding about SI. I'm not saying there aren't some people that do it for attention, but I can assure you I am not one of those people. Take the time to find out. Help those people that are not doing it for attention. Don't give ultimatums because those never work. Remember, it has been a secret for so long, it can continue to be. And if you think you can just "check people" before bed or something, remember this. There will always be places you would never think to look. Sure, it's more painful, but then again, who said we were in this for the comfort of it all.

CHAPTER 13

Screening and Assessment of Juvenile Offenders with Mental Health Disorders

"Why does everyone ask me the same questions over and over again?"

Todd, 14

Protocols and processes for the accurate screening and assessment of juvenile offenders with mental health disorders are essential if juveniles are to receive adequate treatment and rehabilitative services. Mental health screening and assessment helps identify which youth are in need of mental health intervention. Screening and assessment also provide information related to which type of treatment strategies may be beneficial for particular youth. Juvenile offenders with mental health disorders are often misdiagnosed or undiagnosed, both of which can result in inappropriate programming and placement of youth. Without proper identification of juveniles' mental health symptoms:

- Appropriate referrals to mental health/medical professionals may not be made

- Effective treatment strategies may not be provided

- There may be an over-or under-reliance on psychotropic medication

Accurate screening and assessment is also critical for the safety and security of juvenile justice facilities. Allowing juvenile offenders

with mental health disorders to remain unidentified can result in increased aggression, assaults and suicidal behavior.

Mental health disorders may go undetected or inappropriately identified in the juvenile justice system for several reasons. First, most juvenile justice professionals have never received training related to identifying signs, symptoms and behaviors related to mental health among adolescent offenders. Within juvenile justice, staff typically focus primarily on youths' criminal, aggressive and oppositional behaviors. Although these behaviors are important and deserving of this attention, they can be related to (and sometimes mask) significant mental health disorders.

Second, mental illness among some juvenile offenders may be undetected due to these youth under-reporting their mental health symptoms. Within juvenile justice, there is often a stigma attached to being labeled "mentally ill." Placement and programming decisions associated with mental health classification may be viewed by juveniles as undesirable, or even aversive.

Third, some juveniles may be misdiagnosed with a psychiatric disorder because they have:

- Manufactured mental health symptoms
- Exaggerated mild mental health symptoms in an attempt to receive a variety of consequences the youth perceive as positive (*e.g.,* increased interaction with staff, psychotropic medication)

Finally, symptoms of intoxication or withdrawal from drugs and alcohol can often appear similar to mental health symptoms, making diagnostic issues among juvenile offenders even more complex.

Mental health *screening* and *assessment* refers to two different processes. Although they are integrally related, they are not the same thing. A mental health screening is a brief procedure used to determine the *possible* presence of a mental health disorder. A screening tool is primarily used to "red flag" juveniles in need of further mental health evaluation. A mental health *assessment* is a more comprehensive diagnostic and treatment planning process that is typically based on initial screening information. A comprehensive mental health assessment may take hours to complete and should be linked to a treatment plan.

 Mental Health Screening

Mental health screening is conducted early in the process of collecting information about youth. It may be accomplished by interviewing youth and/or by using a mental health checklist or questionnaire. Mental health screening in juvenile justice should be brief and should take no more than 30 minutes to complete. Screening tools should be simple enough for a variety of professionals (including nonmental health/medical professionals) to administer, or for youth to complete on their own with little to no assistance. Ideally, they would be available in different languages (or facilities should have access to someone who can translate a tool). If a mental health screening identifies juveniles

as having possible mental health symptoms, the youth should receive a more extensive evaluation. Further evaluation should investigate the nature and degree of these symptoms, as well as determine whether specialized treatment services are necessary. Mental health screenings are not designed to provide a mental health diagnosis and should not be used for that purpose.

Screening all juveniles for mental health disorders upon entry to juvenile justice facilities can serve a variety of purposes:

- Identify youth with mental health disorders in need of services
- Assist in placement decisions
- Assist in programming and management decisions
- Help prevent a crisis situation
- Assist with transition issues
- Obtain/maintain compliance with national standards
- Collect important data
- Access additional funding

Identify Youth With Mental Health Disorders In Need Of Services

Juvenile justice facilities should be aware if they are housing mentally ill youth in need of special services as soon as possible. If juveniles are in need of immediate mental health services, transferring the youth to a psychiatric facility or the emergency room of a local hospital may be necessary. If acutely mentally ill youth (*e.g.* suicidal, psychotic, intoxicated, those withdrawing from drugs) remain in juvenile justice facilities, additional supervision and formal monitoring by staff may be necessary (*e.g.,* documented observation by staff every ten minutes, one-to-one staffing). If youths' mental health symptoms are less urgent, staff can refer the youth to a mental health/medical professional for further evaluation.

Assist In Placement Decisions

Some incarcerated youth with mental health disorders may require placement in particular housing units and/or in special "safe" rooms. Some juvenile justice facilities have units or cottages specifically designated for youth with "special needs," including youth with mental health disorders. Further, some facilities have special rooms that are particularly devoid of ways for youth to injure themselves. Decisions about whether youth should or should not have a roommate can also be affected by information gathered from a mental health screening tool.

Assist In Programming And Management Decisions

Certain mental health signs or symptoms among juvenile offenders may be identified by a mental health screening tool. In these situations, certain modifications may need to be made regarding the youths' juvenile justice and treatment programming. For example, youth who appear to be severely cognitively impaired may not be able to fulfill all of the behavioral expectations required within a facility's token economy program (e.g., point or level system).

The juveniles still must have behavioral expectations and must be held accountable for those expectations. But modifications may be necessary to increase the likelihood that the youth can successfully achieve them, given their intellectual limitations (e.g., complete three chores versus six chores, attend four hours of school versus six hours of school, attend two treatment groups versus five treatment groups). Other modifications to programming that may be necessary for juveniles who "red flag" on a mental health screening tool include:

- Providing additional reminders about facility rules

- Providing written instructions for complex tasks

- Allowing additional time to complete written assignments

Once they become aware that youth may have a mental health disorder, juvenile justice professionals are often more creative in their management strategies. Staff are also less likely to automatically view unusual youth behavior as manipulative and oppositional.

Help Prevent A Crisis Situation

Even when juvenile offenders do not report urgent psychiatric concerns on a mental health screen, the information gathered can be used at a later time to help prevent a crisis situation. Some youth report psychiatric symptoms on a mental health screening tool that are not serious enough to warrant action on the part of a juvenile justice facility. This mental health information can be beneficial in the future if these youth are placed under high levels of stress, and/or their circumstances become more negative.

For example, juveniles screened for mental illness upon admission to juvenile justice facilities may deny current suicidal ideation but report engaging in a suicide attempt two years ago. An awareness of such behavior can prompt juvenile justice professionals to more closely observe, interact with and support the youth if they are given bad news unexpectedly (e.g., long juvenile justice sentence, death of close friend or family member, breakup of romantic relationship).

Regardless of whether youth are stable upon admission to a juvenile justice facility, staff should know if juveniles have:

- Experienced hallucinations in the past

- Engaged in self-injurious behavior

- Had a history of taking psychotropic medication

- Made a previous suicide attempt(s)

This type of information alerts staff that the youth have a history of mental health symptoms and describes the type of symptoms experienced. If juveniles' psychiatric symptoms recur while the youth are incarcerated, staff are more

Screening and Assessment of Juvenile Offenders with Mental Health Disorders

likely to recognize these symptoms as soon as they arise. Staff can then refer the youth to a mental health/medical professional. Using mental health screening tools, therefore, can help juvenile justice professionals be more proactive when juveniles experience mental health-related difficulties, rather than reacting to the youths' problematic behavior once it reaches crisis proportions.

Assist With Transition Issues

Information gathered from a mental health screening tool can also be beneficial for community supervision staff (probation and parole). Obtaining information about youths' mental health status, suicidal behavior, previous mental health treatment, current and previous psychotropic medications, and the like, is crucial to providing appropriate aftercare services. Knowing youths' previous treatment provider(s)—as well as with which types of interventions the youth have already been involved—helps probation/parole staff link the juveniles to mental health services in the community upon release from a facility.

In addition, youths' mental health status can greatly impact their interpersonal relationship with their probation/parole officer, as well as their compliance with community supervision agreements and orders. Issues related to youths' mental health should always be integrated into probation/parole supervision plans. Using the information collected on a mental health screening tool can be a first step in guiding this process.

Obtain/Maintain Compliance With National Standards

The American Correctional Association (ACA, 1991a, 1991b, 2002) contains standards regarding the health screening of all individuals immediately upon arrival at juvenile justice facilities. At a minimum, health screenings should always include an inquiry into "mental health problems," "suicidal behavior," "past or present treatment or hospitalization for mental distur-

bance or suicide," "use of alcohol and other drugs," as well as detailed information about youths' use of substances.

These health screenings should also include the observation of juveniles' behavior, including their mental status, state of consciousness, and general appearance. These types of questions are the recommended *minimum*. Some juvenile justice agencies gather significantly more information about youths' previous and/or current mental health status.

Collect Important Mental Health Data

Most juvenile justice agencies do not have prevalence estimates related to the number of youth with mental health disorders under their care. Even though they are interested in this type of information, gathering prevalence data is difficult if staff are unclear as to how to identify mentally ill youth. When all youth entering juvenile justice facilities receive a mental health screening, data is continuously being collected regarding the mental health symptoms of these juveniles. Obtaining answers to the following questions can facilitate the identification of what resources and services are most needed to effectively manage and treat this population of juveniles:

- How many youth with mental health disorders reside in a particular juvenile justice facility?

- What are the most common types of psychiatric symptoms seen among these youth?

For example, this type of information can guide decision-making about the number of staff (line, medical and mental health) necessary to care for these youth at various locations. Mental health resource decisions must be associated with need so that mentally ill youth most in need of services have ready access to them. Additionally, residential programming, types of treatment groups provided, and diversity of services offered should be influenced by avail-

Juvenile Offenders with Mental Health Disorders: Who Are They and What Do We Do With Them?

able mental health data. Policies and procedures related to suicide, self-injurious behavior, psychotropic medication, and crisis intervention are also likely to be affected. Presenting data to policymakers about the prevalence, characteristics and multi-system needs of juvenile offenders with mental health disorders can also result in significant policy changes related to the provision of care to this complex population.

Access Additional Funding

Most juvenile justice facilities report needing additional funding for mental health services. Government bodies and agencies are more likely to allocate money and resources for mental health services when convinced that there is a significant need for these services. Data collected from a mental health screening tool can significantly influence individuals/ committees as they make decisions regarding the distribution of funding resources. Juvenile justice agencies can demonstrate a significant need for mental health resources by having statistics related to the characteristics of the mentally ill youth in their care.

Currently, most legislative bodies, grantors, foundations and the like are more strongly swayed by objective data (regarding the number and types of mentally ill youth involved with juvenile justice) than by emotional anecdotes related to these youth. Providing these decision-makers with information related to the percentage of youthful offenders with Attention-Deficit/Hyperactivity Disorder, Major Depression, Bipolar Disorder, or Posttraumatic Stress Disorder within juvenile justice agencies/ juvenile justice facilities can be persuasive. Providing figures related to the number of incarcerated youth who present with suicidal ideation—or a previous suicide attempt—can be alarming to individuals unfamiliar with juvenile offenders who have mental health disorders. These individuals are also often surprised by the percentage of juvenile offenders who have been prescribed psychotropic medication and/ or have been hospitalized for psychiatric reasons. When agencies/facilities try to procure funding for mental health services, providing objective data about the complex needs of these youthful offenders can be very educational, as well as persuasive.

————

All youth entering the juvenile justice system should be screened for mental health disorders. This screening should be completed at the earliest point possible after involvement with the system (Peters & Bartoi, 1997). Although an initial mental health screening is critical, continuing to screen youth as they progress through the system is also important. Youth should receive a mental health screening each time they are admitted to a new juvenile justice placement—whether it is a short-term detention facility, long-term training school, work camp, ranch, boot camp or group home.

Mental health screenings also should be conducted throughout youths' stay at residential programs if the youth display a dramatic change in behavior and/or mental health symptoms are suspected. Previous mental health screening information can be helpful to community supervision staff. But they should also conduct their own mental health screening due to the change in youths' circumstances as the youth transition back into the community.

At a minimum, a mental health screening in juvenile justice should include (but not necessarily be limited to) the key areas of:

- Current/previous mental health symptoms (*e.g.*, depression, hyperactivity, hallucinations, self-injury)

- Current/previous suicidal thoughts/ behavior

- Current/previous mental health treatment (*e.g.*, inpatient, outpatient, psychotropic medication)

- Recent drug and alcohol use

- Cognitive/intellectual limitations

- Recent traumatic event(s)

Screening and Assessment of Juvenile Offenders with Mental Health Disorders

- Current/previous aggressive or violent thoughts and behavior
- Degree of insight regarding need for treatment
- Observation of juveniles' behavior (*e.g.,* mental status, appearance, speech)

Juvenile offenders may have both a mental health disorder and a substance use disorder. *(Please see Chapter 10 for additional information about screening juveniles with co-occurring mental health and substance use disorders.)*

If youth are overtly intoxicated or extremely agitated when admitted to a juvenile justice facility, mental health screening should be delayed until staff can elicit compliance and obtain more reliable results. However, these juveniles should remain in an area where they can be observed by staff. Juvenile offenders should not be placed with the general population of youth until a mental health screening has been completed.

Juvenile justice professionals who are not familiar with mental health disorders may be reluctant to inquire about symptoms of mental illness. Often, this reluctance is due to being uncomfortable with youth who display unusual or bizarre behavior. For instance, staff may not know how to respond to youth who cut themselves or who talk in sentences that make no sense. Staff training on mental health issues, close working relationships between juvenile justice and mental health staff, and practice asking mental health-related questions are essential and can help ease awkwardness. The more knowledgeable staff become about the mental health symptoms of juveniles, the more natural this type of questioning becomes.

 MENTAL HEALTH ASSESSMENT

A mental health assessment is a comprehensive evaluation designed to obtain specific information about youths' mental health issues. A mental health assessment typically occurs after juveniles are identified as having a possible mental health disorder, and identified issues are explored on a more in-depth basis. Formal diagnostic criteria are used to establish whether a mental health disorder is present, and if so, the scope and severity of the disorder. Juveniles are typically queried about their thoughts, feelings, behavior, and functioning. In addition to issues related specifically to mental health, other important areas of youths' lives are explored. A comprehensive mental health assessment may take hours to complete and provides the foundation for treatment planning. Clinicians conducting these types of evaluations are typically well trained in the area of mental health and have experience working with adolescents—particularly adolescents involved with the juvenile justice system. Mental health assessments are in-depth evaluations that may include:

- A clinical interview
- Tests of cognitive and intellectual functioning
- Personality tests
- Other measures of youths' behavioral and emotional adjustment

In addition to using specialized assessment tools, clinicians should gather information from a variety of individuals who can report on the juveniles' functioning and behavior (e.g., the youth, juvenile justice professionals, teachers, case managers, health care providers, mental health providers, substance abuse treatment providers, recreation staff, vocational supervisors). Obtaining information from family members/caretakers is essential.

Information from a mental health assessment is typically summarized in a written report. Ideally, this report identifies:

- The nature and severity of the youths' disorder
- Youths' mental health diagnosis
- Other psychosocial problems that need to be addressed

Juvenile Offenders with Mental Health Disorders: Who Are They and What Do We Do With Them?

- Strengths/resiliencies of the youth
- Recommendations for treatment

Mental health assessment reports should be written in a manner that is understandable to youths' family/caretakers, as well as to professionals in related disciplines (e.g., education, substance abuse, juvenile justice, child welfare). The reports, therefore, should contain minimal, to no, mental health jargon. Youth always should receive face-to-face feedback after participating in a mental health assessment. Too many juvenile offenders have sat through several hours (sometimes even days) of mental health testing without being provided with information about the results of the evaluation. Feedback to youth does not need to be detailed and in-depth; it should be communicated in such a way that the youth can understand it. Juveniles should have the opportunity to ask questions and clarify anything about the test results that remain confusing to them.

Mental health assessments often include (but are not limited to) the following key areas:

- Current/previous mental health symptoms (e.g., depression, hyperactivity, hallucinations)
- Current/previous suicidal thoughts/ behavior
- Current/previous mental health treatment (e.g., inpatient, outpatient, psychotropic medication)
- Current/previous drug and alcohol use
- Current/previous drug and alcohol abuse treatment (e.g., inpatient, outpatient)
- Relationship between mental health symptoms and substance use
- Cognitive/intellectual limitations
- Recent/previous traumatic event(s)
- Current/previous aggressive or violent thoughts and behavior
- Level of emotional distress or functional impairment

- Home environment/relationships with family and/or caretaker
- Family history of mental health and substance use disorders
- Abuse and neglect
- Out-of-home placements
- School/vocational history and status
- Health/medical issues
- Delinquent behavior/juvenile justice involvement
- Peer/romantic relationships
- Coping/problem-solving abilities
- Current support system
- Hobbies/interests
- Strengths/resiliencies
- Degree of insight regarding need for treatment/level of motivation for treatment
- Observation of juveniles (e.g., behavior, mental status, appearance, speech, thought processes, mood, affect)

Many juvenile offenders are only in contact with the juvenile justice system for brief periods of time (e.g., pre-trial detention). In addition, extensive psychological evaluations of all youth entering the system could be difficult and expensive. Therefore, screening and assessment for mental health disorders should be time-efficient and cost-effective. That said, mental health screening and assessment still needs to be thorough enough to:

- Identify youth with mental health disorders
- Provide information about the nature and severity of youths' mental health disorder(s)
- Provide practical information for the development of an individualized treatment plan

Mental health assessments should always be linked to a treatment plan. Determining a psychiatric diagnosis without making recommendations for intervention is not helpful for individuals who work with mentally ill youth. It is also a waste of valuable resources to conduct mental health assessments with juveniles only to have the results placed in the youths' file—with no influence on treatment planning and juvenile justice supervision. Results from mental health assessments should be integrated into juveniles' programming, treatment and supervision plan.

Mental health assessments with juvenile offenders can be complex and challenging. These youth often present with a variety of issues related to mental health, substance abuse, educational difficulties, family conflict, health concerns, and so forth. Taking into account the multi-dimensional aspects of these youth, as

---

INFORMATION FROM JUVENILE JUSTICE SCREENING AND ASSESSMENT TOOLS CAN PROVIDE HELPFUL INFORMATION TO MENTAL HEALTH PROFESSIONALS WHEN THEY ARE CONDUCTING A MENTAL HEALTH ASSESSMENT.

---

well as the multiple determinants of their symptoms and behavior can be difficult and time-consuming. Consequently, results from a mental health assessment may not be as clear-cut and straightforward as recipients of the resulting report would like them to be. If the outcome of a mental health assessment is not clear, the clinician who conducted the evaluation should be contacted for clarification. However, the lack of clarity may be associated with the mixed clinical picture presented by the youth.

The discussion above refers to *clinical* mental health assessments. Some youth receive *forensic* assessments. Forensic evaluators are mental health professionals who work for the court. Information is collected to help the court/judge make appropriate decisions about

the youth (versus helping design intervention plans for youth). This information is not meant to be used for juvenile justice programming, and resulting reports are not designed to be shared with juvenile justice personnel (*e.g.*, facility staff, community supervision staff).

Juvenile Justice Screening and Assessment

The juvenile justice system provides a continuum of services with varying levels of intervention. The system is required to identify the proper security level for each youth (*e.g.*, probation versus more restrictive setting, community-based facility versus training school, moderate security versus maximum security facility). Inappropriate matching of youth to security level can result in the placement of nonviolent juveniles in overly restrictive settings. In addition, it can result in an increased risk to the community if violent/high risk youth are placed in settings that are unable to manage their behavior. Further, inequity can result if youth with the same offense and risk are placed at different levels of restriction.

To properly classify youth and refer them for appropriate placement and services within the system, juvenile justice professionals often use special screening and assessment tools. Risk assessment and needs assessment tools, as well as youths' juvenile justice history, can influence decision-making related to:

- Where youth will reside
- The type of programming in which youth will be involved
- The type of specialized treatment services (if any) youth will receive

Information from juvenile justice screening and assessment tools can provide helpful information to mental health professionals when they are conducting a mental health assessment. Integrating juvenile justice and mental health information can provide a more comprehensive and holistic view of juvenile offenders with mental health disorders. Also, information

232

Juvenile Offenders with Mental Health Disorders: Who Are They and What Do We Do With Them?

about youths' juvenile justice history may be related in some way to youths' mental health disorder.

The following are some key areas of juvenile justice information that should be integrated with mental health information about youth:

- Current offense
- Prior arrests
- Prior juvenile detention and/or training school admissions
- Sanctions received during incarceration in juvenile detention and/or training schools
- Incidents of isolation, seclusion, and/or restraint during incarceration
- Status offenses (*e.g.,* running away, truancy)
- Drug-related offenses
- Violent offenses
- Time spent on community supervision and any violations
- Family history of criminal involvement/ incarceration

RISK ASSESSMENT

Risk assessment within juvenile justice typically refers to the process of estimating the likelihood that youth will continue their involvement in criminal behavior. This type of assessment provides information to juvenile justice staff to assist them in deciding which level of security/ supervision is appropriate for particular youth. Decisions based on a risk assessment can occur throughout the juvenile justice system: arrest, intake, detention, prosecution, disposition and placement (OJJDP, 1995). Judges typically consider offender risk when determining whether youth should be committed to a juvenile justice facility or placed on probation. Upon commitment to a facility, juvenile justice professionals might assess youths' level of risk to determine the appropriate intensity of placement and services.

Staff must assess the likelihood of juveniles escaping, harming themselves, assaulting staff or peers, or being victimized by others. Decisions also need to be made about transitioning youth back into the community. Some secure facilities use risk assessment instruments to help determine which youth are least likely to return to criminal behavior and are thus eligible for a group home—or other less restrictive placement. Many community supervision professionals also rely on risk assessment tools. Parole and probation resources are limited, so identifying those youth who pose the greatest risk to the community and allocating resources accordingly is important.

Historically, risk assessment and classification within juvenile justice have been informal, highly discretionary procedures. These tools were typically given by juvenile justice professionals with varying philosophies, different levels of experience, and different criteria for making decisions.

During recent years, juvenile justice agencies have adopted more formal procedures for decision-making, including standardized risk assessment instruments and structured classification systems. This practice provides greater objectivity, consistency and structure to the assessment and decision-making process. It also helps the system to allocate resources more efficiently, with the most serious and chronic offenders receiving the most intensive and intrusive interventions.

Risk assessment instruments in juvenile justice typically contain a limited number of factors found to be related to recidivism (*e.g.,* age of first adjudication, number of prior arrests, problems in school)—although various tools contain different numbers and combinations of items. Pre-determined decision rules are usually used to classify offenders based on a total risk score (*e.g.,* youth with scores of 22 or higher are placed in a maximum security facility).

The ability to predict whether an individual youth will engage in future criminal behavior is difficult at best, so risk assessment tools classify juveniles according to information based on groups of offenders. In addition, many of the studies investigating which variables are most closely associated with recidivism have typically included Caucasian males. Factors predictive of recidivism among female juveniles, as well as youth from various racial/ethnic minority groups may differ from those predicting recidivism among a Caucasian male population. Further, mental health factors may play a more significant role in the prediction of recidivism among some groups of juveniles but not others (Wierson & Forehand, 1995). Therefore, risk assessment scores should not be used as the sole criteria when making placement decisions for an individual youth (OJJDP, 1995).

Some juvenile offenders with mental health disorders may be placed in a restrictive setting (or receive a high level of supervision) due to factors other than their criminal behavior. Current/previous mental health symptoms (*e.g.*, impulsivity, aggression, suicidal behavior), current/previous mental health treatment, substance use, current/previous substance abuse treatment, and the like, are items included on some juvenile justice risk assessment tools. Juvenile offenders with mental health disorders often have the above risk factors. Therefore, they can receive moderate-to-high risk scores even when their criminal history or current criminal behavior is not severe. Resulting juvenile justice placements may not be appropriate for youth who are determined to be high-risk due to mental health issues versus other factors related to delinquent behavior.

NEEDS ASSESSMENT

A needs assessment within juvenile justice typically refers to the process of identifying the factors that are most critical for the rehabilitation of a particular juvenile offender. Using needs assessment tools prompts juvenile justice professionals to consider a variety of areas (*e.g.*, physical health, education, social skills, peer relationships, family relationships, mental health, substance abuse) when developing service plans for youth. Results from these

types of measurement tools help staff determine which interventions or programs would be most beneficial for an individual youth (*e.g.*, social skills training, anger management, remedial education, substance abuse treatment, family therapy) and also influence resource allocation. Because one of the primary goals of a needs assessment instrument is to describe youths' functioning (strengths and deficits) versus to predict an outcome (*e.g.*, danger to community), most of these measures are not based on research. In fact, many juvenile justice agencies have designed their own needs assessment forms. Individual items on a needs assessment tool should be clearly defined to reduce subjective interpretation by different juvenile justice professionals.

The current risk assessment and needs assessment tools used in juvenile justice are a great improvement over what was used in the past. However, much more research needs to be conducted to establish the reliability and validity of these instruments.

Collaborating on Mental Health Screening and Assessment

Historically, mental health professionals and juvenile justice professionals have been operating independently in their screening and assessment of juvenile offenders with mental health disorders. This practice was common regardless of youths' status within juvenile justice during the time screening or assessment took place (*e.g.*, pre-arrest, arrest, probation, detention, training school, parole).

In most settings, even today, mental health and juvenile justice professionals meet separately with youth to acquire necessary information. Each of these individuals scores and interprets the data/information collected from juveniles and then writes separate reports. This procedure usually results in separate rehabilitation/treatment recommendations for juvenile offenders who have a mental health disorder. Ironically, mental health assessments and needs

234

Juvenile Offenders with Mental Health Disorders: Who Are They and What Do We Do With Them?

assessments in juvenile justice often target similar, if not exactly the same, areas of concern.

Increasing the integration of mental health and juvenile justice information at the time it is collected can be beneficial to all parties involved. Ideally, substance use information is integrated as well. Many of the various screening and assessment tools used within the juvenile justice, mental health and substance abuse systems contain the exact same questions (*e.g.*, suicidal behavior, substance use, aggression, previous treatment, psychotropic medication). Coordinating the gathering of this type of information can reduce the amount of time to screen or assess juveniles, as well as decrease the amount of paperwork required. Reducing question redundancy across systems also may improve the reliability of information collected. Many youth become frustrated and annoyed when repeatedly asked similar questions by different professionals.

After collecting important information related to youths' functioning, mental health and juvenile justice professionals may communicate little, if at all, about overlapping findings or shared treatment goals related to particular offenders. Fortunately, this situation is improving within some juvenile justice agencies, but many continue to operate with minimal collaboration between the juvenile justice and mental health systems.

Juvenile justice professionals report that access to mental health information related to youth (*e.g.,* mental health status, previous mental health treatment, suicidal behavior) helps them to manage mentally ill juveniles in their custody more effectively.

In addition, mental health professionals typically report that their evaluations of youth would be greatly enhanced if they had more access to youths' juvenile justice information (*e.g.*, recent criminal behavior, juvenile justice status, juvenile justice history). The sharing of this information is essential. Involvement with juvenile justice and the experience of symptoms

(mental health and/or substance use) are related for a significant number of juvenile offenders who have mental health disorders. Increased coordination and integration of the results from juvenile justice, mental health and substance abuse screening and assessment tools can result in more effective communication between these key systems. It also can result in comprehensive treatment plans that take into account the various aspects of youths' difficulties. In addition, important information obtained during previous mental health screenings and assessments should be communicated across the different areas of the juvenile justice system as youth move through the continuum of care. This practice helps facilitate juveniles' seamless transition into a facility and out into the community when the youth are released from a secure setting.

Special Issues in Screening and Assessment

OVERRIDES

The scoring of many screening and assessment tools involves the totaling or combining of several items into specific scales or a total score. Most juvenile justice agencies have policies dictating what actions should be taken if youth score above or below a particular cutoff point on a certain screening or assessment tool (*e.g.*, place youth on suicide watch, transfer youth to a hospital, house youth on a special needs unit, refer youth for psychotropic medication, place youth in a highly restrictive area of the facility). Sometimes, individuals administering or scoring a screening or assessment tool do not believe that juveniles' resulting score accurately represents the attributes of those particular youth.

For example, a 15-year-old juvenile may be classified as high risk to re-offend due to scoring above the predetermined cutoff on a risk assessment tool. But the youth's high score may be due to a serious criminal offense that occurred six years earlier, when the youth first began using drugs. This juvenile typically would receive several points for committing a serious crime, having a history of substance use, and being arrested at a young age. The staff member conducting the assessment may become aware that the juvenile has successfully participated in several treatment programs, is currently a straight-A student, has been clean and sober for three years, and is involved in numerous church and community programs. Even if the youth's current charge is fairly minor (*e.g.*, trespassing), he may score in the high-risk range based on his previous history. The staff member may want to override the juvenile's score on the risk assessment tool and place him in a less-restrictive category.

Within juvenile justice, overrides can occur with mental health screening and mental health assessment tools as well as risk assessment tools. Overrides typically occur when examiners do not think the results from a mental health screening or assessment tool accurately represent youths' true mental health status.

For example, juveniles may have been intoxicated during the evaluation or may have vehemently denied all problems and issues, even the most benign. Some youth from diverse racial, ethnic or cultural backgrounds may not fully understand all of the mental health questions asked of them. Language issues can be significant barriers if English is not youths' primary language. Also, some youth have been raised not to discuss personal issues outside of the family, even with mental health professionals. Juvenile offenders may appear to be severely mentally ill based on the results of a mental health instrument, but an evaluator may strongly believe that the results are inaccurate. In contrast, an evaluator may question youths' mental health screening or assessment if it looks too "clean." The clinician may believe that the juveniles are hiding or covering up psychiatric symptoms. In either case, an evaluator will probably attempt to override the decision dictated by the youths' objective scores.

Closely monitoring the use of overrides associated with screening and assessment tools is important for juvenile justice agencies. Fortunately, most juvenile justice agencies allow only specified staff to supersede predetermined decisions and actions related to these types of instruments. One advantage of allowing overrides is that relevant factors associated with individual youth can be considered during points of decision-making, even if they are not captured on a screening or assessment instrument. This can be beneficial when juveniles' scores seem either erroneously high or low.

Overrides also allow staff to include their observations in the decision-making process. For example, during the screening or assessment process, intuitive and/or experienced staff members may notice signs that youth are intentionally trying to conceal certain information—or are trying to embellish and exaggerate certain issues. Staff instincts need to be represented in some way. Having the option of overriding screening and assessment scores can be beneficial in select cases. But experts recommend that no more than 15 percent of decisions be the result of overrides (OJJDP, 1995). Otherwise, juvenile justice agencies run the risk of having their screening and assessment process become subjective and inconsistent. Too many decisions may be based on various staff members' differing philosophies and/or level of experience.

Reassessment

Juveniles often need to receive periodic reassessments (*e.g.*, mental health diagnosis, treatment services, juvenile justice programming, level of supervision, management strategies) to determine whether current services are still appropriate or are in need of modification. Adolescence itself is associated with changes in cognitive, emotional, and physical growth and development.

In addition, the life circumstances, mood states and behavior of juvenile offenders in particular can change dramatically over time. Some juvenile offenders are reluctant to verbalize distress or problematic issues during initial

Juvenile Offenders with Mental Health Disorders: Who Are They and What Do We Do With Them?

screening and assessment opportunities. These youth may be more comfortable disclosing this type of information at a later time once they have:

- Adjusted to a juvenile justice environment
- Developed a higher level of trust in an examiner

Some juvenile justice agencies conduct reassessments of youths' level of risk and/or needs on a regular basis (*e.g.*, every 90 days). Mental health screenings also should occur periodically, particularly if juveniles are experiencing high levels of stress and/or if staff notice dramatic changes in youths' mood or behavior. Juvenile offenders who have been diagnosed with a mental health disorder should receive a comprehensive mental health evaluation every few years to assess whether:

- Their psychiatric diagnosis remains accurate
- Adjustments are needed in their treatment plan

A comprehensive reassessment may need to occur even sooner if there is reason to believe that a previous mental health evaluation was unreliable or invalid. Results from any reassessments should be integrated into juvenile offenders' supervision and treatment plan.

Referrals

Youth identified during a mental health screening process as requiring additional assessment should be referred for a more in-depth mental health evaluation. There also should be a process in place for juvenile offenders who do not "red flag" on an initial mental health screening tool but who may need to be referred for a mental health evaluation at a later time (*e.g.*, if they demonstrate behaviors of concern).

Additionally, juveniles should be able to refer themselves for a mental health evaluation if they experience emotional or behavioral distress or impairment. Any adult who interacts with juvenile offenders should have access to the mental health referral process (*e.g.*, line

staff, community supervision staff, teachers, family members, clergy, substance abuse counselors, unit supervisors, vocational supervisors, health care providers), as they may be the first to notice a change in youths' behavior. A referral does not necessarily guarantee that juveniles will receive a mental health evaluation. Therefore, specific procedures should be in place for reviewing all mental health referrals, including how decisions are made about which youth will receive additional mental health assessment.

Mental health referrals play a significant role in the assessment of juvenile offenders with mental health disorders. This situation is true regardless of the results of youths' initial mental health screening upon admission to a juvenile justice facility. Because juveniles' mental health symptoms can change considerably over time, ongoing monitoring of their behavior is critical. When juvenile justice professionals notice youth behaviors of concern and/or juveniles become distressed, intervening before problems become any worse is important. Referring youth to mental health/medical professionals is one step in the possible prevention of significant mental health issues.

Mental health referrals are most helpful when they are stated in objective, behavioral terms. Alerting a supervisor or mental health/medical professional that youth are "whacked out," "acting crazy," or "seem weird" does not convey much useful information. These terms can bring particular juveniles to the attention of an evaluator. However, behavioral descriptions of youth, such as "cannot sit still," "is talking about suicide," "seems nervous," "is not eating," "says the devil is talking to her," help an evaluator determine where to focus an assessment.

Specific, behavioral descriptions are critical, given the usual limitations on time and resources of most mental health professionals in juvenile justice. Juvenile offenders who refer themselves to a mental health professional should be encouraged to phrase their concerns in a similar fashion. Staff can help youth identify the specific thoughts, feelings or behaviors of concern to juveniles if they are unable to do this by themselves.

Within facilities, juvenile justice professionals, teachers, recreational staff and vocational supervisors interact continuously with youth. These individuals are in an ideal position to recognize unusual behaviors or changes in juveniles' functioning. Their input to an evaluator (*e.g.*, psychologist, social worker, psychiatrist, nurse) is critical and should be encouraged. Some juveniles behave differently during one-on-one assessments with a mental health professional than they do in a unit with peers, in the classroom, or in the gymnasium. To obtain an accurate picture of youths' functioning, clinicians conducting mental health assessments need descriptions of juveniles' behavior in several different situations. A variety of staff have this type of information. Therefore, a referral process needs to be in place so that a number of individuals can convey information to clinicians in an easy and time-efficient manner.

Individuals Who Conduct Mental Health Screening and Assessment

Any professional (*i.e.*, juvenile justice, medical, mental health) conducting mental health screening and assessment with juvenile offenders should possess the knowledge and skills to do so—especially when screening and assessment tools require specific training before using them. Depending on the particular tool being used, this type of training may be simple and brief , or time-intensive and cumbersome. In addition, individuals conducting screenings and assessments of mental health symptoms should have some knowledge about:

- The type of mental health information they are soliciting
- Developmental issues of childhood and adolescence

- Stressors of incarceration
- How substance use can be related to mental health symptoms
- How medical issues can be related to mental health symptoms

Clearly, juvenile justice professionals who administer a brief mental health screening tool at intake do not need to have the same level of mental health knowledge as psychologists administering a comprehensive set of mental health assessment tools. But it is essential that an individual's knowledge and training be commensurate with the task at hand.

In addition, mental health professionals conducting comprehensive assessments of juvenile offenders should have knowledge about, and experience with, this particular population of youth. Some juvenile justice agencies employ mental health professionals in their facilities, whereas others refer offenders to mental health professionals in the community. Either way,

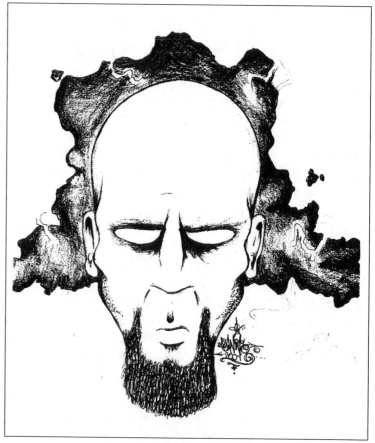

Juvenile Offenders with Mental Health Disorders: Who Are They and What Do We Do With Them?

these mental health professionals should have experience evaluating adolescents, particularly high-risk adolescents and/or those involved with the juvenile justice system. Assessing juvenile offenders can be particularly challenging for a multitude of reasons, including:

- The presence of multiple presenting problems
- The interrelationship of mental health and substance use disorders
- Rebellious or anti-authority attitudes
- Multi-determined causes of difficulties
- Unconventional lifestyles
- Effects of juvenile justice status on mental health
- Stressors specific to incarceration

Clinicians unfamiliar with this population of young people often focus on youths' aggression and criminal behavior, leaving underlying mental health issues uncovered. Or, they may not detect important psychiatric symptoms due to sophisticated juveniles knowing how to distract professionals from discovering key mental health issues. If they have been involved with mental health professionals in the past, some juvenile offenders can be very aware of how the mental health system operates. Many of these youth know exactly what to say to facilitate admission to a psychiatric hospital or to receive a prescription of psychotropic medication. These youth also typically know what not to say in order to avoid involvement with mental health treatment services. Clinicians responsible for assessing juvenile offenders with mental health disorders need to be aware of these dynamics.

In addition, assessments by mental health professionals should be objective and unbiased. Some mental health providers specialize in working with individuals who have particular psychiatric disorders (*e.g.*, Attention-Deficit Hyperactivity Disorder, Bipolar Disorder, Conduct Disorder). However, this expertise should not significantly influence the results of mental health assessments of particular offenders. Assessment information should be collected, scored, interpreted and reported in an impartial manner, based solely on the data collected for individual youth. Juvenile justice professionals commonly express frustration and disappointment with mental health professionals who repeatedly diagnose most youth with the exact same mental health disorder—despite the diversity and dissimilarity of symptoms they exhibit. Many juvenile offenders have similar issues, and some professionals use templates to write their reports. However, mental health assessments always should be individualized. Writing mental health reports that contain the same language, diagnosis and recommendations for every juvenile assessed is poor practice, unethical, and a misuse of mental health resources.

Strength-Focused Assessment

When collecting screening and assessment information from juvenile offenders, adults can be tempted to focus primarily on the areas of youths' lives that are in need of improvement. Further, when talking to the families/caretakers of these juveniles, professionals often concentrate on the families'/caretakers' areas of difficulty as well. But even if mentally ill youth and/or their families/caretakers are experiencing significant problems, each of them has assets that can help improve the quality of their lives.

During a mental health screening or assessment, professionals should avoid language that implies something is wrong or bad. For example, many clinicians ask youth and/or their family/caretakers about problems the juveniles may have at home, in school or in relationships.

Using words such as "challenges" instead of "problems" can help youth and their family/caretakers feel more supported during this type of questioning. Rather than asking only about where the youth have had difficulty in the past, clinicians should inquire about the areas in which the juveniles have achieved or excelled.

Screening and Assessment of Juvenile Offenders with Mental Health Disorders

Juvenile offenders with mental health disorders are much more than their pathology, diagnosis or label. Many youth in juvenile justice, as well as their families/caretakers, have experienced tragedy and crisis in their lives. It is often because of their strengths and resiliencies that these individuals have survived—physically and emotionally. These assets should be identified and explored during mental health assessments.

A strength-focused assessment often requires creative questioning. If youth have had difficulty with academic achievement and have a history of poor grades, clinicians should ask about other aspects of the youths' school experience. For example, do the youth have friends at school? Or have they continued to apply themselves in the classroom even when they were frustrated and/or the schoolwork was difficult for them? These are important skills for juveniles to possess. Are the youth involved with any extra-curricular activities, sports teams and the like? Inquiring about other aspects of the school experience—in addition to academic achievement—can be particularly helpful for juvenile offenders who may already feel inadequate and incompetent due to their poor grades.

Identifying youths' talents and capabilities is an essential part of any assessment of juvenile offenders. Questions about problem areas should be balanced with inquiries about hobbies, interests and things about themselves youth feel good about. If juveniles are unable to verbalize their positive qualities, asking the youth why other people like them can be helpful (*e.g.*, friends, teachers, relatives, juvenile justice staff). Taking this broader view of youth and their functioning demonstrates to juveniles that adults are interested in knowing all about them.

Juvenile offenders' past experiences with social service, mental health and juvenile justice professionals may have reinforced the idea that the youth are "bad" and/or that something is "wrong" with them. Focusing on youths' abilities and achievements (no matter how small) helps youth view themselves from a broader, more inclusive perspective. However, taking a strength-based approach does not entail overlooking delinquent behavior or ignoring issues that are causing distress to youth or those around them. Those issues are critical. But assessments should be balanced, which includes drawing attention to the ways in which juveniles are doing well or have done well in the past.

When youth with mental health disorders come into contact with the juvenile justice system, their family/caretakers may feel hopeless about the youths' behavior and future. The juveniles may feel hopeless as well. Asking how youth and their family/caretakers have survived hardships and difficulties in the past is important. Learning about times when the juveniles were functioning more effectively, as well as assessing what factors contributed to the their previous successes, is crucial in truly understanding the youth. This information also can be valuable when developing treatment strategies. Many families/caretakers of juvenile offenders have histories of involvement with social services and the juvenile justice system. They may have had numerous experiences in which professionals pointed out what they were doing wrong in raising their children. Taking a strength-based approach helps youth and their family/caretakers feel less hopeless. Acknowledging their positive characteristics can increase the likelihood of youth/families/caretakers engaging in the assessment process, as well as actively participating in treatment interventions. Youths' emotional and behavioral strengths can be measured informally or with a standardized, norm-referenced tool (Epstein, 1999).

Culturally Sensitive Assessment

Attention to cultural issues should be a part of all mental health screening and assessment of juvenile offenders. Failure to identify youths' positive attributes may be due to an acceptance of cultural/racial stereotypes (intentional or unintentional). When clinicians gather informa-

240

Juvenile Offenders with Mental Health Disorders: Who Are They and What Do We Do With Them?

tion from youth (as well as their families/ caretakers) from a culture or race different from their own, strengths and resiliencies may not be identified. Certain questions may be avoided or deemed unnecessary during an interview. When areas of juveniles' (and their family's/ caretaker's) lives are dissimilar to the professional conducting an assessment, differences can be misinterpreted as "problems" or "deficits" when that is not the case. In fact, differences specific to youths' race/ethnicity or their cultural traditions actually may enhance the juveniles' ability to cope.

Conducting valid and reliable assessments with youth (including their families/caretakers) who are different than themselves is important for clinicians. Otherwise, treatment recommendations will not reflect juveniles' true intervention needs. The likelihood of obtaining accurate assessment information from youth increases when they feel respected and understood by the examiner. Being culturally sensitive about the types of questions asked and the instruments used, increases the likelihood that juvenile offenders and their families/caretakers will actively participate in assessment activities and carry out any resulting recommendations.

Professionals should consider the following issues whenever conducting mental health screening and assessment with juvenile offenders from diverse ethnic/racial/cultural backgrounds (Suzuki & Kugler, 1995):

- Inappropriate content with screening and assessment tools
- Inappropriate norms
- Language discrepancies
- Examiner bias
- Measurement of different constructs
- Differences in ability to make predictions
- Variations in test-taking behavior

INAPPROPRIATE CONTENT WITH SCREENING AND ASSESSMENT TOOLS

Juvenile offenders from various racial/ethnic/ cultural groups may not understand certain test questions if a test reflects the values, lifestyle and culture of middle-class Caucasians. For example, youth—such as African-American youth from the inner city, Caucasian youth from a rural community, youth who emigrated from Mexico—may lose valuable points if they do not recognize certain words or phrases used on a test (e.g., do not recognize the word lanai on an intelligence test although they know what a terrace/balcony is; when asked to answer a question related to a cup and saucer on an intelligence test, they confuse the word saucer with a flying saucer/UFO, so answer incorrectly).

INAPPROPRIATE NORMS

Many mental health screening and assessment tools have been standardized to populations primarily consisting of Caucasian individuals of middle-class status. When juveniles take a standardized and norm-referenced test, their score is compared to the "norm" group. The youths' scores are then ranked (i.e., 30th percentile) or placed in a range (i.e., below average range of intelligence) depending on how they measure up to individuals in the comparison group. The scores of the norm group may not serve as an appropriate comparison group for individuals from different racial/ethnic/cultural groups.

LANGUAGE DISCREPANCIES

Juvenile offenders of different races/ ethnicities/cultures may not fully understand the language used by an examiner during an interview (or testing), and the examiner may not completely understand the youth. Examiners can be confused by youths' use of slang or phrases specific to their culture or community. Language discrepancies not only can interfere with the building of rapport but also can result in misinterpretation of youths' answers. Some of the more popular mental health assessment tools have been translated into various languages. But these non-English versions of the tests typically have not been validated in the same manner as the English version. If English is not youths' primary language, an interpreter may be necessary to translate the interview and assessment material. However, not all words and concepts can be translated directly into and from English, particularly in the realm of a mental health assessment.

EXAMINER BIAS

When examiners are unfamiliar with juveniles from diverse cultures, races and ethnic groups, misinterpretation of youth behavior can result. This situation can be compounded when there is an over-reliance on stereotypes from the media. Examiner bias is evident when behaviors exhibited by juveniles (or lack thereof) are misconstrued as pathological, when, in fact, they are well-accepted, and sometimes expected, in youths' culture (e.g., not engaging in direct eye contact, not disclosing personal information to strangers, talking about spirits). In contrast, an examiner may mistakenly dismiss juveniles' psychiatric symptoms by automatically attributing them to cultural differences.

MEASUREMENT OF DIFFERENT CONSTRUCTS

Many screening and assessment instruments were developed primarily for middle-class Caucasian individuals. Therefore, the tools may not necessarily measure the same characteristics (e.g., depression, anger, hyperactivity, intelligence) when used with individuals from different racial/ethnic/cultural backgrounds.

DIFFERENCES IN ABILITY TO MAKE PREDICTIONS

Specific screening and assessment tools are often used to predict particular outcomes (e.g., suicide, violence) among youth. Tests that make valid predictions for middle-class Caucasian youth may not be valid when making predictions for youth from other ethnic/racial/cultural minority groups. In addition, the definition of a "successful" outcome may differ for juve-

niles from various ethnic/racial/cultural minority groups.

VARIATIONS IN TEST-TAKING BEHAVIOR

Juveniles from various ethnic/racial/cultural minority groups may not be familiar with the assessment process in which they are participating. They may not understand the benefit of:

- Working quickly on certain tasks (i.e., timed tests)
- Guessing when they do not know an answer
- Asking for clarification if they do not understand a question

Certain cultures value test-taking skills more highly than others, so some youth have additional practice in this arena. Juveniles' motivation, determination and ability to perform under stress during the assessment process can greatly influence examination results.

Professionals conducting mental health screenings and assessments with juvenile offenders from various racial/ethnic minority groups must pay attention to cultural issues. But evaluators do not necessarily need to be of the same race or background as minority youth. However, these professionals should have knowledge of the important issues, values and beliefs of the juveniles' culture and community. They also need to be able to recognize various terms used by youth and if they are unable to do this, to ask for immediate clarification. In addition, evaluators should be aware of the issues involved in using standardized assessment tools with minority youth.

Because many of these measures have not been "normed" on youth from racial/ethnic/cultural minority groups, it is critical that all test results be integrated with culturally sensitive interviews. Information gathered from thorough clinical interviews and mental health-related measurement tools can be beneficial when appropriately administered and interpreted. Having knowledge of the potential

242

Juvenile Offenders with Mental Health Disorders: Who Are They and What Do We Do With Them?

limitations when youth from diverse racial/ethnic/cultural groups are assessed and taking appropriate precautions can increase the reliability and validity of the information collected.

Most mental health providers believe in the importance of taking cultural factors into account when evaluating individuals from minority groups. However, a large proportion of these professionals report a high need for additional training in this area. Some mental health providers have not received any culturally focused training at all (Ramirez, Wassef, Paniagua, & Linskey, 1996).

The potential limitations associated with the testing of juvenile offenders from various racial/ethnic/cultural minority groups are relevant to all types of testing. This would include screening and assessment instruments related to risk, needs, mental health and substance abuse.

 SCREENING AND ASSESSMENT INSTRUMENTS

When choosing mental health screening and assessment tools to be used with youth involved in the juvenile justice system, agencies should consider:

- If reading is required, is the reading level appropriate for the population of youth being assessed?
- What background or training is required to administer the instrument?
- Who administers the instrument?
- How long does it take to administer, score and interpret the instrument?
- Does the amount of time it takes to administer, score and interpret the instrument fit with the context of where the youth is being tested?
- What type of information is provided by the instrument?
- How will results from the instrument be used?

- Where will the test results be kept and who will have access to them?
- Is the instrument/or the questions on it culturally appropriate?

Most juvenile justice agencies have a process in place in which youth are screened for a few critical mental health issues. Although the tools used vary in their format and specific wording, most have questions about suicide, hallucinations and current psychotropic medication. These questions are often embedded in general health-screening forms and are typically asked by medical professionals during juveniles'

STANDARDIZED TESTS ARE SUPPOSED TO BE CONDUCTED UNDER STANDARD CONDITIONS SO THAT ALL YOUTH ARE GIVEN THE TEST IN SAME MANNER. THE GOAL IS, AS MUCH AS POSSIBLE, TO PROVIDE A FAIR AND UNBIASED COMPARISON AMONG ALL JUVENILES WHO TAKE A PARTICULAR TEST.

---

basic health screening. Some agencies ask questions related to above areas, as well as additional areas associated with mental health, during routine intake procedures. Juvenile justice professionals typically conduct these types of screenings. The mental health questions may be part of a more comprehensive screening form that assesses a variety of psychosocial issues. Or it may be included in a measure specifically designed to collect information about juveniles' mental health status (*e.g.,* Mental Health Juvenile Detention Admission Tool/MH-JDAT; Washington State Detention Managers Association & Boesky, 2000). Some juvenile justice agencies use standardized, norm-referenced screening and assessment instruments that have been developed specifically to measure one or more psychological constructs (*e.g.,* depression, trauma, anxiety, hyperactivity).

Standardized and Norm-Referenced Screening and Assessment Instruments

Standardized tests in the area of mental health are typically designed to measure one or more aspects of youths' functioning (*e.g.*, intelligence, personality, mood, skills, behavior) in an objective manner. These types of instruments are often referred to as "norm-referenced" tests because the instruments are standardized to a clearly defined group, the norm group (Sattler, 1988). Scaled scores are developed so that specific juveniles' scores on a test can be compared to those of individuals in the norm group. This practice helps evaluators determine whether youth have more or less of a certain psychological construct in comparison to others who are similar to them (*e.g.*, same age, same gender). Standardized tests are supposed to be conducted under standard conditions so that all youth are given the test in same manner. The goal is, as much as possible, to provide a fair and unbiased comparison among all juveniles who take a particular test. Some standardized mental health assessment tools require specific training, so only certain individuals are able to administer them.

Many standardized and/or norm-referenced tools have a great deal of research associated with the development, scoring and interpretation of the test. This information helps evaluators determine which tools are the most reliable and valid tools to use. Just because a screening or assessment instrument is standardized and/ or norm-referenced, however, does not guarantee that it is a reliable or valid tool for particular youth in particular circumstances. Although some mental health instruments have broad and inclusive norm groups with which to compare juvenile offenders' score(s), many do not. Most screening and assessment tools used with juvenile offenders do not include a norm group of youth involved with juvenile justice. Therefore, juvenile offenders' test scores on most mental health assessment instruments are compared to the scores of youth who are not involved with the juvenile justice system. Similar concerns arise regarding youth from various racial/ethnic/cultural minority groups, females, very young offenders, cognitively delayed youth, inner-city youth, youth from rural communities, and the like. Their scores may be compared to youth who are very different from themselves.

In addition, testing conditions for juvenile offenders may not be similar to the testing conditions experienced by youth in the norm group. Most nonoffending youth are evaluated in a clinician's office, which is typically quiet and free of interruptions. In contrast, it is not unusual for juvenile offenders to be assessed in noisy environments with several interruptions. Further, the juveniles may be aware that their test results could potentially affect disposition decisions (*e.g.*, transfer to adult criminal justice system, transfer to psychiatric facility, declared incompetent to stand trial), which can also influence test performance. *(Please refer to Chapter 7 for additional information about possible issues that can interfere with juvenile offenders' performance on standardized tests.)*

When used properly, standardized tests can be extremely helpful when professionals conduct mental health screening and assessment with juvenile offenders. These tools typically can be administered in a fairly short period of time and have the potential to provide a wealth of information about youth. Also, the information collected from these tools is often more reliable and valid than the opinions and informal judgments made by individuals who come into contact with juveniles. These types of measurement tools also allow determination of how youth are functioning in comparison to others. In addition, these tools can be used to assess juveniles over time to establish whether treatment strategies result in desired outcomes.

Evaluators administering mental health screening and assessment tools should be aware of the strengths and limitations of the tool(s) they are using and the population for whom it

244

Juvenile Offenders with Mental Health Disorders: Who Are They and What Do We Do With Them?

was developed. These considerations should be taken into account during all phases of the assessment process, including test administration, scoring, interpretation and the reporting of results. Mental health screening and assessment tools are not designed to be used in isolation. They should not be the sole criterion for making decisions about the mental health diagnosis or treatment of juveniles. Information from these tools should be supplemented with information from:

- An interview with youth
- Previous records
- Information from collateral sources who are familiar with the youth
- Observations of the youths' behavior

The following is a list of some of the most common standardized mental health instruments used in the screening and assessment of juvenile offenders. This list is not exhaustive by any means. Each of the following tests varies regarding the amount of time required for administration, evaluator expertise required for administration, and cost. No one test is superior to the others. The decision about which mental health screening and assessment instrument(s) to use will depend on several factors, including:

- The type of juvenile justice setting
- An agency's resources
- The level of detail of information required

One of the instruments or a combination of several instruments can be used. Using the same, or similar, screening and assessment instruments within an entire juvenile justice agency—as well as within key partnering agencies—can facilitate more efficient and effective communication within and across systems.

MENTAL HEALTH MEASURES

- The Children's Depression Inventory (CDI) (Sitarenios & Kovacs, 1999)
- The Beck Depression Inventory-II (Steer, Kumar, Ranieri, & Beck, 1998)

- The Reynolds Adolescent Depression Scale (RADS) (Reynolds, 1987)
- The Minnesota Multiphasic Personality Inventory-Adolescent Version (MMPI-A) (Butcher *et al.*, 1992)
- Millon Adolescent Clinical Inventory (MACI) (Millon, 1983)
- Symptom Checklist –90-Revised (SCL-90-R) (Derogatis, 1983)
- The Brief Symptom Inventory (BSI) (Derogatis & Melisaratos, 1983)
- Child Behavior Checklist (CBCL) (Achenbach, 1991)
- Childhood Trauma Questionnaire (CTQ) (Bernstein, Ahluvalia, Pogge, & Handelsman, 1997)
- Trauma Symptom Checklist for Children (TSC-C) (Briere, 1996)
- Conners Parent Rating Scale-Revised (CPRS-R) (Conners, Sitarenios, Parker, & Epstein, 1998a) and Conners Teacher Rating Scale-Revised (CTRS-R) (Conners, Sitarenios, Parker, & Epstein, 1998b)
- Revised Children's Manifest Anxiety Scale (RCMAS) (Reynolds & Paget, 1983)

INSTRUMENTS THAT MEASURE MENTAL HEALTH AND SUBSTANCE ABUSE

- The Massachusetts Youth Screening Instrument-Second Version (MAYSI-2) (Grisso & Barnum, 2000)
- The Diagnostic Interview Schedule for Children Version 4 (DISC-IV) (Shaffer Fisher, Lucas, Dulcan, & Schwab-Stone, 2000)
- The Problem Oriented Screening Instrument For Teenagers (POSIT) (Latimer, Winters, & Stinchfield, 1997)
- Personal Experience Inventory (PEI) (Winters, Stinchfield, & Henly, 1993)
- Comprehensive Addiction Severity Index for Adolescents (CASI-A) (Meyers, McLellan, Jaeger, & Pettinati, 1995)

Screening and Assessment of Juvenile Offenders with Mental Health Disorders

- The Teen-Addiction Severity Index (T-ASI) (Kaminer, Bukstein, & Tarter, 1991)
- The Child and Adolescent Functional Assessment Scale (CAFAS) (Hodges & Wong, 1996)

Intelligence tests (*e.g.*, Wechsler Intelligence Scale for Children, 3rd Edition/WISC-III, Stanford-Binet Intelligence Scale, 4th Edition) and projective personality tests (*e.g.*, Rorschach Inkblot Test, Thematic Apperception Test/TAT) are also sometimes used during mental health screening and assessment of youth involved with the juvenile justice system. These instruments must be administered by trained individuals and are beyond the scope of this chapter. In addition, screening for suicidal thoughts and behavior is an essential part of mental health screening and assessment for juvenile offenders. (*Please refer to Chapters 7 and 11 for additional information about intelligence (IQ) testing and suicide assessment.*)

Self-Reported Information

Within the juvenile justice system, much of the information collected about youths' mental health symptoms comes directly from juveniles' self-report. Direct interviews with youth rely on this method of data collection, as do many mental health screening and assessment tools. Adolescents, particularly older adolescents, can provide fairly accurate descriptions of their thoughts, feelings and behavior. Clearly, they are the only ones who truly know what they are thinking and feeling. Also, some of their behavior can go unnoticed by others; sometimes, it is purposely hidden from them. In general, most youth who experience mental health symptoms, including strange or unusual thoughts and behavior, answer honestly if directly asked about them (Herjanic & Reich, 1982; Verhurst & van der Ende, 1992).

However, some juvenile offenders may falsely report their thoughts, feelings and behaviors during mental health screening and assessment. This reporting may or may not be done intentionally. Youth may inadvertently provide inaccurate information if they are intoxicated, do not have good memories, or are unable to verbally describe their internal experiences. Other youth may deliberately provide false information. These juveniles may purposely minimize their mental health symptoms, or may manufacture or exaggerate them.

POTENTIAL REASONS JUVENILE OFFENDERS MAY MINIMIZE MENTAL HEALTH SYMPTOMS

- Do not want to be seen as weak or vulnerable by peers
- Do not want to be seen as "weird" or "crazy"
- Do not want to talk to a mental health professional, nurse, doctor, juvenile justice supervisor, etc.
- Do not want to take psychotropic medication
- Do not want to participate in additional mental health assessments
- Do not want to be sent to a psychiatric hospital
- Do not want to be placed in a specialized treatment unit or in a special "safe" room
- Do not want to attend specialized treatment groups
- Do not want to be placed on any type of precautionary levels, with staff intensively observing them
- Do not want anything to lengthen the amount of time they have to reside in a juvenile justice facility
- Do not want staff to intervene with their suicide plan
- Want the screening/assessment to be over as quickly as possible

POTENTIAL REASONS JUVENILE OFFENDERS MAY EXAGGERATE OR FABRICATE MENTAL HEALTH SYMPTOMS

- Want to talk to and spend time with as many staff members as possible

Juvenile Offenders with Mental Health Disorders: Who Are They and What Do We Do With Them?

- Want mind-altering psychotropic medication
- Want peers to think they are "crazy" or "weird," so they will be left alone
- Want to be sent to a psychiatric hospital (*e.g.*, co-ed, less restrictive, less security, etc.)
- Want to be placed in specialized treatment unit (*e.g.*, co-ed, different programming, etc.)
- Want to be placed in a special room (*e.g.*, no roommate, located near staff)
- Want to attend treatment groups (*e.g.*, time out of their room, activities, etc.)

It is not difficult for youth to "fake mentally ill" or "fake nonmentally ill" on most self-report mental health tools if youth are motivated to do so. Many mental health screening and assessment tools contain items where it is obvious what is being measured. Obvious items are particularly common among screening tools that juvenile justice agencies develop themselves. Some standardized and norm-referenced instruments have tried to address this issue. On a number of these tools, youth are unable to determine which way they should answer a question (*e.g.*, to appear mentally ill or not appear mentally ill) just by taking an item at face value. A few of these tools even include special items or scales to detect whether juveniles are answering the test questions honestly—or whether they are minimizing problems, exaggerating problems or answering questions in a random fashion.

Some juvenile offenders may actually appear worse on self-report measures when reassessed at a later time. Once they feel more comfortable in a particular setting and/or with certain staff, these youth may be more willing to reveal personal information.

Improving the Accuracy of Self-Reported Information

Most youth in the juvenile justice system answer self-report questions as truthfully as they are able. However, the following steps can be taken to increase the chances of obtaining accurate self-report information:

- Conduct the screening/interview in a private environment where interruption is unlikely
- Ask questions in matter-of-fact tone.
- Portray a nonjudgmental attitude, regardless of youths' answers
- Preface the screening with a discussion about what will be done with the results
- Discuss limits of confidentiality before beginning the screening
- Review any documentation or records on the youth to guide questioning
- Do not confront the youth during the screening if they report engaging in negative behaviors
- If possible, have someone the juveniles know and trust conduct the screening
- If juveniles have difficulty remembering exactly when certain symptoms, experiences or behaviors occurred, developing a timeline with important events of their lives (*e.g.*, birthday, Christmas, last time they were incarcerated, a big concert) can provide some historical anchors and help them be more specific

Due to the potential limitations of self-reported mental health information from juvenile offenders, evaluators should supplement screening and assessment results with additional sources of data. Reviewing previous records (including prior mental health evaluations) can provide essential information, as can observing youths' behavior. In addition, gathering information from individuals who are familiar with youth (*e.g.*, family/caretakers, arresting officers, juvenile justice staff, teachers, treatment staff, case managers, community supervision staff) is often beneficial. These collateral sources can often provide valuable and fairly accurate information about juveniles (Abikoff, Courtney, Pelham, & Koplewicz, 1993;

Comtois, Ries, and Armstrong, 1994; Herjanic & Reich, 1982; Verhulst & van der Ende, 1992). However, the accuracy of their reporting can diminish if:

- They are questioned about ambiguous symptoms
- They are questioned about behavior that is not readily observed
- Oppositional behaviors co-occur with youths' mental health symptoms

 COMMUNITY ASSESSMENT CENTERS

Comprehensive evaluations of youth in the juvenile justice system are much more likely to occur when there is coordination and coop-eration among a variety of child-serving agen-cies. Community Assessment Centers (CAC's) continue to develop across various parts of the country in order to more effectively and efficiently screen and assess youth involved with the juvenile justice system. Although they may differ in their specific practices, most of these facilities are centralized, multi-agency, assessment and case management systems. Juvenile justice, mental health, substance abuse, education, social and health services all work collaboratively to assess and evaluate the needs of youth who are brought to the center.

One of the goals of Community Assessment Centers is to identify and intervene with high-risk youth so they can avoid entering the juve-nile justice system. For those youth who have already become involved with the juvenile justice system, a primary goal is to prevent them from becoming more entrenched in criminal behavior—by identifying their service needs and meeting these needs in an efficient and effective manner.

Where Community Assessment Centers exist, these facilities typically serve as the entry point for youth who are likely to become in-volved with the juvenile justice system—or who have already been charged with an offense.

Some key elements of CAC's include (Oldenettel & Wordes, 2000):

- 24-hour-a-day/seven day a week operation
- Central location for law enforcement officers to take youth
- Mental health, substance abuse and social service agencies are often located on the same premises
- Immediate screening and clinical assessment for youths' placement and service needs
- Development of individualized treatment plans based on assessment results
- Continual communication and integration between treatment providers and juvenile justice professionals
- Ongoing case management to coordinate and monitor services youth are receiving
- Statistics collected about the prevalence of youth entering the centers, their service needs, and their treatment progress
- Computer links between key agencies working with youth

Several potential benefits to having key agencies work together to assess, treat, and monitor juveniles at risk for involvement, or who are already involved with the juvenile justice system include:

- Consistent and coordinated response to juvenile crime
- Law enforcement is allowed to spend their time more efficiently and effectively
- Time between arrest and assessment is reduced
- More comprehensive assessments
- Information can be passed on to courts in a timely manner
- Time between assessment and access to treatment is reduced
- Youth are referred to treatment services that match their needs

248

Juvenile Offenders with Mental Health Disorders: Who Are They and What Do We Do With Them?

- Avoidance of unnecessary detention of youth
- Availability of collaborative funding opportunities
- Increased information sharing and communication between key agencies
- Reduced duplication of information
- A more holistic approach to case management/treatment planning is used
- Comprehensive risk assessment increases public safety
- Increased opportunities for family involvement exist
- Coordination and integration between various youth-serving agencies is facilitated
- A more seamless transition of youth into and through the juvenile justice system

Currently, most communities do not have Community Assessment Centers. However, juvenile justice agencies can still collaborate with mental health and substance abuse systems to develop more coordinated and integrated screening and assessment processes.

———

Identifying juvenile offenders with mental health disorders is critical. Without proper screening and assessment of youths' mental health symptoms, positive treatment and management outcomes are unlikely, if not impossible.

Screening and Assessment of Juvenile Offenders with Mental Health Disorders

CHAPTER 14

Treatment of Juvenile Offenders with Mental Health Disorders

"They keep telling me I need mental health treatment, but nobody gives it to me."

Deshawn, 17

Juvenile offenders with mental health disorders need mental health treatment. Just as juvenile justice provides medical services to youth with external physical injuries, the system should also be responsive to youths' internal mental health symptoms. As obvious as this may appear, the provision of mental health treatment within the juvenile justice system can be fraught with challenges. The preceding chapters in this book have described various strategies staff can employ when supervising and managing juvenile offenders with a various mental health disorders. Many of the strategies are designed to *manage* youths' behavior while they are incarcerated, and are focused on keeping youth, their peers, and juvenile justice professionals safe. These strategies also help:

- Maintain orderly living units
- Facilitate opportunities for juveniles to be successful
- Develop important skills in juveniles
- Stabilize juveniles' emotions and behavior

However, most youth with mental health disorders need more intensive *treatment* to ensure that stabilization of mood and behaviors—as well as skill retention—are maintained for extended periods of time. The ultimate goal is to help juvenile offenders with mental health disorders:

- Experience few to no mental health symptoms
- Discontinue delinquent activity
- Function successfully in the community upon release

Treating juvenile offenders with mental health disorders can be complex and challenging. This population of youth has issues related to delinquent behavior *and* mental illness. For some juvenile offenders, these two issues are very much related. For others, mental health symptoms and offending behavior co-exist, but do not significantly influence each other. Either way, both issues need to be addressed in treatment. In addition, a significant percentage of juvenile offenders with mental health disorders also have a co-occurring substance use disorder. Therefore, substance use issues must be taken into account during treatment planning as well.

Some mental health treatment can be provided while youth are incarcerated, but a great deal of it will occur when the youth are released back into the community. Effective mental health treatment typically involves the active participation of a variety of individuals and systems working together around the specific needs of particular juveniles.

The population of juvenile offenders with mental health disorders is heterogeneous, and the treatment needs of these youth vary considerably. Some juveniles are too acutely mentally ill to be held in a juvenile justice facility. These youth should be managed in a psychiatric facility, where there is increased access to mental health resources. Further, most juvenile justice facilities are not adequately equipped to manage youth with chronic and serious mental health disorders who are in need of intensive, long-term mental health services. Juveniles who have less serious mental health symptoms can be managed fairly effectively with good behavior management, psychotropic medication, and the variety of programs and groups offered within juvenile justice facilities; however, this is only true if staff are properly trained, and sound policies and procedures regarding mentally ill juvenile offenders have been developed. Most of these youth will require continued mental health treatment once they are released and return to the community.

The treatment needs of mentally ill youth do not change just because they enter a juvenile justice facility. Many juvenile offenders receive mental health treatment in the community before, during, or after periods of incarceration. In fact, a number of young offenders have long histories of involvement with the mental health system, including one or more psychiatric hospitalizations. Some mentally ill offenders have participated in numerous treatment programs with a variety of mental health providers. But only a few of them have experienced much success. Unfortunately, the juvenile justice system is frequently the "last stop" for juvenile offenders with mental health disorders, espe-

cially when youth are perceived as "untreatable" or appropriate mental health services are difficult to access.

Many juvenile justice professionals argue that *security* issues and *treatment* issues are incompatible with one another within juvenile justice agencies. Although the population of youth in juvenile justice facilities is similar to that of psychiatric hospitals (Cohen *et al.*, 1990), underlying philosophies and available mental health resources are different within these two settings. A primary responsibility of juvenile justice facilities is to manage issues related to the custody and control of the offenders in their care. Safety and security issues are of utmost importance. However, juvenile justice facilities must also respond to the mental health needs of youth in their care. Although these objectives may appear to conflict, they are integrally related. Safety and security are seriously compromised when the needs of juvenile offenders with mental health disorders remain untreated. In addition, the likelihood of providing effective mental health treatment within juvenile justice is significantly compromised when youth are housed in environments that are not safe and secure. Both issues must be addressed simultaneously.

Because they are responsible for managing juvenile offenders with mental health disorders, juvenile justice facilities should provide youth with access to mental health services. The American Correctional Association standards for correctional facilities recommend: "Written policy, procedure, and practice provide for juvenile access to mental health counseling and crisis intervention services in accordance with their needs" (ACA, 1991a, b, c; 2002). Juvenile justice facilities are not mental health facilities or psychiatric hospitals, and given the nature of their resources, should not be expected to function in that capacity. However, developing and implementing protocols for providing mental health services while youth are incarcerated, as well as when under community supervision (probation, parole), is critical and essential.

Providing effective mental health treatment to incarcerated juveniles with mental health disorders benefits:

- Mentally ill youth
- Other youth in a living unit
- Juvenile justice professionals
- A juvenile justice facility as a whole

When appropriately treated, juveniles with mental health disorders are able to manage their emotions and behavior more appropriately and consistently. They are less likely to be distressed and self-destructive (*e.g.*, suicidal, self-injurious), and their ability to participate in facility programming, as well as function successfully, is significantly increased. Living units run more smoothly and safely when youth with mental health disorders are effectively treated.

Left untreated, some mentally ill juvenile offenders are difficult to manage and can be destructive to themselves, staff, peers, and property. They can be unpredictable, irritable, and unwilling to comply with facility rules. Staff working with mentally ill juveniles who have not received appropriate treatment can easily become frustrated, irritated, confused, frightened, or exhausted. In addition, the other youth may be irritated with or afraid of peers with a mental health disorder, particularly if they are sharing a room. Providing effective mental health treatment also reduces the chances of a lawsuit related to the care of this population, something which has become increasingly common in recent years.

There is much variation among the mental health professionals associated with juvenile justice facilities. ACA standards for juvenile facilities recommend: "An adequate number of qualified staff members (*e.g.*, psychiatric nursing, psychiatry, psychology, and social work) should be available to deal directly with juveniles who have severe mental health problems as well as to advise other correctional staff in their contacts with such individuals" (ACA, 1991a, b, c; 2002).

Mental health professionals who work with incarcerated juvenile offenders can either be employees of juvenile justice agencies or private contractors. However, these individuals should have the appropriate education, training, and experience to work with this clinically complex population of youth. Mental health staff should also be certified or licensed by the state in which they are providing mental health services. When juvenile justice agencies use unqualified mental health professionals—those who are unfamiliar with issues related to normal adolescent development, juvenile offenders, or the effects of substance use—misdiagnosis and inappropriate treatment recommendations are likely.

Mental health professionals should play a key role in:

- Mental health evaluations
- Crisis intervention
- Individual counseling
- Treatment groups
- Staff training
- Psychotropic medication

However, these individuals should also be involved in decisions regarding:

- Individualized treatment plans
- The placement of youth on/off intensive monitoring (*e.g.*, suicide watch, mental health watch)
- Treatment programming
- Isolation/restraint of youth

Due to the high numbers of mentally ill juvenile offenders in the system, juvenile justice and mental health professionals must work closely together. They must continuously communicate about individual youth and programs as a whole.

Juvenile justice facilities also vary widely with regard to the type of mental health assistance available to the youth in their care. Most facilities offer crisis intervention for juveniles who are psychotic or suicidal. The majority also offer some form of medication management for youth who are taking psychotropic medication.

Juvenile Offenders with Mental Health Disorders: Who Are They and What Do We Do With Them?

Some facilities also provide mental health evaluations, individual counseling, and/or group counseling to mentally ill youth. However, others do not provide any of these services. Even when they exist within corrections, mental health services may be provided only to a small number of youth or be delivered in a fairly cursory manner. Currently, a significant number of juvenile offenders remain unidentified and untreated.

Juvenile justice facilities may provide mental health treatment services in-house or may transport youth to mental health providers in the community for needed services. Some facilities have special cottages or units that specifically house juveniles with mental health disorders and/or those who are cognitively impaired. These specialized programs may have additional staff resources, more flexible programming, and various treatment services, although some do not. Because of some of the challenges that exist in the management of mentally ill juveniles within juvenile justice facilities, there has been a recent desire to create specialized forensic mental health programs. These specialized programs generally integrate components of psychiatric hospitals and maximum-security correctional units. They are typically designed for the most aggressive and/or impaired mentally ill offenders.

A juvenile justice facility's decisions regarding mental health programming and resources tend to be based on:

- The typical "length of stay" at the facility
- The type of facility (*e.g.*, pre-adjudication detention center, training school, boot camp, group home)
- Staff resources
- Relationships with community mental health programs
- Philosophy regarding mental illness
- Geographical location
- Liability issues

- Prevalence of mentally ill youth in a particular community/jurisdiction

Regardless of any of these factors, all juvenile offenders with mental health disorders should have access to mental health services during periods of incarceration. Written policy, procedure and practice should exist so that incarcerated youth receive crisis intervention services and mental health counseling in accordance with their needs (ACA 1991, 2002). Treatment should be provided in both group and individual formats. And youths' mental health issues should be integrated into aftercare plans. This does not mean that juveniles should be detained or committed to juvenile justice facilities *in order to* receive mental health services; that should never be the case. However, once detained or committed on the basis of offense-related behavior, the needs of mentally ill juveniles should be addressed.

 Effective Treatment for Mentally Ill Juvenile Offenders

Initial reviews of several studies on the treatment of juvenile offenders resulted in the conclusion that "nothing works." Evaluations of different types of treatment programs demonstrated little, if any, behavioral improvement among these youth. There was also little evidence that one type of treatment program was more effective than any other program. When these studies were evaluated more carefully, however, researchers noticed that several of the studies suffered from methodological flaws (*e.g.*, no comparison group, small numbers of youth, lack of adherence to the protocol of a treatment program).

Closer inspection of these studies also revealed some well–designed treatment programs that *did* demonstrate effective results in changing the behavior of juvenile offenders. Since that time, evaluations of treatment programs have improved and are growing in number. More work needs to be done on what specific types of treatment work best for particular juvenile offenders, in what setting, and for how long. But results of recent studies indicate that in general, several intervention strategies have been shown to be effective with young offenders (Lipsey, 1992; Lipsey & Wilson, 1998; McGuire & Priestley, 1995). A number of components related to effective treatment for juvenile delinquency are also effective components in the treatment of mental health disorders among youth.

The treatment of juvenile offenders with mental health disorders is a multifaceted endeavor—it consists of much more than focusing solely on youths' criminal behavior *or* mental health symptoms. Psychological or psychiatric treatment can positively influence mental health symptoms, but does not necessarily influence offending behavior. By the same token, treatment specifically targeting delinquent behavior is not likely to have a great influence on youths' mental health disorder. The most effective treatment approaches for mentally ill offenders should target youths' mental health symptoms, as well as their criminal thinking and behavior. Due to the often numerous and diverse needs of this population, effective treatment must also encompass the multiple areas of juveniles' lives in which they are experiencing distress and difficulty functioning. Treatment should be comprehensive and may need to target psychological, biological, familial, social, environmental, academic, vocational and substance-related issues.

Although treatment programs for juvenile offenders vary in specifics, the following treatment components have been shown to have positive outcomes with juvenile offenders. However, much more research is needed to determine exactly what components work with which particular youth, especially female offenders. Much of the research focused on treatment interventions with juvenile offenders has been conducted with males. Because differences exist between male and female adolescents, whether the same treatment

approaches are as effective for both populations remains unclear. This issue is currently being addressed, but it is too soon to draw any firm conclusions (Covington, 1998). *(Please see Chapter 15 for additional issues about female juvenile offenders.)*

Some of the following treatment strategies can be easily provided to youth while in residential care. Others are more easily provided while youth are in the community. And some can be easily provided in either context. Juvenile offenders with mental health disorders typically require a combination of various treatment components, individually tailored to their particular strengths and needs.

Behavior Management Programs

Effective behavior management programs can result in positive behavioral change among juveniles with mental health disorders. These programs are typically based on sound theoretical premises regarding how individuals learn new behaviors and maintain them over a period of time. A primary focus is providing reinforcement to juveniles when they engage in positive behavior and ignoring or disciplining juveniles when they engage in negative behavior. Programs implementing key principles of *behavior modification*, particularly contingency management (*e.g.*, point systems, level systems), can effectively teach youth new prosocial behaviors during their residence in juvenile justice facilities.

Many juvenile offenders with mental health disorders have lived in environments that were unstable, inconsistent, and even chaotic. As much as they appear to rebel against authority and rules, these youth often respond well to highly structured environments that are predictable and organized around logical consequences. Juvenile offenders do not necessarily have to agree with all rules and expectations of a residential program. But they tend to be more motivated to adhere to rules when aware of the rationale behind what is expected. Effective

Juvenile Offenders with Mental Health Disorders: Who Are They and What Do We Do With Them?

behavior management programs clearly tell youth exactly what they need to do to receive positive consequences (*e.g.*, points, privileges, advancement within a level system) and exactly what behaviors will result in negative consequences. As juvenile justice professionals respond with positive or negative consequences, youth receive continuous feedback about their behavior.

Juvenile justice facilities are an optimal setting in which to implement behavior modification programs. Adults continuously observe youth. Also, staff have significant control over what youth can and cannot do, as well as where they can and cannot go. Although most juvenile justice facilities have implemented some type of behavior management program for youth, not all of these programs are effective. For example, some juvenile justice facilities have such extensive and complex behavior modification programs that the staff administering the program (and the youth trying to fulfill the behavioral expectations) are confused.

Behavior management programs should be simple enough for staff to administer and for juvenile offenders to participate easily in. When this is not the case, both become frustrated and less motivated to involve themselves fully in a program. A number of facilities have behavior management programs that are highly subjective—one staff member reinforces the exact behavior that another staff member has recently punished. Or, behavior that is acceptable during the day shift is completely unacceptable during the evening shift. This inconsistency can be confusing for youth and is unlikely to result in positive behavioral change.

Effective behavior management programs are designed so that rewards or punishment are presented or withdrawn *contingent* upon the occurrence of certain behaviors. Token economies, such as point systems and level systems are examples of *contingency management* programs. Youth engage in certain prosocial behaviors (*e.g.*, complete chores, attend school, participate in treatment groups) to receive a speci-

fied number of points or move to a higher level within the system, both typically associated with increased incentives (*e.g.*, later bedtime, more independence at the facility, increased access to personal property).

These types of programs are most effective when the behaviors that are encouraged, as well as discouraged, are clearly specified and communicated to youth. When behaviors are observable, objective, and measurable, both youth and staff will be able to determine whether or not a behavior occurred. Juvenile offenders can be hyperaware of fairness and justice issues as related to how they are treated. Therefore, staff can decrease the likelihood of youth becoming upset and angry if behavioral expectations are unambiguous and observable.

Consistency is another critical aspect of an effective behavior management program. As much as possible, youth should receive the same consequences (positive or negative) *each* and *every* time they engage in a specified behavior—a challenging task in juvenile justice facilities due to different staff working different shifts. Regardless, providing swift and consistent consequences that have value for youth is essential to changing juvenile behavior.

Effective behavior management programs are not designed to control or dominate juveniles. These programs should be developed to help youth learn and maintain skills and behaviors that allow them to control themselves better. Effective behavior management programs typically result in safer and more efficient living units. But, the ultimate goal is also to teach juveniles behavioral skills that have a larger impact upon the youths' lives. Most behavior management programs in juvenile justice rely heavily on *disciplining* youths' negative behavior by taking away something positive (*e.g.*, deducting points within a token economy, decreasing privileges, removing youth from an activity, separating youth from peers) or by providing something negative (*e.g.*, placement in a room with minimal to no stimuli, unpleasant chores, reprimands).

Just as important, in fact even more so, is *reinforcing* youth when they engage in positive behavior. Reinforcement can occur by providing juveniles with something positive (*e.g.*, points within in a token economy system, extra time on the telephone, later bedtime, fun activity, praise) or by taking away something negative (*e.g.*, letting them out of their room early, allowing them to forgo an aversive task or chore). The most effective behavior management programs reinforce juveniles more often for positive behavior (no matter how small) in comparison to how often they are punished for negative behavior. A 4:1 ratio of reinforcement to punishment has been suggested for juvenile offenders (Gendreau, 1994). However, most facilities have yet to achieve this ideal ratio.

The same behavioral contingencies used in a living unit should also be used throughout the other areas of juvenile justice facilities (*e.g.*, school, gymnasium, cafeteria, vocational program). This type of continuity and consistency helps youth to generalize positive and prosocial behavior to a variety of locations, with different individuals. The goal is not for juveniles to behave a certain way in a unit in order to receive points. The goal is to help youth learn prosocial behaviors, as well as provide incentives for youth to continue engaging in these behaviors upon release. Therefore, parents/caregivers and community supervision staff should be aware of the specific expectations of juveniles' residential behavior management plan (*e.g.*, psychotropic medication compliance, no profanity, no fighting, completion of chores, participation in treatment groups, completion of homework assignments) when the youth return to the community. The more that parents/caregivers and probation/parole staff can maintain contingencies in the community that are similar to what was provided in the residential program, the greater the likelihood that youth will sustain positive behavioral changes.

Effective behavior management programs also allow for a significant amount of interaction between youth and staff. Token economy systems should be centered on staff providing feedback to youth about their behavior. Youth should be praised for positive behavior and made aware of what changes need to be made to correct negative behavior. "Points" and "levels" should be recorded in order for juveniles to have a visual representation of the consequences they receive. However, explaining to youth why they receive particular positive or negative consequences is also important. This type of feedback should be provided several times a day, if possible. At the very least, staff should meet with juveniles once daily to review the youths' behavior.

Some token economy programs may need to be modified for juveniles with mental health disorders, especially if the juveniles are consistently unsuccessful with the standard program. Youth with severe cognitive limitations or serious mental health disorders (*e.g.*, psychotic thinking, extreme hyperactivity, intense depression) may not be able to achieve the same criteria as higher-functioning youth. Juveniles with a modified behavior management program should still be held accountable for fulfilling behavioral expectations, but the specific expectations should be tailored to match youths' individual needs and capabilities.

Most juvenile justice professionals need additional training in effective behavior management strategies. Although nearly all juvenile justice agencies provide some training in "behavior management" to new staff when they are hired, this training is usually simplistic and too brief. Effective behavior management is a key factor in well-run, safe, and secure juvenile justice facilities. Positive treatment outcomes are unlikely if the foundation of good behavior management is missing. Particularly in relation to juvenile offenders with mental health disorders, well-meaning staff are often unaware of how they may inadvertently reinforce behavior such as:

- Suicide threats/behaviors
- Self-injury

Juvenile Offenders with Mental Health Disorders: Who Are They and What Do We Do With Them?

- Aggression
- Reports of hearing voices

Juvenile justice professionals must fully understand concepts such as positive and negative reinforcement, positive and negative punishment, shaping, extinction, and so forth. Without this knowledge, influencing behavior change among mentally ill juveniles for a sustained period of time will be difficult for staff.

Juvenile justice professionals have a tremendous influence on youths' behavior. Every interaction they have with youth can reinforce appropriate or inappropriate behavior. Juveniles soon discover how to obtain one of the most sacred resources in juvenile justice facilities: attention from staff. Behaviors that ensure youth will obtain staff attention include:

- Verbally or physically assaulting peers
- Flooding their room
- Cutting themselves
- Making suicide threats
- Smearing feces

Staff are mandated to respond to these behaviors, which may reinforce the juveniles' behavior if they were primarily seeking a reaction from staff. However, these behaviors also can reflect the presence of a mental health disorder. Appropriate referrals to mental health professionals—and collaborative relationships between juvenile justice and mental health staff—are critical in the effective management of youth who engage in these behaviors. However, staff awareness of the contingency patterns present in a living unit and the role staff can play in inadvertently reinforcing these negative behaviors is just as critical. Once they understand how their behavior influences juveniles' behavior, staff can intentionally reinforce youth *not* to engage in the above behaviors. Staff can purposely provide extra attention to juveniles when they do not engage in these behaviors versus only when they do. Without a solid foundation of the principles of behavior manage-ment, this expectation is unrealistic for most staff—negative behaviors are dramatic and naturally draw extra staff attention.

In addition, juvenile offenders with mental health disorders can be some of the most challenging youth to manage in juvenile justice facilities. Staff must frequently be strategic and creative in their supervision approaches with these youth. Without proper training in the principles of behavior management, ineffective treatment plans may be developed. This typically results in frustration and hopelessness for both mentally ill juveniles and the staff committed to helping them.

Although a strong behavior management program is critical to the treatment of juvenile offenders with mental health disorders, it is a necessary, but not sufficient treatment component. Most juveniles with mental health disorders also require intervention strategies that are more specifically focused on other problematic areas of youths' lives (*e.g.*, mental health symptoms, interpersonal relationships, academic/vocational skills, anger control). *(Please see Chapters 3 and 5 for additional information about behavior management strategies.)*

Cognitive-Behavioral Skill-Based Programs

Cognitive-behavioral treatment approaches use techniques and strategies related to changing youths' thinking patterns and behavior. An underlying assumption is that juveniles' behavior is significantly influenced by their thoughts and perceptions. Youths' reaction to a situation is based more on their *evaluation* or perception of an event, rather than what actually occurs during an incident. When juveniles' perceptions are distorted or inaccurate, maladaptive reactions (*e.g.*, anger, disappointment, sadness) and behaviors (*e.g.*, aggression, suicidal behavior, withdrawal) can result.

Aggressive youth consistently have been found to have an *attributional bias*, interpreting neutral or ambiguous social situations as hostile (Dodge, Price, Bachorowski, & Newman, 1990).

Treatment of Juvenile Offenders with Mental Health Disorders

Aggressive youth often misperceive the intentions of others, thinking that those around them have hostile or malicious intent when they do not. Because these juveniles often believe they are being disrespected or attacked, they tend to react aggressively to defend themselves. In fact, many aggressive juveniles feel justified in their aggressive behavior based on their *perception* of an incident as provocative.

For example, suppose two juveniles are walking down a crowded hallway and one of the youth accidentally bumps into the other. A juvenile with an attributional bias might react with anger and verbal threats—sending a message that he is the tougher of the two and unwilling to tolerate being "dissed." If the other youth does not share this attributional bias, he is likely to be confused at this reaction. In his mind, the two boys accidentally ran into each other due to the crowding in the hallway. Juvenile justice professionals are often amazed at how aggressive youth have misinterpreted things staff have said or when these youth react angrily to a neutral request. This type of reaction is often due to youths' distorted perception of what and how something was stated. Cognitive-behavioral treatments attempt to educate juveniles about how their thoughts affect their emotions and behaviors. These treatments typically focus on helping youth identify and modify their inaccurate perception of social cues. In addition, contingency management techniques are usually incorporated to teach youth self-regulation skills, as well as new ways of coping and behaving.

Although there are many skill-based programs to match a variety of juvenile offender treatment needs, most have several key factors in common. Many of these programs use strategies such as:

- Modeling prosocial behavior for youth
- Role-playing with youth
- Having youth practice new skills
- Providing youth with specific feedback regarding their demonstration of new skills

Treatment sessions typically focus on helping juveniles develop more prosocial and skillful responses during difficult interpersonal situations (from the youths' lives or hypothetical situations). Several interpersonal problem-solving processes may be targeted including:

- Taking another person's perspective
- Using self-statements to regulate behavior
- Generating alternative solutions to a problematic situation
- Considering the consequences of particular actions

Aggression Replacement Training (ART) and social-cognitive training have both been shown to be effective with juvenile offenders (Goldstein and Glick, 1987; Guerra & Slaby, 1990). Aggression Replacement Training is designed to teach youth a variety of new and more prosocial skills. Key treatment areas for juvenile offenders include:

- Modifying angry responses (being able to control anger)
- Improving moral reasoning skills
- Learning a broader range of interpersonal behaviors

Effective social skills programs typically concentrate on changing youths' thoughts and beliefs about the legitimacy or necessity of using violence to achieve goals, especially interpersonally. This type of treatment strategy is typically structured and skill-based. Juveniles are taught new and specific responses to use when interacting with others, particularly when involved in conflict-laden situations. Training sessions should involve interpersonal situations that are similar to or directly from juvenile offenders' community and lifestyle. Otherwise treatment engagement is likely to decrease if youth do not find hypothetical social situations realistic and relevant. Moreover, juveniles' new anger management skills need to be applicable in a juvenile justice facility, as well as in the community to which the youth are returning.

Dialectical Behavior Therapy (DBT) is a cognitive-behavioral treatment that can be effective for juvenile offenders with mental health disorders, particularly those youth who are repeatedly suicidal and/or self-injurious. The treatment approach was developed for individuals suffering from Borderline Personality Disorder. But the psychosocial skills training component is applicable to juvenile offenders who have difficulty regulating their emotions, interpersonal difficulties and poor coping skills. DBT psychosocial skills groups consist of activities and discussions about various interpersonal situations and youths' ineffective emotional reactions and behaviors in these situations. Juveniles are taught practical coping strategies to help regulate their emotions and behavior, as well as specific skills to help them be more interpersonally effective (Linehan, 1993).

Cognitive-behavioral skill-based interventions can be provided in an individual or group setting. Due to limited resources, many juvenile justice agencies rely on group treatment because it can be both time and cost-effective. Many juvenile offenders take suggestions from same-age peers more seriously than those from an authority figure. These youth have reported feeling as if the other group members (versus adults) could better "relate" to what the youth was experiencing. Adults who lead treatment groups with juveniles can obtain a great deal of information from observing the group members interact with one another. They can then use these interactions to help demonstrate treatment concepts. Group members can role-play scenarios with each other and provide feedback to one another about their performances.

Although group work has its benefits, it can also have its challenges. Depending on the particular members involved, treatment groups of juvenile offenders can quickly become chaotic and disorganized, particularly if several youth are vying for the group's attention. In addition, some seriously mentally ill juveniles may monopolize group sessions (sometimes unintentionally), resulting in the other youth becoming annoyed or bored. Cognitively delayed juveniles may not be able to grasp treatment concepts as quickly as their peers and may fall behind and become frustrated.

Further, juveniles who are bored or frustrated during treatment groups can become distracted or disruptive, which can negatively influence the entire set of youth. There is some evidence that peer group interventions with delinquents can actually *increase* problem behavior and negative life outcomes in adulthood (Dishion, McCord, & Poulin, 1999). The decision to use a group format should be carefully considered with specific attention given to the number and constellation of individual group members. All professionals leading treatment groups for juvenile offenders should be adequately trained to do so.

Effective skill-based treatment approaches are competency-based. Just *attending* treatment sessions is not enough for juveniles. Active participation is required, and youth must be able to *demonstrate* the new skills learned.

Family-Focused Treatment Approaches

Family-focused treatment approaches do not treat juvenile offenders in isolation, and treatment sessions typically involve youth, their families/caregivers, and sometimes their siblings. Treatment is based on the notion that juveniles' difficulties are largely a function of disordered relations within the family system. A therapist typically meets with an entire family unit and focuses on the interactions

DEPENDING ON THE PARTICULAR MEMBERS INVOLVED, TREATMENT GROUPS OF JUVENILE OFFENDERS CAN QUICKLY BECOME CHAOTIC AND DISORGANIZED, PARTICULARLY IF SEVERAL YOUTH ARE VYING FOR THE GROUP'S ATTENTION.

Treatment of Juvenile Offenders with Mental Health Disorders

among all family members. Increasing positive interactions among the family members is essential. Professionals providing family-focused treatments emphasize communication skills, clarification of family roles and boundaries, conflict resolution/negotiation, and modification of the family system to improve the behavior of youth. Specific intervention strategies typically focus on the interactions (especially those that are maladaptive) among juveniles and other family members. Parents are educated about behavior management strategies and assisted in developing behavior modification plans for their children. The behavior modification plans emphasize the reinforcing of adaptive behaviors and the ignoring or disciplining of maladaptive behaviors. Some family-oriented approaches focus heavily on the communication patterns of family members. Others focus more on effective behavior management skills.

Functional Family Therapy (FFT) is an outcome-driven, family-focused treatment approach. It can be implemented in youths' homes, in clinics or in schools. This treatment is centered on motivating juveniles and their families/caregivers to make positive changes by pointing out and developing the unique strengths of the families. FFT strategies help family members view themselves in a more positive light, while teaching them specific ways to improve their functioning (Alexander *et al.*, 1998). Targeting risk and protective factors, following a structured treatment plan, and using empirically sound intervention strategies are emphasized throughout treatment.

In addition, the interpersonal functions of youth and families'/caregivers' behavior are explored. Communication training, parenting skills training, and behavioral contracts are used and specifically tailored to the needs of particular families. Monitoring progress and modifying treatment plans to increase the likelihood of positive outcomes is stressed. Family Functional Therapy also includes a strong emphasis on helping youth and their families/caregivers

maintain treatment gains in the "real world" after formal treatment has ended. Therapists must be both active and supportive. As they help family members modify interpersonal skills with each other, therapists also help family members focus on achieving specific behavioral goals.

―――――――

Regardless of the specific approach used, mental health treatment with juvenile offenders should involve youths' families/caregivers. Although this involvement can be challenging when juveniles are incarcerated, every effort should be made to engage families/caregivers during assessment, treatment planning, and implementation of treatment services. The chance of positive outcomes and maintenance of treatment gains is much higher when significant individuals in youths' lives are involved in the juveniles' treatment.

Substance Abuse Treatment

Many juvenile offenders with mental health disorders also have a co-occurring substance use disorder. Youths' mental health and substance use disorders can be interrelated in a variety of ways (*e.g.*, worsening, imitating, producing, covering up symptoms). When working with juvenile offenders who have co-occurring disorders, clinicians should assess and treat the juveniles' mental health and substance use disorders simultaneously in an integrated fashion. *(Please see Chapter 10 for additional information about the assessment and treatment of co-occurring mental health and substance use disorders.)*

Psychotropic Medication

During the past decade, there has been a significant increase in the use of psychotropic medication with juvenile offenders who have mental health disorders. Psychotropic medication is being prescribed to youth at younger and younger ages (Zito, *et al.*, 2000). Seeing some juvenile offenders taking two, three, or even four (or more) different types of medicines at

Juvenile Offenders with Mental Health Disorders: Who Are They and What Do We Do With Them?

the same time is not unusual. Much more research is needed concerning the use of psychotropic medication with youth. The empirical efficacy of many medications currently prescribed to juvenile offenders remains unknown. Even for the medications that have demonstrated beneficial effects, the mechanism of action for those medicines is often unclear. In addition, there are few to no studies on the long-term effects of psychotropic medications when taken during the adolescent years. Moreover, studies related to the use of psychotropic medication among juvenile offenders, a population with a host of possible complicating factors, is significantly lacking.

Decisions about whether to prescribe psychotropic medication to juvenile offenders should be based on a weighing of the risks and benefits for particular youth. Psychotropic medication should be considered if juveniles are:

- In significant distress
- In danger of harming themselves or others
- Experiencing considerable impairment in their ability to function

Medication should not be prescribed solely because juveniles' behavior is loud or annoying. Additional factors that should be taken into account before psychotropic medication is prescribed include:

- The duration, severity and intensity of youths' mental health symptoms
- Whether youth are willing to take psychotropic medication
- Whether there is adequate time to monitor youths to ensure there are no untoward effects from the medication
- Whether youth are willing to continue taking the medication when they return to the community (especially if youth are residing in a short-term facility)
- Youths' willingness to refrain from using alcohol and drugs while taking the

medication (especially if youth are residing in the community)

- Whether a responsible adult is present to administer the medication properly (especially if youth are residing in the community)

It is easy to see why the decision to place juvenile offenders on psychotropic medication is complicated and should be carefully considered. Psychotropic medication should be viewed as an adjunct to other treatment modalities and considered only when less intrusive approaches have been tried and been unsuccessful.

Medications commonly prescribed to juvenile offenders with mental health disorders include, but are not limited to:

- Stimulants (Ritalin®, Dexedrine®, Adderall®, Concerta®)
- Tricyclic Antidepressants (Elavil®, Tofranil®, Pamelor®)
- Selective Serotonin Re-uptake Inhibitors/ SSRIs (Prozac®, Zoloft®, Paxil®, Celexa®)
- Atypical Antidepressants (Desyrel®, Wellbutrin®, Effexor®)
- Mood Stabilizers (Lithium®, Depakote®, Tegretol®)
- Antipsychotics (Risperdal®, Thorazine®, Trilafon®, Zyprexa®)

Psychotropic medication is only one possible component of an effective treatment plan for juvenile offenders with mental health disorders and should never be used in isolation. Medication can address the acute mental health symptoms that interfere or inhibit youths' ability to function successfully in a living unit, in school or within interpersonal relationships. When administered appropriately, psychotropic medication can help stabilize youths' behavior so that they are better able to participate in the various juvenile justice and mental health interventions available to them.

For example, youth with Attention-Deficit Hyperactivity Disorder may be unable to sit still

Treatment of Juvenile Offenders with Mental Health Disorders

and focus during treatment groups. Psychotic juveniles may be too confused to interact with peers. And depressed youth may be so preoccupied with thoughts about death and dying that they cannot concentrate in school. Some juvenile offenders with significant mental health disorders have difficulty participating in token economy programs or skill-based treatment groups due to difficulty regulating their emotions and behaviors.

Psychotropic medication can help these youth better control their feelings and actions, enabling the youth to participate, and be successful, in psychosocial interventions. However, for medication to be effective, juveniles must take it as prescribed for a specified amount of time—without combining it with alcohol or other substances of abuse. Too often, medications are thought to be ineffective with particular youth because the juveniles stopped taking the medicine prematurely or a physician changed the youths' medication too hastily. Some medications, such as the selective serotonin reuptake inhibitors, can take four to six weeks before therapeutic effects are evident.

Juveniles receiving psychotropic medication should be educated about important issues related to their medicine. First and foremost, youth should be told:

- The reasons why a particular medication(s) has been prescribed for them

- What positive behavior changes are expected to occur from taking the medication(s)

- How the medication(s) works within their body—in a brief, simple way

Many mentally ill juvenile offenders taking psychotropic medication have not received this type of information. Youth should also be educated about the risks and benefits of taking a particular type of psychotropic medication, since not all medicines are the same. The potential side effects of the medication, as well as how common or rare they are, should be carefully discussed with youth so the juveniles are not surprised if they begin to have unusual bodily experiences.

Juvenile offenders with mental health disorders vary in their attitudes about taking psychotropic medication. Some take their medicine consistently and without problems because the youth recognize the benefits of the medication on their behavior. Other youth may not recognize the benefits, but take their medication as prescribed because:

- The youth believe, "The doctor knows what is best for me"

- The youth have been taking medication for so many years that they do not question it

- The youth do not want to receive sanctions from staff for refusing to take it

Some juveniles take their medication fairly regularly, but occasionally refuse to take it for a few doses or a few days. However, these youth typically resume their medication regimen again. A subset of youth refuse to take their medication on a regular basis, which can be frustrating for both juvenile justice and mental health staff. Medication refusal also can have negative consequences for juveniles' mental health symptoms, as well as youths' physical health.

There are a variety of reasons that juveniles might refuse to take their psychotropic medication, including, but not limited to:

- They do not want to be viewed as "crazy" by the other youth

- Peers harass them and try to steal their medication (so they can ingest it in hopes of getting "high")

- The side effects are bothersome and physically uncomfortable

- Previous treatment with medication was unsuccessful

- They do not think the medication is currently helping them

- They think the medication is making their behavior worse

262

Juvenile Offenders with Mental Health Disorders: Who Are They and What Do We Do With Them?

- They cannot swallow pills
- They want to experience a feeling of control in an environment with limited opportunities for independent decision-making
- They are adolescents with a natural striving for autonomy
- Their parents are opposed to the medication and have told the youth not to take it
- They are psychotic and believe that the medication will harm them

Juvenile justice facilities can take some actions to try to reduce the influence of some of these factors. For example, to reduce some of the embarrassment or stigma attached to taking psychotropic medicine, it is best to:

- Not shout mentally ill youths' names aloud in front of peers when it is time for them to take their medication
- Not require youth to go to a very public and visible area to take their medication

When possible, parents/caregivers should be involved when youth are prescribed psychotropic medication. If parents/caregivers need education about a particular medication, this information should be provided. Inquiring about and discussing juveniles' perceptions of how prescribed medication is impacting their behavior involves youth in the treatment regimen and can increase medication compliance. Monitoring juveniles' behavior before *and* after taking psychotropic medication and providing feedback to the youth about any behavioral change can be helpful. Ensuring that youth completely swallow their pills (versus "cheeking" their medication) can reduce opportunities for peers to obtain substances that are prescribed for someone else. It can also help prevent youth from overdosing on their psychiatric medication. If youth have difficulty swallowing pills, staff can crush them or find out whether a liquid form of the medication is available. Youths' freedom is limited within a juvenile justice setting. Therefore,

refusing to take prescribed medication is one way some juveniles choose to experience a sense of power over their lives. Allowing them to have options and make choices in other areas of their programming and treatment can reduce the need for youth to exert their independence around medication.

Many mentally ill youth, and the juvenile justice professionals supervising them, are unaware of the potential side effects associated with various psychotropic medications. Some of the side effects are mild, while some are more severe. Further, some side effects may dissipate or completely diminish after youth have taken a particular medication for several weeks and their bodies have adapted. All staff working with youth who take psychotropic medication (particularly staff who interact with these youth on a continuous basis) should receive basic training on the most common side effects associated with this type of medicine. Medication side effects such as increased irritability, lethargy and restlessness can result in juveniles receiving negative reactions from staff, as well as sanctions. In addition, staff commonly assume that youth are refusing psychotropic medication as a purposeful attempt to be oppositional or create a power struggle. Oftentimes, there are other reasons underlying juveniles' decision not to take prescribed medication—and avoiding negative side effects is one of the most common.

Potential side effects associated with psychotropic medications include, but are not limited to:

- Headaches
- Insomnia
- Weight gain/loss
- Nausea
- Drowsiness
- Heart palpitations
- Constipation
- Akathesia (inability to sit still, rocking, fidgeting, tapping feet continuously)
- Dry mouth

- Dizziness
- Orthostatic hypotension (a decrease in blood pressure when standing up, possibly resulting in youth fainting)
- Skin rashes
- Dystonia (spasms of tongue, neck and jaw)
- Irritability
- Blurred vision
- Loss of appetite
- Tardive dyskinesia (involuntary face, limb or trunk movements)
- Priapism (sustained painful erection)

The experience of side effects from psychotropic medication is extremely variable. Some side effects are fairly common, while others occur only among small numbers of juveniles. Some youth experience several symptoms at one time, whereas other youth experience no side effects at all. Specific side effects differ depending on the type of medication prescribed and the physiological system of the juveniles ingesting the medicine. For example, some juveniles can tolerate particular medication without associated problems, yet others may experience strong side effects from the same type of medication. Juveniles who experience medication side effects do not always associate their bodily symptoms with their psychotropic medicine, so they may not report them to mental health/medical staff. Youth who repeatedly complain of health-related problems should be taken seriously. Problems such as the following should be further explored:

- Repeated complaints of headaches or stomachaches
- Frequent requests to get a drink of water
- Unexplained weight loss or weight gain
- Displays of strange muscle movements
- Unusual/bizarre behavior

Even though drowsiness is a common symptom of some psychotropic medications, juveniles should be able to awaken in the morning and should not fall asleep during school or treatment groups. If juvenile offenders are taking psychotropic medication, staff should inquire about "strange" or "unusual" things happening with the youths' bodies on a regular basis. Unpleasant side effects should be reported to mental health/medical personnel, and the youth should be evaluated. Reducing the dosage or changing to a different, but comparable, medication may alleviate any problems. It is certainly understandable why adolescents experiencing uncomfortable side effects might refuse to take their medication for a while. However, abruptly stopping psychotropic medication can be dangerous for youth. The discontinuance of psychotropic medicines should always be done under the supervision of a medical professional.

Juvenile justice facilities should have policies and procedures in place regarding the prescribing of psychotropic medication to youth. Because some psychotropic medications can have serious, and even lethal, side effects, specific policies should also be developed regarding the medical monitoring of youth on medication. The monitoring of liver, kidney and heart functioning is required with the use of certain medications, and juveniles' physical safety is significantly compromised if proper procedures are not followed. In addition, specific policies related to providing involuntary medication during emergency situations should also be developed. Physicians prescribing medication should make every effort to collect information about youths' history of psychotropic medication. They should review previous medical records, as well as consult with past treatment providers. Nursing staff can often facilitate the gathering of this information if a physician is unable to do so due to time limitations.

Medical staff should be responsible for administering medication to juvenile offenders. Due to limited resources, however, some juvenile justice facilities rely on juvenile justice professionals to administer medication. These

264

Juvenile Offenders with Mental Health Disorders: Who Are They and What Do We Do With Them?

staff should be properly trained (including routine refresher courses) on issues related to psychotropic medication. This type of training should include, but not be limited to:

- The various classes of psychotropic medications
- Side effects associated with the medications
- Responding to youth who have an acute negative reaction to medication
- Ensuring youth have truly ingested the medication
- Effectively handling medication non-compliance.

There is some evidence that individuals from different racial and ethnic cultures may respond differently to psychotropic medication. These different responses may be due to biological differences, various cultural views toward medication to treat mental illness, and/or the relationship between youth and their treatment provider (Herrera *et al.*, 1999). Clinicians should always consider cultural issues when prescribing psychotropic medication to juvenile offenders, as well as when youth regularly refuse to take their medication. In addition, there is some evidence that psychotropic medication may be prescribed less frequently to minority youth in comparison to their Caucasian peers (Zito, Safer, dosReis, & Riddle, 1998).

Family-Style Group Homes

Family-style group homes are one model of community residential placements that have been shown to be effective with juvenile offenders. These programs typically accommodate a small number of youth, and adult supervisors serve as surrogate parents, known as "teaching parents." The adults not only provide structure and discipline, but also attention, nurturance, and support typical of the parental role. Within effective programs of this type, supervisory staff consistently adhere to a structured behavior management program—including the use of a token economy in which juveniles can earn points for appropriate behavior and lose points for inappropriate behavior.

In addition to reinforcement from external sources, there is a focus on helping youth learn to manage their own behavior, based on internal resources. For example, juveniles are allowed to serve as peer managers, as well as provide input into the design and implementation of the program. A variety of services and programs are typically available to residents in this type of group home, including individual and group counseling, and several skill development training programs (*e.g.*, communication, negotiation). Educational/vocational support and achievement are also emphasized. The most successful programs of this type are comprised of adult personnel with extensive training and experience who are committed to using effective behavioral treatment strategies (Bedlington, Braukmann, Ramp, & Wolf, 1988; Braukmann & Wolf, 1987).

Recreational Sports/Physical Activity

In recent years, a great deal of attention has been given to the positive effects of physical exercise on mental health. Vigorous exercise can enhance self-esteem, decrease depression and provide an overall sense of well-being. In addition, anxiety and tension are frequently reduced after exercising. These results may be due to:

- Feelings of accomplishment and success
- A sense of control over one's body
- The inducement of relaxation
- Distraction from various stresses

Exercise also changes some of the chemicals in the brain, particularly those that play a role in mood-related disorders.

A considerable number of juvenile offenders suffer from mental health disorders with components of depression, anxiety and irritability. Therefore, engaging in physical exercise can provide them with a variety of benefits (MacMahon, 1990). Moreover, many of these youth feel they have little control over their lives, especially when they are incarcerated.

Providing mentally ill juveniles with opportunities to be active and to participate in recreational activities is important. Recreation gives these youth a chance to demonstrate success in prosocial activities, as well as burn off high levels of energy that are common during the teenage years. Team sports, in particular, allow juveniles to interact with peers without criminal activity or drug use being the focus of the interaction. Exercise also can help mentally ill juvenile offenders sleep better at night.

Good Nutrition

The way youth eat can affect their behavior. Although the exact influence of food intake on aggression and antisocial behavior is not known, some studies have shown promise with this type of intervention strategy. Studies of several juvenile justice facilities across the United States demonstrated that changing the diet of young people can decrease antisocial behavior (Schoenthaler, 1985; Schoenthaler, 1987). Youth who participated in these studies had the following changes made to their diet:

- Cereal was not pre-sweetened
- Syrup was washed off canned fruit
- Fruit juice replaced Kool-Aid and soft drinks
- Honey supplemented table sugar
- Whole wheat bread replaced white bread
- Brown rice replaced white rice
- Fresh produce replaced processed food (only when they could get it at similar prices so cost was not a factor)
- Healthy snacks (*e.g.*, fresh fruit, fresh vegetables, nuts, cheeses, fruit juices, whole grain crackers) replaced high-sugar/high fat snacks (*e.g.*, ice cream, potato chips, candy bars, pastries)

Positive behavior change was observed among the juvenile offenders, including a 47 percent decrease in antisocial behavior. When youth were fed the healthier diet, reductions were seen among the following behaviors: theft,

violence, insubordination and hyperactivity/ "horseplay." One of the juvenile justice facilities wanted to be sure the positive behavior changes were due to the healthier diet (rather than other factors), so the facility returned to the old diet. Antisocial behavior increased 54 percent within the first six months (Schoenthaler, 1985).

Nutrients affect those areas of the brain that regulate mood and behavior, including the cerebral cortex. Providing juvenile offenders with healthier foods, less sugar and more nutrients appears to help them think more clearly and may increase their ability to control their behavior. Studies monitoring the nutrient intake of incarcerated juveniles found that (Schoenthaler, 1987):

- Youth who consumed the most nutrients were the best-behaved
- Youth lowest in nutrient consumption were the worst-behaved
- Youth whose nutrient intake was in the middle displayed average behavior

Just modifying youths' diet is unlikely to result in long-term behavior change for juvenile offenders with mental health disorders. Providing more nutritious meals to these youth, however, may help them to better regulate their emotions and behaviors. This improved regulation, in turn, can result in these youth increasing their participation in (and taking greater advantage of) various mental health and juvenile justice treatment programs.

The aforementioned intervention strategies and treatment components can be beneficial for all juvenile offenders, including those who have mental health disorders. However, helping youth maintain treatment gains once the formal "treatment period" is over remains a significant challenge. A primary goal when treating juvenile offenders is helping youth to function more effectively in a variety of situations and contexts—not just while under juvenile justice supervision. Not surprisingly, emotional and behavioral change within a juvenile justice

Juvenile Offenders with Mental Health Disorders: Who Are They and What Do We Do With Them?

facility is no guarantee of continued emotional and behavioral change in the community. In truth, maintenance of treatment gains among juvenile offenders is often the exception rather than the rule. Despite clinically sound treatment principles and programs, youth often have difficulty generalizing what they have learned in an institution and/or community treatment program to their "real world" circumstances. This challenge has begun to be addressed by recent treatment approaches that are designed to take place within youths' natural environment.

Community-Based Interventions

Community-based interventions deliver treatment services in youths' natural environment in order to facilitate long-term changes in the juveniles' "real life." Multisystemic Therapy (MST) is one approach that has demonstrated short and long-term positive outcomes for juvenile offenders. It has been shown to have positive effects on youth who have severe psychiatric disorders, as well as youth with substance use disorders (Borduin, *et al.,* 1995; Henggeler *et al.,* 1999; Henggeler, Melton, & Smith, 1992; Pickrel & Henggeler, 1996). Although MST is family-centered, it also emphasizes the other social networks with which youth and their families/caregivers interact (*e.g.,* school, neighborhood, church, peers). Primary goals of MST are to:

- Improve parenting/caregiver skills
- Increase positive interactions between family members
- Increase youths' association with prosocial peers
- Decrease youths' association with deviant peers
- Increase youths' involvement in prosocial activities
- Improve youths' school/vocational functioning
- Broaden the support network for the entire family unit

MST interventions are present-focused and action-oriented. An assessment of juveniles' family/caregiving environment and their particular social context drives all treatment planning. Behaviors chosen for change are specific and concrete. And intervention strategies highlight and utilize the strengths of the family unit and their particular environment. Treatment is monitored continuously and modifications are made to treatment plans when progress is not evident. Family members/caregivers are empowered to meet their own treatment needs and to interact effectively with various systems and agencies. These skills help families/caregivers maintain positive treatment outcomes even after formal MST treatment is completed.

Multisystemic Therapy incorporates cognitive-behavioral skills training, Family Functional Therapy, and various approaches used in marital/couples therapy. Treatment is highly structured and targets for change are detailed and easy to understand. The emphasis is on:

- Creating change
- Building on strengths
- Responding to youths' needs in the essential areas in which they function (*e.g.,* individual, family, peer, school, neighborhood, community)

Fundamental to this approach is the assumption that the engagement and motivation of families/caregivers, school personnel and community members is critical to effective treatment.

Treatment Strategies That Do Not Work for Juvenile Offenders

Given the type of treatment components shown to be beneficial, it should not be surprising that the following treatment strategies have had limited to no success in the treatment of juvenile offenders (McGuire & Priestley, 1995):

- Psychodynamic therapy (emphasis primarily on childhood events, subconscious processes, achievement of insight)

- Client-centered therapy (emphasis primarily on empathy, unconditional positive regard, building esteem)
- Psychotropic medication with no psychosocial adjuncts
- Punishment-based programs (*e.g.*, boot camps, shock incarceration)
- Incapacitation (emphasis primarily on removing youth from others)

In the few instances where boot camps demonstrate some positive outcomes for juvenile offenders, intervention strategies consist of much more than military style, boot camp programming. These programs offer treatment-related activities such as educational assistance, individual and group counseling, and substance abuse treatment services. The programs also emphasize continued supervision and intervention services when youth return to the community. That being said, boot camps are typically not appropriate placements for juvenile offenders with mental health disorders. Even with "treatment" related services and comprehensive aftercare, these programs are usually too physically and emotionally intense for juveniles with serious emotional and behavioral issues. Committing juveniles with mental health disorders to a boot camp may not only exacerbate mental health symptoms, but can prevent the youth from gaining access to appropriate psychological or psychiatric treatment.

Conclusions Regarding Effective Interventions

The most beneficial treatment programs for juvenile offenders with mental health disorders offer ongoing, long-term intervention in numerous areas of youths' lives. Continuing to search for a magic pill or a single treatment approach that works well with all mentally ill juveniles is too simplistic. Effective mental health treatment for juvenile offenders begins with a comprehensive assessment of youth and their families/

caregivers—so that treatment can be individualized to their particular strengths and needs.

Treatment should be culturally relevant and provided in the natural environments in which juveniles interact. When choosing intervention strategies, the following factors about youth should be taken into account:

- Age
- Cognitive abilities
- Developmental maturity
- Gender
- Ethnicity
- Community in which they reside
- Juvenile justice status

EFFECTIVE MENTAL HEALTH TREATMENT FOR JUVENILE OFFENDERS BEGINS WITH A COMPREHENSIVE ASSESSMENT OF YOUTH AND THEIR FAMILIES/CAREGIVERS—SO THAT TREATMENT CAN BE INDIVIDUALIZED TO THEIR PARTICULAR STRENGTHS AND NEEDS.

Even when youth receive treatment in a group setting, their individual needs still must be taken into account and each juvenile's progress should be monitored. In addition, the presence of the following family/caregiver characteristics should also be considered:

- Mental illness
- Substance abuse
- Child abuse or neglect

Successful outcomes are possible for this complex population of youth when treatment is comprehensive and intervention occurs at several levels (*e.g.*, individual, family, peer, community) and within several systems (*e.g.*, health, juvenile justice, substance abuse, educational, vocational, medical) for an extended period of time. Intervention strategies should be structured and focused on specific changes

Juvenile Offenders with Mental Health Disorders: Who Are They and What Do We Do With Them?

related to youths' emotions and behavior. Treatment should be monitored, and when progress is not being made, treatment plans should be modified. Effective programs exist that encompass many of the necessary components for treating the needs of juvenile offenders with mental health disorders (Bowler, 2001; Kamradt, 2000).

Effective treatment for juvenile offenders with mental health disorders begins with early intervention—at the first signs of mental health-related symptoms. Ideally, these services should be provided by the mental health system *before* youth become involved with juvenile justice. For some juvenile offenders, appropriate and early mental health intervention in the community helps prevent juvenile justice involvement altogether.

Currently, the treatment needs of many mentally ill youth are not being met by the mental health system; some of these individuals are entering the juvenile justice system. These youth may be correctly diagnosed with a psychiatric disorder, misdiagnosed or undiagnosed. A significant number have been unsuccessfully treated for their mental health disorder, and some have never received any mental health treatment at all. If youth are detained in a juvenile justice setting, a variety of intervention strategies can be implemented to stabilize youths' mental health symptoms, as well as foster their growth and development. However, these efforts must be continued and broadened once the juveniles are released back into the community. Without continuity of mental health care, prolonged treatment gains are unlikely, if not impossible.

Characteristics that Complicate Treatment

Even when agencies utilize treatment strategies that have been shown to be effective, several potential issues can make treating juvenile offenders with mental health disorders particularly challenging. Whenever the following characteristics are present, they need to be specifically addressed in youths' treatment plans:

- Lack of stable housing
- School will not allow youth to return
- Lack of a supportive adult
- Association with deviant peers
- Family members with mental illness/ substance abuse
- Cognitive limitations
- Youths' avoidance of school/vocational involvement
- Multiple psychiatric diagnoses
- Multiple drugs of abuse
- Removal of youths' typical coping strategies (*e.g.*, substance use, aggression, sex, running away) before replacing with new ones
- Recurrent suicidal and/or self-mutilating behavior
- Gang involvement
- Abusive or neglectful family members
- Abusive romantic partner
- Pregnancy or being the parent of small child/children
- Repeated incarcerations
- Potential for violent behavior
- Criminal activity by family members

 ## Enhancing Motivation with Mentally Ill Juvenile Offenders

The vast majority of juvenile offenders with mental health disorders do not refer themselves for treatment services. Parents/caregivers, teachers, probation/parole officers, judges, or juvenile justice facility staff typically bring youth to the attention of mental health professionals. In fact, many juveniles do not perceive their mental health symptoms and/or behavior as problematic. Not surprisingly, this can significantly impact youths' motivation and willingness to engage in mental health treatment interventions, and can serve as a major barrier to successful outcomes. Even if youth are initially motivated toward treatment, their commitment to behavior change often fluctuates during the course of an intervention.

Motivational Interviewing/Motivational Enhancement Therapy (Rollnick & Miller, 1995) is one approach that addresses issues of denial and poor motivation, and can be beneficial in the treatment of juvenile offenders with mental health disorders. This approach assumes that youths' internal motivation significantly influences their ability to change their behavior. Therefore, a primary task of treatment providers is to create an environment that supports and reinforces juveniles' own motivation and commitment to change. This approach has been shown to be effective around issues of substance abuse. But the approach also can be used with issues related to mental health and juvenile offending. The approach focuses on five basic principles to help facilitate youths' decision to change their behavior, comply with treatment recommendations, and remain committed to behavior change:

EXPRESS EMPATHY
Treatment providers truly try to understand juveniles' lives, thoughts, feelings, and behavior by viewing the world as the juveniles view it. Clinicians accept youth as they are, listen without judgment, and normalize juveniles' ambivalence about wanting to change their behavior.

DEVELOP DISCREPANCY
Treatment providers help juveniles become aware of the disparity between what their lives are like in the present, in comparison to what kind of lives they would like to have. Clinicians gently point out the ways in which youths' current behavior may be moving them away from the goals youth have set for themselves. Highlighting some of the negative consequences associated with juveniles' current behavior can be helpful.

AVOID ARGUING
Taking a confrontational approach with juvenile offenders can result in youth arguing the opposite position, resisting helpful advice, and/or prematurely terminating treatment. With many juvenile offenders, the more authority figures tell them what they need to do or how they need to change, the more defensive the youth become. The motivational interviewing approach avoids telling youth what to do. Instead, treatment providers help juveniles identify the negative consequences of the behavior in need of changing, and begin to devalue the positive aspects of it. Clinicians do not focus on having youth "break through their denial" or "admit" to anything. Instead of facing denial head-on, clinicians work around it. A primary goal is for juveniles to realize the benefits of changing their behavior and develop justifications in support of making this change.

ROLL WITH RESISTANCE
The manner in which treatment providers respond to youths' "resistance" is critical in this approach. Rather than confronting juveniles about their opposition to change, clinicians work with youth at wherever they are in terms of change. Treatment providers may need to use a variety of different strategies before getting youths' "buy in." The focus is on eliciting solutions from the juveniles rather than telling them what they should or should not do. This way youth cannot argue with the clinicians' suggestions. When youth are hesitant about changing their behavior, treatment providers explore and normalize the juveniles' feelings of ambivalence. In addition, positive steps toward behavior change that youth are already taking are continuously reinforced.

SUPPORT SELF-EFFICACY
To take the necessary steps to make behavioral changes, juveniles must believe they currently possess the ability to change their behavior. Many juvenile offenders have previously been told they are "untreatable" or "treatment fail-

ures". These youth typically need a great deal of encouragement and support, and should be reinforced for even thinking about making difficult changes. Clinicians inquire about successful changes youth have made in the past and highlight the positive skills they possess that can facilitate behavior change in the present. Without the hope of success, there is little motivation for juveniles to continue working on their problems.

Motivational interviewing is a practical approach that shows promise with populations which have significant treatment needs, including individuals with both mental health and substance use disorders (Swanson, Pantalon, & Cohen, 1999).

 ## Barriers to Mental Health Treatment

About 20 percent of youth in the general population have a diagnosable mental health disorder. However, only one in five of these youth receive treatment from the mental health system (Burns, *et al.*, 1995). A variety of barriers can interfere with juveniles' access and use of effective mental health services. Many of these barriers are present, and sometimes intensified, in relation to juvenile offenders. Particular characteristics of youth, families/caregivers, as well as systems/agencies can potentially hinder juvenile offenders from receiving and/or complying with mental health treatment.

Youths' own beliefs and behaviors can potentially hinder access to effective mental health treatment. Most juvenile offenders with mental health disorders do not seek treatment on their own and are referred by a significant adult in their life. Juveniles may not think that there is anything wrong with their behavior and may resist the notion that they have a "problem." Even if they can see where their behavior is causing them difficulty, they may not want to make necessary changes.

For instance, some youth have such a long history of anger and aggression that they cannot

conceive of giving either of them up. These youth may regard anger and aggression as essential factors for their physical and emotional survival. In addition, drug and alcohol use may be a central component of how and with whom juveniles choose to spend their time. Even if youth are willing (or are coerced) to enter treatment, most treatment programs are highly structured—with restrictions placed on the youths' behaviors and activities. This type of environment can be threatening to juveniles who have been without significant adult direction and who have established noncompliant and oppositional response patterns. The youth may avoid important treatment activities or drop out of a treatment program altogether.

Issues related to youths' *families/caregivers* might make the implementation of mental health treatment more challenging. For example, families/caregivers may not be very motivated to participate in their children's mental health treatment. This reluctance could be due to a variety of factors, including:

- The presence of multiple family stressors
- A real or perceived sense of racism or ethnic bias
- Parental mental illness/substance abuse
- Frustration/burnout from years of working on their youths' mental health issues
- Feeling blamed/criticized by the mental health or juvenile justice system in the past

In addition, juveniles' families/caregivers may not be able to financially afford mental health treatment for their children. Even when treatment is offered at no cost within juvenile justice facilities, families/caregivers may not be able to participate due to costs associated with transportation and/or childcare. If youths' families/caregivers are non-English speaking, they may need to have a bilingual treatment provider, which may not be possible. In addition, families/caregivers may avoid participating in mental health treatment sessions with their

Treatment of Juvenile Offenders with Mental Health Disorders

children due to the stigma attached to mental illness. These individuals may be uncomfortable sharing personal information with a stranger—regardless of whether they are trained mental health professionals. This reluctance can be particularly strong if family members are afraid of specific issues being uncovered (*e.g.*, abuse, neglect, parental mental illness, parental substance use). Some parents/caregivers of juvenile offenders have inconsistent histories of trust in their own relationships with adults, which can impact how they view and interact with treatment providers.

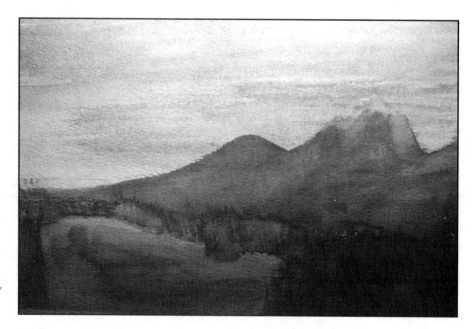

Even if youth and their families are motivated and committed to participating in mental health treatment, *system/agency* barriers can make treatment difficult to implement. Obstacles can exist whether youth are receiving mental health services within a juvenile justice facility or out in the community. For example:

- Many juvenile justice facilities do not have enough mental health personnel to provide the level of treatment many of these youth require.

- Some mental health providers are reluctant to work with juveniles who are angry and hostile until their anger is under control. Ironically, this problem may be the primary reason the youth requires treatment. When juvenile offenders display angry/hostile emotions during treatment, they are often viewed as noncompliant, labeled untreatable, and prematurely terminated from programs.

- Confidentiality laws (which are designed to protect youths' rights) can hinder the communication between professionals from different systems and agencies.

- Some treatment providers working with juvenile offenders have not been trained to work with adolescents, are unaware of important developmental issues, and have minimal experience working with this complex population.

- Mental health programs often use a model in which clinicians diagnose and design treatment plans with minimal input from youth and their families/caregivers. Instead of supporting their strengths and empowering the youth and their families/caregivers, this practice creates a sense of alienation or increased dependence on experts.

- If juvenile offenders are receiving treatment for both mental health and substance abuse, they may receive conflicting treatment recommendations. For example, many mental health treatment approaches rely on youth taking responsibility for their actions and actively changing their thoughts, feelings and behavior. Youth also may be prescribed psychotropic medication. Both of these strategies may be at odds with a substance abuse treatment approach that

272

Juvenile Offenders with Mental Health Disorders: Who Are They and What Do We Do With Them?

relies on youth accepting they are "powerless" over their drug and alcohol use. Further, some substance abuse programs discourage the use of any type of chemical substance, including psychotropic medication.

- Many treatment programs exclude mentally ill juvenile offenders because of "safety" concerns (*e.g.*, sexual victimization, arson, aggression).

- There is typically minimal collaboration between mental health and juvenile justice systems.

- Depending on available resources, there can be extensive waiting lists to access mental health services.

- Most mental health treatment occurs in artificial settings (*e.g.*, juvenile justice facility, mental health clinic, treatment provider's office, psychiatric hospital) rather than youths' homes, schools, or communities. Newly taught skills may not be maintained long-term if the juveniles do not practice them in home and community settings with peers and family members.

- Mental health and juvenile justice providers often do not provide strong incentives to help engage and involve juveniles' families/caregivers in treatment.

- Few treatment programs have been specifically designed for youth of color and/or females who have mental health disorders.

- Daytime appointments are often difficult to keep given the school and work schedules of youth and their parents/caregivers.

- There are often limited "follow-up" mental health services once formal treatment is over, resulting in little to no ongoing contact with youth.

- If youth are required to obtain mental health treatment at a residential/inpatient

program, it may be located a far distance from the juveniles' home. Attending family treatment sessions or visiting youth at a treatment facility can be difficult for family/caregivers if it is outside of the juveniles' community.

- Separate funding sources typically exist for mental health and juvenile justice services, making coordination and integration of these services difficult.

- Youth with mental health disorders are often released from juvenile justice facilities without reliable mental health treatment services in place.

- Lack of accessible, affordable, mental health care in the community (inpatient and/or outpatient) makes accessing mental health treatment difficult for youth and their families/caregivers.

Integrated, community-based mental health treatment approaches that are based on empirically supported intervention strategies attempt to overcome these potential barriers. To be effective, these approaches need to be culturally relevant, flexible and focused on family/caregiver engagement and youth compliance. Collaboration and integration between key agencies and systems are critical.

 KEY TREATMENT ISSUES

Crisis Intervention Plans

Some incarcerated juvenile offenders with serious mental health disorders require crisis intervention services. Crisis response plans should be developed for severely mentally ill juveniles, as should backup plans in case an initial response is not effective. There should be clear policies and procedures about:

- Involuntary medication
- Seclusion and restraint
- Transfer to an emergency room at a local hospital/inpatient psychiatric facility

Treatment of Juvenile Offenders with Mental Health Disorders

If crisis situations typically result in transfer to an outside facility, agreements should be in place with all hospitals that may be used during a psychiatric emergency—well before a crisis occurs. Criteria for offenders' admission and discharge from a hospital should be explicit and unambiguous. Any behavior that automatically results in youths' expulsion from a hospital unit also should be made clear.

Treatment Coordination

Many juvenile offenders with mental health disorders participate in a variety of treatment programs (*e.g.*, individual counseling, group counseling, anger management, substance abuse, sexual offending). In addition, the youth may be involved with a school counselor, tutoring, a vocational program, an afterschool recreation program or a mentoring program. These different services may be provided consecutively or all at the same time. The coordination of juveniles' various treatment efforts and components is essential. Each intervention strategy will probably focus on a slightly different aspect of youths' behavior. Even so, all professionals providing treatment to the juveniles should have a holistic view of the youth and an awareness of other treatment services the youth are receiving. Continual communication and collaboration between the various treatment providers can greatly facilitate service integration.

Treatment Continuity

Continuity of mental health treatment, or the lack thereof, significantly influences positive outcomes for youth. Mentally ill juvenile offenders commonly have been involved with the mental health system before their involvement with juvenile justice. If youth have a mental health treatment provider in the community, that provider should remain in communication with the juveniles while they are in a juvenile justice setting. Incarceration is often the time when mentally ill youth are in the greatest need of support, and having a consistent relationship

with significant adults is essential. Ideally, treatment providers should come to a juvenile justice facility to meet with the youth. But if that is not feasible, phone calls are also beneficial.

Along the same lines, mentally ill juveniles should have an appointment set up with mental health agencies/providers in the community—so the youth have appointments with clinicians immediately upon release. This practice should be routine, unless there is a justifiable reason not to link youth with previous providers (*e.g.*, juveniles did not like their provider, treatment strategies were harmful). Previous treatment providers are familiar with the youth and have already developed a relationship with them. Also, previous agencies typically have past records of mental health evaluations, as well as treatment progress notes, which means not having to start over (which can be frustrating for youth).

In addition, continuity of treatment is critical *within* the juvenile justice system itself. Many mentally ill youth are involved with several aspects of the system: juvenile court, probation, a detention center, a training school, a group home, parole, and so forth. Each of these settings may have conducted mental health screenings and assessments with youth, as well as implemented various treatment strategies. Important mental health information should follow youth as they move through the juvenile justice continuum—with new treatment approaches integrating assessment information and intervention strategies that have come before. Too often, juvenile offenders receive fragmented and uncoordinated mental health services within juvenile justice because each faction of the system starts anew.

Treatment Expectations and Noncompliance

Even if youth and their families/caregivers are initially engaged in mental health treatment, it is not unusual for compliance to diminish after a period of time. At the outset of treatment for

Juvenile Offenders with Mental Health Disorders: Who Are They and What Do We Do With Them?

juvenile offenders, representatives from both the mental health and juvenile justice system should identify potential areas of noncompliance. The representatives should then agree upon associated consequences should any of the potential circumstances arise. Care should always be taken when deciding how to respond to juveniles' noncompliance with mental health treatment. Juveniles may:

- Stop attending treatment sessions
- Refuse to take their psychotropic medication
- Engage in behaviors specifically prohibited by their treatment plan

In most cases the mental health system, versus the juvenile justice system, should provide the *initial* consequence if youth fail to comply with treatment agreements (Griffin, Hills & Peters, 1996). The therapeutic relationship between the mental health professional/agency, the youth, and their families/caregivers is likely to be negatively affected if the juvenile justice system automatically responds each time difficulties arise during the youths' mental health treatment. Treatment providers always should investigate the possible reasons for juveniles and/or their families/caregivers beginning to detach from treatment and help remedy any problematic situations.

Treatment providers, as well as juvenile justice professionals, should not focus exclusively on youths' mental health symptoms. Although concentrating on the juveniles' symptoms is essential during treatment, exploring what else may be occurring in the youths' lives is also important. Juvenile offenders usually grapple with typical adolescent issues in addition to working on their juvenile justice treatment plan. Many youth in treatment are expected to develop a variety of new skills simultaneously including:

- Regulating their emotions
- Controlling their behavior
- Reconnecting with family members

- Socializing with positive peers
- Avoiding deviant peers
- Attending school regularly
- Avoiding drugs and alcohol

The cognitive, biological and emotional changes that accompany the adolescent years can be challenging for any youth. But they can be particularly so for juvenile offenders with mental health disorders. Juvenile justice and mental health treatment providers can forget too easily about the variety of demands placed on teenagers in addition to the juvenile justice and mental health treatment responsibilities often required of youth. School responsibilities or juvenile justice requirements may be so time-consuming that they interfere with youths' ability to attend mental health treatment sessions, or vice versa. Juveniles' families/caregivers or friends may try to convince the youth that they do not have a mental health disorder. Not surprisingly, some juveniles become overwhelmed and increasingly frustrated while participating in mental health treatment.

Because mentally ill juvenile offenders are likely to have requirements placed on them by both the mental health and juvenile justice systems, it is important not to overburden them. All professionals working with these youth should talk with the juveniles, their families/caregivers, and each other to prioritize which goals are most important and meaningful. Many juvenile offenders with mental health disorders have had difficulty maintaining positive behavior change, as well as consistently committing to treatment, in the past. Placing too many treatment expectations on youth too quickly can set the juveniles up to fail. Creating conditions in which youth can succeed in treatment is critical to successful outcomes.

Maintaining Treatment Involvement

Once youth and their families/caregivers make a commitment to participate in treatment, they must be continually reinforced in their involvement. Otherwise, they are likely to drop out if treatment becomes difficult. The juvenile justice system often tends to focus more on sanctioning youth for noncompliance with treatment versus rewarding them for their participation. Reinforcing juveniles and their families/caregivers for even the smallest efforts in mental health treatment is important. Reinforcement is particularly important at the beginning of a treatment program, when participants might be hesitant to involve themselves.

Juvenile justice agencies should routinely evaluate what types of positive incentives are available to youth and their families/caregivers. Although verbal praise and acknowledgment are always helpful, sometimes more tangible rewards are also necessary. Even the biggest, toughest or oldest juvenile offenders can appear touched and moved after:

- Receiving a certificate of achievement
- Participating in some form of a graduation ceremony

Many juvenile justice facilities and community supervision programs have discovered creative and effective ways to reinforce the offenders in their custody, even when resources are limited. Incentives for youth and their families/caregivers do not need to be expensive or elaborate. The following incentives can been used to increase motivation to attend treatment sessions, particularly when individuals begin to feel tentative about it:

- Supplying food during treatment sessions
- Providing extra time for the youth and their families/caregivers to visit with each other after sessions are over
- Offering free movie tickets
- Allowing youth to play a video game after sessions

A reduction in juvenile justice supervision (*e.g.*, fewer restrictions, earlier release) also can be a powerful motivator to continue treatment involvement for both youth and their families/caregivers. Because individuals differ greatly in what they find rewarding, it is important to ask each juvenile (and their family/caretakers) what positive incentives would be most motivating for them.

Exploring what negative sanctions are most commonly used when youth or families/caregivers do not comply with treatment is also important for juvenile justice agencies. Evaluating how effective (or ineffective) these penalties have been in the past is particularly important. Although commonly used sanctions may prompt youth and their families/caregivers to attend treatment sessions, the sanctions may or may not result in these individuals participating in the treatment process. There are definitely some juvenile offenders with mental health disorders—as well as families/caregivers—who would not be involved with mental health treatment if it were not mandated by the juvenile justice system. Although many of these

> REINFORCEMENT IS PARTICULARLY IMPORTANT AT THE BEGINNING OF A TREATMENT PROGRAM, WHEN PARTICIPANTS MIGHT BE HESITANT TO INVOLVE THEMSELVES.

individuals participate in treatment because they "have" to—at least they are involved. Even when forced, some juveniles and families/caregivers eventually see encouraging results, including more positive family interactions and increased prosocial behavior on the part of the youth. These results can alter these individual's views toward treatment and can result in increased participation of their own accord.

Relying solely on negative consequences and sanctions can alter the behavior of youth and their families/caretakers for the short term. But positive incentives must be present if the goal is to truly motivate and engage these individuals. A combination of incentives and penalties can be effective in maintaining youth

Juvenile Offenders with Mental Health Disorders: Who Are They and What Do We Do With Them?

and their families'/caretakers' involvement in mental health treatment. However, the number of positive consequences should always be higher than that of negative consequences—a feat that is often difficult to accomplish within juvenile justice as it is currently designed.

Who Should Provide Treatment

Many juvenile justice agencies use both mental health and juvenile justice professionals in the implementation of various treatment programs. There is some evidence that using mental health professionals results in more beneficial treatment effects (Lipsey & Wilson, 1998). This finding may be related to juvenile justice professionals having a dual role (custody and treatment) or having less formal training in treatment issues. Having mental health professionals provide as much of the treatment services as possible is optimal. However, these types of decisions are often based on resource availability. In situations where mental health professionals provide much, or all, of the treatment services to youth, juvenile justice staff should still participate and play a role in service delivery (*e.g.*, sit in on treatment groups, co-lead treatment activities).

If they are expected to provide treatment (*e.g.*, individual counseling, treatment groups) to juvenile offenders with mental health disorders, juvenile justice professionals should receive proper training and support. Too often, juvenile justice staff is expected to conduct a variety of treatment groups based on instructions from a manual, with no other preparation or training. Whether required to provide individual or group treatment with youth, juvenile justice staff should first receive training on interpersonal and developmental issues. They should also be trained in the identification and management of mentally ill juveniles. This way, staff can interact and respond to youth in a way that fosters their growth and development, without reinforcing negative behaviors. Providing juvenile justice professionals with treatment manuals and no accompanying supervision or training is

likely to result in frustration for the staff and the juveniles receiving services. Staff should be provided with whatever tools are necessary to provide effective treatment interventions, be supervised closely, and be supported for their efforts.

Relapse Prevention

Treating juvenile offenders with mental health disorders is a long-term and ongoing process. Even when youth make progress in treatment, there probably will be times when youths' mental health symptoms return or worsen. Therefore, a significant part of mental health treatment should focus on situations most stressful for juveniles and on developing the skills to cope with those situations.

Immediate action should be taken if:

- Mentally ill youths' symptoms begin to worsen
- There is a return of symptoms after youth have been symptom-free for a while

Treatment providers, family members/caretakers, and juveniles should not panic, but should collectively explore what needs to happen to help the youth return to their previous level of functioning. The reemergence of previous symptoms or behaviors should not be viewed as a treatment failure, but as a signal to reevaluate or reinstate mental health treatment strategies. Issues related to substance use, psychotropic medication compliance, current level of expectations, and exposure to high-risk situations should each be examined. Any positive actions youth take to reduce the severity of relapse should always be acknowledged and reinforced.

 INformATION SHARiNG ANd IssuES of CONfidENTIAliTY

Because juvenile offenders with mental health disorders often require services from multiple systems, professionals from various disciplines (*e.g.*, juvenile justice professionals, community

Treatment of Juvenile Offenders with Mental Health Disorders

supervision staff, mental health providers, substance abuse providers, educators, vocational supervisors, child welfare workers, recreation specialists, health care providers) must communicate with one another. Given the limited resources of many agencies, difficult-to-meet deadlines, and large caseloads, interagency communication often falls to the bottom of the list of priorities. However, successful treatment outcomes for mentally ill juveniles are unlikely without the sharing of important information.

Mental health professionals and juvenile justice professionals each have their own area of expertise. Both realms of knowledge are critical and necessary for achieving success with juvenile offenders who have mental health disorders. When juvenile justice staff are challenged by particular mentally ill youth, mental health providers may be able to provide insight into the juveniles' behavior, as well as suggest possible intervention strategies.

Conversely, mental health providers may become increasingly frustrated with particular youths' noncompliance or uncommunicative behavior during treatment sessions. Juvenile justice professionals may be able to recommend effective strategies they have used with those youth to increase their motivation and compliance. There is no need for each system to struggle in isolation with challenging juvenile offenders who have a mental health disorder—an all too-common dynamic.

In order to do their job effectively, juvenile justice professionals often require particular mental health information about youth they are supervising. For example, knowing the following can significantly influence the supervision/management strategies staff employ with youth:

- Youth made a recent suicide attempt
- Youth are currently depressed
- Youth often hear voices
- Youth were recently raped

When they are unaware of youths' mental health status, juvenile justice staff may instinctively attribute juveniles' mental health symptoms to the juveniles being manipulative or intentionally oppositional. Problems can also arise if staff have no knowledge of youths' low level of cognitive (or emotional) functioning. Staff may place expectations on the juveniles that are at a level too high for them to achieve. This situation typically results in negative sanctions for the youth, as well as frustration for both parties.

In addition, some juvenile justice facility staff are responsible for dispensing psychotropic medication to youth. Staff should have knowledge about the medications they are distributing, behaviors the medications are treating, and any possible side effects. Additionally, when they are aware of youths' mental health status, juvenile justice staff can incorporate relevant mental health issues into the juveniles' treatment/supervision plan.

Along the same lines, mental health professionals can provide more effective treatment services when they have important information about youths' juvenile justice involvement. Knowing youths' juvenile justice status can help treatment providers develop more comprehensive mental health treatment plans that incorporate relevant juvenile justice issues. The following juvenile justice information can be particularly helpful for professionals providing mental health treatment services to juvenile offenders:

- Youths' current offense
- Youth's previous juvenile justice involvement
- Youths' recent behavior in a juvenile justice facility or under community supervision
- Aggressive or violent behavior
- Length of time youth are under juvenile justice supervision
- Length of time the juvenile offenders are required to be in treatment
- Youths' motivation for treatment

Juvenile Offenders with Mental Health Disorders: Who Are They and What Do We Do With Them?

- Consequences of not complying with treatment requirements
- Any requirements regarding reports of the youths' treatment progress

Before youth are released from a residential facility, mental health agencies and treatment providers in the community should be provided with relevant information about juveniles' mental health disorder. Many mentally ill juvenile offenders receive a variety of mental health services during periods of incarceration. The following information can be beneficial to community mental health providers who will be working with mentally ill juvenile offenders upon release:

- Mental health assessments
- Treatment strategies that were effective and ineffective
- Discharge summaries
- Community transition plans
- Areas of treatment that still need to be addressed

Confidentiality

Laws and regulations regarding confidentiality have been developed to protect the privacy of individuals who participate in mental health treatment. The intent is for juveniles' personal mental health information to remain private and confidential. It is hoped that youth will feel more comfortable seeking and participating in mental health treatment if they know their personal information will not be shared with others and/or used against them.

Although intended to benefit a youth, confidentiality laws and regulations can potentially interfere with effective communication between various professionals and agencies. This type of interference can occur when it is not clear what types of information can and cannot be discussed—and to whom the information can be disclosed. There are both federal and state laws/regulations regarding the confidentiality of mental health information.

Juvenile justice and mental health agencies should be aware of the current rules under which they are operating.

Confidentiality laws/regulations can be somewhat confusing. They generally state that information related to juveniles' mental health status, as well as associated mental health assessment and treatment, is to remain confidential. But there is often some flexibility related to juvenile justice facilities.

For example, some state regulations allow disclosure of mental health records "to a facility in which a minor resides" (*i.e.*, juvenile detention center, training school, group home). If laws/regulations do not automatically allow the release of mental health information, youth can provide written permission for the information to be released. The most common way of providing this permission is by signing a "release of information" form. If juveniles are old enough to consent to treatment without parental permission, they are old enough to sign a release of confidential information form without parental permission. All juvenile justice agencies should routinely use "consent for release of information" forms. Even with written permission, however, mental health information should be disclosed only to juvenile justice professionals who need the information to effectively monitor, supervise, or treat the youth. And only pertinent information should be communicated.

There are certain circumstances in which mental health information can be released without youths' written consent. Juvenile justice professionals who suspect child abuse or neglect are typically mandated to report their suspicions and do not need juveniles' permission to do so. In addition, confidential mental health information can usually be disclosed during a medical emergency. When there is an immediate threat to the health of juveniles and they require immediate medical attention, written consent is typically not required.

Even though juveniles can authorize disclosure of mental health information, this does not

Treatment of Juvenile Offenders with Mental Health Disorders

mean mental health providers/agencies are *obligated* to provide it. If professionals holding confidential information do not think disclosure is in the best interest of youth, they can withhold the information. As one can imagine, this situation can cause animosity and conflict between various systems. Withholding confidential information after written permission has been given by youth should be reserved for exceptional circumstances.

Interagency agreements can help guard against problems related to the release of confidential information. Each system should have clear policies regarding what type of information should be released and to whom. Policies should also clearly delineate what type of information will not be released, even when written permission has been given to do so. The process of releasing mental health information should be manageable and efficient. The process should be routinely explained to juvenile justice and mental health staff at all levels to reduce confusion and potential barriers to communication.

Most confidentiality issues are related to the release of information from mental health providers. But juvenile justice professionals also have restrictions related to the type of information they are allowed to release. Juvenile justice professionals (*e.g.*, facility staff, probation/parole officers) often collect important information from mentally ill youth, as well as interact with them on a regular basis. Therefore, these professionals usually have information that can be helpful for treatment providers. As with the mental health system, there are restrictions regarding juvenile justice staffs' ability to communicate youths' mental health information to individuals working outside of the juvenile justice system. All juvenile justice agencies should familiarize themselves with state laws (as well as court policy and local agency policy) regulating the release of confidential information.

 ### Transitioning Juvenile Offenders With Mental Health Disorders Back Into the Community

Regardless of the level of mental health treatment provided in secure/residential settings, juvenile offenders with mental health disorders typically require mental health services in the community to make long-term positive outcomes. Links will need to be made with the various individuals, agencies and systems from whom youth require services. These may include:

- Family/caregivers
- Community mental health center
- Child welfare
- Substance abuse treatment program
- Educational/vocational programs

Well before youth are ready to leave a juvenile justice facility, important contacts should be made and transition planning begun.

Some juvenile offenders with serious mental health disorders require specialized residential placements or specific intervention services immediately upon release from a facility. Some examples include:

- Inpatient psychiatric hospital
- Day treatment program
- Therapeutic foster care
- Intensive home-based treatment

Families/caregivers may need crisis intervention services or access to respite care. Some families/caregivers may not have the capacity or the willingness to take care of mentally ill juveniles upon their release from incarceration. Although out-of-home placements have frequently been utilized in the past with this population, every effort should be made to connect youth with family members. Placing youth with "strange relatives" instead of "relative strangers" can be beneficial for many juvenile offenders with mental health disorders—even if those family members are distant

280

Juvenile Offenders with Mental Health Disorders: Who Are They and What Do We Do With Them?

relatives or do not live nearby. In addition, physical health and psychotropic medication management in the community are often critical for the maintenance of treatment gains and also need to be secured. Community resources such as churches, afterschool programs, and advocacy groups can play a significant role in the successful reintegration of a juvenile offender back into the community.

Many juvenile justice agencies need to engage in assertive outreach to community agencies (including community mental health centers), and develop incentives for them to become involved with juvenile offenders who have mental health disorders. Community agencies are often unfamiliar and uncomfortable collaborating with the juvenile justice system. It is important for them to have an understanding of:

- The policies and procedures under which the juvenile justice system operates
- The characteristics of the youth in the system (including their many strengths)
- The type of collaborative relationship desired

Many community agencies are fearful that large numbers of juvenile offenders with mental health disorders will be "dumped" upon them. These agencies are usually concerned that they will not have the necessary resources (financial and otherwise) to manage the youth. Juvenile justice agencies must emphasize their continued involvement with youth, as well as their accessibility. Collaborative funding options should also be explored.

The Denver Juvenile Justice Integrated Treatment Network is a model of how communities can forge effective links with the multiple systems affecting juvenile offenders with mental health treatment needs (Field, 1998).

Effective community coordination and collaboration involves the organization of a variety of public and private agencies, as well as various service providers that are willing to work together to care for juvenile offenders with mental health disorders. Because the needs of these youth are often multiple, services are typically required in a variety of domains including: mental health, education, medical, vocational, familial, recreational, substance use, peers, housing and transportation. A wide variety of agencies and organizations should be enlisted to increase the likelihood that youth and their families/caregivers receive services that are:

- Relevant to their values and lifestyle
- Provided close to their home.

Aftercare and Continuing Care Services
"Aftercare," also known in some jurisdictions as "continuing care," services are provided to juvenile offenders after release from a residential facility. Services are focused on helping youth readjust to residing in the community. Extra supervision and monitoring is usually provided to youth of "high risk" status.

Depending on how long youth have been incarcerated, the move from a residential facility back into the community can be challenging. Although juvenile offenders may be excited to experience more freedom and choice, there are also more responsibilities placed upon the youth. The community offers many temptations that were minimally present or completely absent in a residential setting. Basic decisions that were made for juveniles in an institution must be made by the youth themselves. Female (as well as male) offenders may be reunited with their young children, adding another set of responsibilities. When they are not adequately prepared for this transition, many juvenile offenders with mental health disorders are overwhelmed upon return to the community. Mental health, substance abuse, and juvenile justice treatment gains may be lost quickly if appropriate support services are not in place.

Usually, the longer they have been incarcerated, the more aftercare/continuing care services youth require—because their change in circumstances is more extreme. Gradually transitioning youth back into the community can be very beneficial. Juveniles can be allowed to make visits to their families'/caregivers' home or reside for a short time in a less restrictive residential setting in the community (e.g., step-down program, group home). Many juveniles who reside in group homes are able to attend school and various treatment services outside of their residence. This practice allows youth to practice functioning with fewer external controls before fully reintegrating back into the community.

Probation and parole staff can play a significant role in youths' mental health treatment. Mandating participation in mental health services is a common requirement in the community supervision plans of juvenile offenders with mental health disorders.

Although positive incentives for treatment compliance are essential, the fear of sanctions for noncompliance can also be a powerful motivator for some juveniles and their families/caregivers. Community supervision staff should be in regular contact with youth and monitoring their involvement in a variety of areas (e.g., home, school, peers). Therefore, these individuals may notice a worsening of youths' functioning, as well as a return or exacerbation of youths' mental health symptoms. If mentally ill juveniles have a co-occurring substance use disorder, probation/parole staff can use drug tests to strengthen youths' motivation to remain clean and sober.

The first few months after release from a juvenile justice facility can be particularly difficult for mentally ill juvenile offenders as they try to:

- Readjust to their home environment
- Reenter school
- Maintain a crime-free lifestyle
- Maintain sobriety despite pressure from peers

Community supervision staff can be particularly helpful during this period by closely monitoring aftercare/continuing care treatment goals. Juvenile justice supervision during this phase can be critical for juvenile offenders with mental health disorders to facilitate treatment compliance. Close supervision can also help these youth refrain from delinquent activity. The Intensive Community-Based Aftercare Program (IAP) is a model of an effective program emphasizing pre-release planning, aftercare monitoring, family involvement, and service delivery (Altschuler & Armstrong, 1996, 1997).

Community Transition Plans

Whether mentally ill youth successfully make use of the gains achieved in secure/residential settings greatly depends on the successful development and implementation of community transition plans (e.g., aftercare plans, continuing care plans). Community transition plans typically outline what services need to be provided once juveniles are released from a residential setting, and a strategy for implementing these services. These plans must address all of the domains and systems from which youth will require support and monitoring. Tailoring a plan to the individual strengths and needs of particular juveniles and their families/caregivers is essential.

Ideally, the development of transition plans should begin as soon as youth enter a residential setting. This practice provides ample time to coordinate needed services before the juveniles are released from residential care. Transition plans should be the result of input from a variety of individuals who are involved with the juveniles' supervision and treatment (e.g., probation/parole officer, parents/caregivers, facility staff, facility treatment providers, community treatment providers, the youth, teachers, vocational supervisors, recreation staff, medical staff). Even if youth and their families/caregivers do not show much interest in the development of these plans, continuing to encourage their participation is essential. This effort helps ensure that transition plans are relevant to the particular cir-

Juvenile Offenders with Mental Health Disorders: Who Are They and What Do We Do With Them?

cumstances of juveniles and their families/caregivers. It also increases the likelihood of youth and family/caregiver support once a plan is implemented.

Community transition plans should be written in clear, objective language that can be understood by juveniles, their families/caregivers, and professionals from a variety of different systems. Plans should specifically address the following areas (when relevant) for specific youth:

- Juvenile justice expectations (*e.g.*, probation/parole requirements)
- Housing/residential plan
- Educational/vocational plan
- Mental health treatment plan (including monitoring of psychotropic medication)
- Substance abuse treatment plan (including strategies to avoid relapse)
- Physical health care plan
- Strengths of youth
- Delineation of responsibilities of various systems (*e.g.*, family/caregiver, child welfare, education, juvenile justice, mental health)
- Specific, objective and measurable outcome goals for each area in which youth (and their families/caregivers) require services
- Specific, objective incentives youth (and their families/caregivers) will receive for continued participation and involvement with the requirements set out in the plan
- Specific, objective consequences for youths' (and their families'/caregivers') noncompliance with the requirements set out in the plan

Even if a great deal of thought and preparation goes into the development of transition plans, successful implementation is heavily dependent on various community systems and agencies coordinating and integrating their services.

Coordinated Case Management

Because juvenile offenders with mental health disorders often need to be linked with a variety of services, the task of re-integrating these youth into the community can be overwhelming. To help ease this burden, some agencies are using case managers to take the lead in building relationships with community providers and connecting youth to relevant services. Case managers' responsibilities often include:

- Linking juvenile offenders with important resources in the community
- Keeping track of youths' treatment progress
- Monitoring youths' compliance with any conditions imposed by the court, mental health providers, and any other relevant agencies

Case managers balance a variety of responsibilities and are typically the "glue" that holds youths' aftercare services together. These individuals may be seen as brokers of services, youth and family advocates, or even therapists. But their main goal is to ensure that all of the systems with which juveniles are involved are "on the same track." Case managers monitor progress of community transition plans and communicate with probation/parole staff, as well as with the various professionals providing services to the youth (and their families/caregivers). As services are provided, old issues may resolve themselves and new needs arise.

Effective case managers continuously reassess the needs and abilities of each juvenile and family/caregiver on their caseload. If youth and their families/caregivers become discouraged in treatment, effective case managers implement strategies to enhance treatment motivation and engagement. Case management works best if it begins when juveniles are initially detained and then follows the youth as they move throughout all phases of juvenile justice supervision.

Resolving the sometimes-conflicting interests of youth, their families/caregivers, the

Treatment of Juvenile Offenders with Mental Health Disorders

juvenile justice system, and mental health providers can be a challenging task. The most effective case managers are those who are knowledgeable about, and comfortable with, youths' families/caregivers and the community, culture and various services in which youth engage. Case managers often help families/caregivers learn to navigate the multiple systems in which their children are involved. This instruction can decrease families'/caregivers' dependence on professionals and increase the likelihood of positive treatment outcome maintenance when a case manager is no longer working with the juveniles.

Case managers have been referred to as "boundary spanners" because of their ability to manage interactions in multiple settings (Steadman, 1992). Case managers are usually employed by the mental health, juvenile justice or child welfare systems. But these professionals could theoretically be employed by any of the key systems with which youth are involved. Due to the challenging aspects of the position, case managers should have:

- Small caseloads
- Few to no other responsibilities outside of their case management activities

Because resources are often limited, designated "case manager" positions do not always exist. In these situations, probation/parole officers, treatment providers or child welfare representatives can take the lead in coordinating the myriad of services for youth. Some suggest that having treatment providers serve in this role is best because they have a great deal of clinical and personal information about juveniles and their families/caregivers. This knowledge places providers in a good position to make referrals to whichever additional services are necessary (Field, 1998). Regardless of who fills the case manager role, it is beneficial to designate one professional as the coordinator of the many services that youth receive, and with whom everyone communicates. Having at least one person aware of each aspect of juve-

niles' treatment/supervision increases the chances that:

- A holistic service plan will be developed
- Any gaps in the service plan will be quickly detected.

 Conclusion

Although juvenile offenders with mental health disorders are a challenging population with a multitude of diverse needs, effective intervention strategies currently exist. However, we need to give up the unrealistic notion that there is a single treatment strategy that will "cure" these youth. Only then we can begin to do what is required to intervene successfully with mentally ill juveniles. Effective treatment starts with a comprehensive assessment of youth and their families/caretakers—so that juvenile offenders in need of treatment can be identified, and so that individually tailored intervention plans can be developed. Effective mental health services are culturally relevant, gender-specific and provided in youths' natural environment. Treatment needs are addressed on an ongoing basis, rather than solely when symptoms and behavior reach crisis proportions.

Mental health treatment can be initiated in juvenile justice facilities. But long-term positive outcomes require that treatment continue after juveniles are released and reintegrated into the community. Short-term detention facilities cannot provide the same intensity of mental health services as long-term residential placements. However, mental health evaluations, symptom stabilization strategies, and appropriate treatment referrals should be provided, when indicated, regardless of youths' length of stay.

The mental health community has not met the needs of many mentally ill youth involved with the juvenile justice system. Therefore, many juvenile justice agencies have begun to provide these services themselves. Some agencies hire their own mental health staff, whereas

284

Juvenile Offenders with Mental Health Disorders: Who Are They and What Do We Do With Them?

others contract with providers in the community. As a result, increasing numbers of juvenile offenders are receiving mental health assessments and interventions upon entering the justice system. This effort is a positive step, but it is a complicated one. Although the juvenile justice system should respond to the mental health needs of the youth in their care, juvenile justice does not want to take the place of the mental health system. For example, some juvenile justice facilities have begun to manage their mentally ill youth so well that community mental health agencies and psychiatric hospitals are no longer an asset to them. In addition, some judges have ordered mentally ill youth into detention facilities (or sentenced them to training schools) to help the juveniles access mental health services when none are available in the community. Both of these situations are unfortunate and should not continue.

One system (mental health or juvenile justice) should not be solely responsible for the treatment of juvenile offenders with mental health disorders. Issues related to funding, staff training, basic philosophy and resource differences make this impossible. Providing effective mental health services for mentally ill juvenile offenders requires that the juvenile justice and mental health systems work together to *jointly* assess, manage and treat this complex population of youth. Coordination, collaboration and integration of mental health and juvenile justice services, as well the development of joint funding opportunities, must occur to achieve long-term positive outcomes. Some agencies have begun to do this, and the results are promising.

CHAPTER 15

Special Issues I: Minority Youth, Female Offenders, Homosexual Youth

"I'm a gay black guy. What chance do I have of making it in here?"

Henry, 15

 Minority Youth in Juvenile Justice

In comparison to the percentage of minority youth in the general population, minority youth are *overrepresented* in the juvenile justice system. This overrepresentation appears to be present at all important decision points within the system (*e.g.*, arrest, intake, detention, adjudication, disposition). For example, African-American youth comprise close to 15 percent of the population of the United States. However, they represent 26 percent of juvenile arrests, 30 percent of delinquency referrals to juvenile court, 45 percent of juveniles detained in delinquency cases, 40 percent of juveniles committed to secure institutions, and 46 percent of juveniles transferred to adult criminal court (Snyder & Sickmund, 1999).

Upon arrest, a greater number of Caucasian youth are released to their parents and have their cases dismissed or handled informally in comparison to African-American youth. More African-American youth are referred to juvenile court. Once referred to juvenile court, African-American youth are more likely than Caucasians to be detained in juvenile detention facilities prior to trial. The discrepancy between rates of pretrial detention among African-Americans and Caucasians is even greater when youth are charged with a drug-related offense. Caucasian youth are more likely than African-American youth to receive probation as a disposition, and African-American youth are more likely to receive out-of-home placements. When they are tried for the same delinquent behavior, minority youth are found guilty more often than Caucasian youth and are more likely to receive longer juvenile justice sentences (Corley, Bynum, Prewitt, & Schram, 1996; Poe-Yamagata & Jones, 2000; Martin & Grubb, 1990).

Disproportionate minority confinement (DMC) exists within most juvenile justice facilities across the nation (Poe-Yamagata &

286

Juvenile Offenders with Mental Health Disorders: Who Are They and What Do We Do With Them?

Jones, 2000; Community Research Associates, 1997). More than two-thirds of incarcerated youth are of minority status; yet, minority youth comprise less than one-third of the population of young people in the United States. Minority youth are overrepresented in public juvenile justice facilities in particular (*e.g.*, federal, state and county institutions). African-American youth are six times more likely, and Hispanic youth are three times as likely, to be committed to a public juvenile justice facility than their Caucasian counterparts.

The bias against minority youth in juvenile justice is often subtle and indirect—although sometimes not. This indirect bias can be especially operative during the first stages of juvenile justice processing. When youth are initially picked up by law enforcement, a decision must be made whether to:

- Release the youth to their families/caretakers
- Escort the youth to a juvenile justice facility (*e.g.*, detention center)

If youth are taken to a juvenile facility, an additional decision needs to be made regarding whether the youth should:

- Remain in custody prior to their preliminary court hearing
- Be released to their families/caretakers

If youth are detained, a judge will make a decision about continued detention of the juveniles, or the juveniles will be released to their familes/caretakers. At each of these important decision points, most individuals working within law enforcement and the juvenile courts try to take into account youths' individual characteristics and situational factors. If asked, most individuals making these decisions probably believe that youths' race does not play a role in their evaluation of juveniles and juveniles' situation. However, youths' race probably does influence the decisions made about arrest, detention and release (Corley *et al.*, 1996). Basing decisions on youths' individual charac-

teristics is admirable and consistent with one of the juvenile court's goals of being responsive to the specific needs of a particular child and his/her circumstances. However, because these decisions may be made subjectively (based on individuals' knowledge and experience working within the system) these decisions are also vulnerable to bias.

Minority juveniles and their families/caretakers are often viewed from a mainstream model of how youth and families are supposed to appear and behave. Therefore, minority individuals may be perceived as dysfunctional and in need of intervention from law enforcement and the courts. For example, decisions related to releasing youth to their families/caretakers versus detaining the youth often consider supervising adults' abilities to manage the juveniles responsibly.

The justice system may perceive single-parent caretakers or individuals of low socio-economic status as less able to provide adequate supervision and care for juveniles—versus two parents of middle-income. Youths' caretakers may be unable to attend juveniles' hearings due to a lack of transportation and/or inability to take time off from work. In these situations, court personnel may decide to detain the youth. Law enforcement or the court may not approve of the way families/caretakers are managing juveniles or maintaining the home environment.

In these situations, the professionals may choose to intervene by removing the juveniles from the home, even if only temporarily. Many minority youth are affected by such situations because they do not have a "traditional" family structure according to middle-class Caucasian norms. This difference does not automatically mean that the youths' situation is inferior to any other, but it may be viewed as such by individuals from the mainstream culture. Most decision-makers are likely unaware of their subtle biases about what is best for children, particularly children whose behavior appears out of control. A lack of familiarity with individuals from different cultures, and stereo-typical thoughts about persons from different races, can result in a reliance on misinformed ideas and beliefs.

In an attempt to reduce subjective bias when processing youth within the juvenile justice system, many jurisdictions have implemented standardized risk assessment tools. These objective tools were developed to provide greater consistency and structure during the decision-making process as youth move through the system. Most risk assessment tools evaluate the presence or absence of a variety of factors shown repeatedly to relate to recidivism (*e.g.*, age of first arrest, academic problems, substance abuse). However, there is evidence suggesting that variables predictive of recidivism for Caucasian youth may be different from those predicting recidivism among minority youth (Wierson & Forehand, 1995). Further, mental health factors may play a significant role in the prediction of recidivism among some racial groups but not others.

A lack of familiarity with, and understanding of, other cultures and races can also affect law enforcement and juvenile justice personnel's perception of particular youth. Minority juveniles' attitude, dress or demeanor may be misinterpreted as appearing disrespectful, arrogant, indifferent or bored to individuals from a different culture. This misconstrued situation can result in youth being detained in juvenile justice facilities versus being released to their families/caretakers. Once law enforcement decides to bring youth to a detention facility, the likelihood increases that the youth will be detained overnight. Once youth are initially detained, the probability increases of continued detention (Wordes, Bynum & Corley, 1994). Each detention stay is recorded in youths' files and is likely to be taken into account if the juveniles are involved in future offenses. Therefore, the consequences of incarcerating minority youth for reasons other than legal ones can have cumulative detrimental effects as the youth move through the juvenile justice system.

Minority Youth and the Mental Health System

Although minority youth are overrepresented in the juvenile justice system, they appear to be underrepresented in the mental health system. Mental illness affects individuals from all ethnic, racial and cultural backgrounds. Unfortunately, there is a dearth of large-scale, quality epidemiological studies investigating the prevalence of mental health disorders among youth from various ethnic, racial and cultural backgrounds. The small amount of prevalence information that is available on mental illness among minority youth is often methodologically limited. Because most studies used different research methods, samples of youth, and definitions of psychiatric disorders, cross-study comparisons can be problematic. Prevalence studies of emotional and behavioral problems among minority youth are critical to better understanding of mental health disorders among youth from various ethnic, racial and cultural backgrounds. Unfortunately, at this point, no firm conclusions can be made.

The Diagnostic and Statistical Manual (*DSM*) appears to be equally valid for adolescents of all races. But studies have shown that ethnicity can play a role in the particular psychiatric diagnoses and type of mental health interventions juveniles receive. African-American and Asian-American individuals are more likely to be diagnosed with Schizophrenia (and other psychotic disorders) in comparison to Caucasians and Hispanics, who are less likely to receive these diagnoses. In addition, Asian-Americans and Caucasians are more likely to be diagnosed with mood and anxiety disorders compared to African-Americans and Hispanics (Flaskerud & Hu, 1992; Kilgus, Pumariega, & Cuffe, 1995). Native American adolescents have been found to have a relatively high level of mental health problems, including Major Depression, Conduct Disorder, and substance abuse (Duclos, Beals, Novins, Martin, Jewett, & Manson, 1998). In addition, refugees from

Juvenile Offenders with Mental Health Disorders: Who Are They and What Do We Do With Them?

other countries often suffer from significantly high levels of psychopathology, including Posttraumatic Stress Disorder and Major Depression (Blair, 1996). One study found a great deal of similarity between African-American and Caucasian youth in relation to mental health symptoms. The only differences noted were African-American youth receiving more diagnoses of Conduct Disorder and Caucasians diagnosed more often with eating disorders (Fabrega, Ulrich, Mezzich, 1993).

There are a variety of reasons why youth of different races may receive different types of mental health diagnoses. Certain mental health disorders may be more prevalent among individuals from certain ethnic or racial backgrounds. Or, mental health professionals may view youth from diverse racial and ethnic backgrounds from an ethnocentric point of view (*i.e.*, according to how a mental health professional's culture views things). Therefore, if youth of another race or ethnicity engages in behaviors that appear *different* to the professional, the youth may be perceived as *pathological*. Consequently, they may be treated as if they had a mental illness. Or these youth may present themselves to mainstream mental health professionals only when their disorders have become severe and in need of immediate intervention. Therefore, the youth are diagnosed more frequently with serious disorders. Other factors, or a combination of factors, may be at play.

Although individuals from all races suffer from mental illness, many minority individuals do not use formal mental health services to the degrees of their Caucasian counterparts (McMiller & Weisz, 1996). Even when suffering from the same psychiatric symptoms or degree of functional impairment, Caucasian youth are more likely to receive mental health services than African-American or Hispanic youth. The following can play a role in hindering minority individuals from accessing formal mental health services:

> ## Although individuals from all races suffer from mental illness, many minority individuals do not use formal mental health services to the degrees of their Caucasian counterparts.

- Language barriers
- Geographical distance
- Discomfort/shame regarding mental illness
- Financial cost
- Lack of knowledge about available resources

In addition, juvenile court judges mandate mental health services more often for Caucasian youth in comparison to their minority counterparts (Garland *et al.*, 2000).

Because juveniles typically do not refer themselves for mental health services, low usage rates may have more to do with the thoughts and behaviors of their families/caretakers. African-American, Hispanic, Asian-American, and Native American parents/caretakers often seek out assistance from informal helping networks (*e.g.*, extended family, members of the religious community, cultural healers, respected elders) for assistance with their children's mental health symptoms. Minority family members/caretakers may be particularly motivated to seek out mainstream mental health services when informal avenues have been unsuccessful, and/or their children's symptoms are severe. This practice of "last resort" may be one of the reasons why African- and Asian-Americans are more often diagnosed with severe disorders such as Schizophrenia and other psychotic disorders.

In contrast to the findings of low usage of mental health services by minorities, some studies have found that African-American youth in particular are actually overrepresented in the mental health system. When the studies are examined more closely, it appears that parents of African-American youth may not voluntarily choose formal mental health services for assistance with their children, especially when initial problems arise. African-American youth are often referred for mental health services not by their parents but by other agencies (*e.g.*, school, social service, juvenile justice; McMiller & Weisz, 1996). It has been suggested that society's tolerance for angry/hostile African-American males is lower than that for angry/hostile Caucasian males.

Consequently, minority youth are more quickly diagnosed with mental health disorders and provided with more restrictive intervention services (Fabrega, Ulrich, & Mezzich, 1993). The higher level of Conduct Disorder diagnoses among African-American youth and the increased number of involuntary commitments to psychiatric hospitals among African-Americans would support this hypothesis. If minority youth and their families/caretakers are coerced into mental health treatment, it is not surprising if they are somewhat cautious, suspicious and less enthusiastic about the intervention services—particularly in comparison to individuals who choose this route of treatment.

Once involved with formal mental health services, minority individuals terminate treatment much more quickly than Caucasians. Effective mental health treatment with juvenile offenders of any race require that youth and their families/caretakers:

- Trust the clinician

- Feel free to express themselves

- Are motivated to work on mutually agreed upon goals

If clinicians do not understand youth and their families'/caretaker's culture and the environment in which they exist (*e.g.*, where they live, how they live, preferred ways of expressing emotion, beliefs about mental illness, family structure, acculturation issues, poverty, racism), youth and their families/caretakers may feel misunderstood, disrespected and frustrated. Given this situation,

discontinuance of treatment is likely. If treatment is mandated, the individuals may attend, but their participation may be minimal. Ironically, prior to accessing mental health services, African-Americans tend to have positive views regarding mental health treatment, sometimes even more positive than Caucasians. However, after receiving services, African-Americans hold more negative views regarding treatment than their Caucasian counterparts (Diala, Muntaner, Walrath, Nickerson, LaVeist, & Leaf, 2000).

When clinicians are unfamiliar with youth and their families'/caretakers' culture, significant bias can result. Reliance on stereotypes and myths can result in clinicians' perceiving dysfunction or pathology among minority youth and their families/caregivers where none exists. Mental health professionals using their own culture and community as the "norm" for expected behavior have misinterpreted the survival behaviors used in inner city neighborhoods as abnormal and in need of treatment.

For example, juveniles' reliance on tough bravado can be viewed as callous, unremorseful and evidence of an antisocial personality. Single mothers of minority juveniles, who may need to be controlling and strict to ensure their children's safety in dangerous neighborhoods, can be viewed as overly harsh and abusive. Religiosity and/or spirituality may be a significant part of minority individuals' everyday lives and culture but may be seen as abnormal or delusional. Seeing visions of deceased relatives after the death of loved ones may be accepted (and even expected) among certain ethnic groups but may be misinterpreted as visual hallucinations.

Unfortunately, some mainstream mental health professionals view the culturally sanctioned behaviors of some minority groups as evidence of bizarre, or even psychotic, thinking. The behaviors are simply dissimilar to the way the clinicians think that individuals should behave. The clinicians may even recommend psychotropic medication and/or some type of out-of-home placement for the youth.

290

Juvenile Offenders with Mental Health Disorders: Who Are They and What Do We Do With Them?

However, misinformation about various cultures can result in clinicians overlooking or dismissing minority youths' true mental health symptoms and attributing them to ethnic or racial differences. Minority juveniles who experience paranoid ideation may be dismissed as just "reacting to years of racism." Abusive management and caretaking practices of minority youths' families/caretakers—or bizarre behaviors on the part of minority youth themselves—may not be taken seriously and attributed to diverse "cultural practices." This lack of proper identification can result in a delay in juveniles receiving a mental health evaluation, or accessing appropriate intervention services.

The Juvenile Justice versus Mental Health System

There is considerable overlap among youth involved with the juvenile justice system and youth involved with the mental health system. Many youth in psychiatric hospitals have engaged in delinquent and dangerous behavior. Some have been in trouble with the law, and a number of these youth have spent time in juvenile justice facilities. Conversely, a significant number of juvenile offenders suffer from psychiatric symptoms. Many have received outpatient and/or inpatient mental health treatment, and some have engaged in suicidal behavior. If the overlap between these two populations is so great, one may wonder how a determination is made regarding which system the youth should be referred.

A number of studies have attempted to assess which factors influence placement in juvenile justice facilities versus mental health facilities. One would assume that youth in juvenile justice facilities are more violent and antisocial than youth in mental health facilities. One also would assume that youth in mental health institutions suffer from more psychopathology and mental health disorders than their juvenile offending counterparts. However, neither situation is necessarily the case.

Studies specifically comparing youth incarcerated in state juvenile correctional institutions and psychiatric hospitals have found that these two sets of youth share many more similarities than differences (Cohen, et al., 1990; Lewis, Shanok, Cohen, Kligfeld, & Frisone, 1980). Incarcerated youth had more accidents and injuries in their medical histories, specifically head and face injuries. However, both groups of adolescents had similar numbers of birth-related complications. Surprisingly, both groups of youth had similar symptoms of mental illness, and the group of incarcerated youth was no more violent than the youth at the psychiatric hospital. Demographic factors, in contrast to mental health factors, often play a larger role in determining whether youth are placed in the mental health or juvenile justice system (Westendorp, Brink, Roberson & Ortiz, 1986).

When comparisons between incarcerated youth and hospitalized youth are examined closely, the influence of race-related factors is undeniable. One study of urban youth from low socioeconomic backgrounds found that the most powerful factor in determining whether youth would be placed in a juvenile justice facility or psychiatric hospital was *race*. African-American youth suffering from psychopathology and violent behavior were more likely to be incarcerated. Caucasian youth suffering from psychopathology and violent behavior were more likely to be hospitalized (Lewis, Balla, & Shanok, 1979). Even after youth have been incarcerated, this type of racial bias appears to exist within juvenile justice facilities. Caucasian girls are more likely to be referred to mental health professionals and/or transferred to treatment units within a juvenile justice facility in comparison to African-American girls who display similar behaviors. Lewis, Shanok, & Pincus (1982) found that Caucasian girls comprised 30 percent of the female population at juvenile justice facilities. But they accounted for more than 80 percent of the female referrals made for clinical evaluations. When they engaged in the same types of troublesome behaviors that initiated referral or transfer to a treatment unit for their Caucasian counterparts, African-American girls were more likely to receive punishments (*e.g.*, placement in a seclusion room). This dynamic was not related to the ethnicity of the adults who made the clinical referrals. Both Caucasian and African-American staff sought more mental health assistance for the Caucasian girls and less mental health assistance for the African-American girls.

Findings related to race bias in the disposition of juvenile offenders are consistent with the notion that:

- Disturbed and angry Caucasian youth are more often seen as "sick" and in need of treatment/mental health services
- Disturbed and angry minority youth are more often seen as "bad" and in need of punishment/juvenile justice intervention

Perhaps to avoid being considered racist or over-pathologizing "normal" cultural behavior, mental health professionals may now be making errors at the other end of the continuum. In an attempt to be culturally sensitive, clinicians may be slow to realize that unusual behavior among minority youth is representative of mental illness. This conservative approach can result in clinicians mistakenly assuming that troublesome mental health symptoms are an expected characteristic of youths' ethnic background. Or that symptoms are a normal response to an abnormal living environment (*e.g.*, dangerous neighborhood, abusive upbringing). Minority juvenile offenders apparently have to exhibit much more dramatic and extreme behaviors reflective of mental illness versus their Caucasian peers—to be perceived as having a mental health disorder and being in need of treatment (Lewis *et al.*, 1982).

Because of this racial bias, the majority of the nation's juvenile justice institutions currently function as psychiatric facilities for undiagnosed and misdiagnosed minority youth in need of mental health intervention. What makes matters even worse is that these men-

tally ill minority youth are typically labeled as bad and in need of punishment. Once labeled in this manner, youths' self-esteem is likely to be negatively affected, as is their chance of accessing quality mental health care in the future. Once minority youth are involved with the mental health system, it is not difficult for them to be transferred to the juvenile justice system. However, once they have been stigmatized by their involvement with juvenile justice, minority youth often find that mental health resources are difficult, if not impossible, for them to access.

Culturally Competent Services

Properly identifying and referring minority youth with psychiatric disorders to mental health professionals is only a first step. When they are provided to juvenile offenders from diverse racial and ethnic backgrounds, mental health services should be culturally competent. Culturally competent services use assessment tools that are culturally appropriate for the individuals who are being evaluated. Clinicians should always be aware that individuals from various cultures might exhibit psychiatric distress in different ways (*e.g.*, depression may be expressed in bodily complaints, suicidal behavior may be exhibited by provoking law enforcement to shoot youth). Interventions should be provided by clinicians who are trained in cultural diversity and who have experience, knowledge and familiarity about youth from diverse racial, ethnic and cultural backgrounds.

Knowing juveniles' race or ethnicity provides little information about the youths' attitudes, family, cultural beliefs, and the like. There is wide variation *between* various ethnic minority groups, as well as *within* ethnic minority groups. Minority juveniles who emigrate from other countries may have issues that are different from those of minority youth born in the United States. Juveniles' conflicts with family members/caretakers may be directly related to differences between youth and their families'/caretakers'

Juvenile Offenders with Mental Health Disorders: Who Are They and What Do We Do With Them?

level of acculturation. Further, youth who identify themselves as biracial may present with additional concerns not experienced by minority youth who are not biracial. Clinicians working with minority youth should take an individualized approach with each juvenile offender and his or her family/caretaker. They should spend as much time as is necessary to understand youths' (and their families/caretakers) particular beliefs, lifestyle, level of acculturation, language usage, and so forth.

MINORITY YOUTH AND THEIR fAMiliEs/ CARETAKERS ARE MUCH MORE likEly TO pARTicipATE iN TREATMENT WHEN THEy HELp dETERMINE iNTERVENTION GOALS, ANd WHEN THE GOALS ARE RELEVANT TO THEIR SPECIfIC NEEds.

Because many minority youth and their caretakers are mistrustful of mainstream mental health services, clinicians should focus on building rapport and allaying any fears regarding treatment. Youth and families/caretakers mandated into treatment through the courts (or social services) may have very different attitudes about mental health intervention than those who sought these services out voluntarily. Depending on the background of minority youth and their families/caretakers, they may need to be educated about the mental health field's knowledge of psychiatric disorders. They may also need to be told about the types of mental health intervention strategies that have been shown to be successful in decreasing distress and functional impairment. Clinicians should integrate youths' and their families'/ caretakers' beliefs about mental illness as well (e.g., spirituality, tribal healing, herbs). Clinicians should continuously empower minority youth and their families/caretakers, focusing on current strengths, as well as those they have exhibited in the past.

When treatment is culturally competent, families/caretakers (as defined by youth and their culture) are viewed as the primary support system. Minority youth and their families/ caretakers usually have informal networks in which they often seek support and assistance. Involving these informal support persons (e.g., extended family, clergy, tribal healers, neighbors) in treatment can help to ease any initial apprehension that youth and their families/ caretakers may have. Because they often play a significant role in the lives of minority youth, these support persons can be critical providers of important information. They can also play a key role with regard to intervention and management strategies for youth. Clinicians should familiarize themselves with the traditional roles that age and gender may play in certain cultures (e.g., youth may be expected to remain in the home to take care of their parents, it may be disrespectful to disagree with an elder in front of others) and respect these roles throughout treatment.

Minority youth and their families/caretakers are much more likely to participate in treatment when they help determine intervention goals, and when the goals are relevant to their specific needs. Clinicians should explicitly ask juveniles and their families/caretakers about priorities for intervention. Concrete issues—such as economics, housing, transportation, child care, school problems, employment, and the like, may need to be addressed before (or at the same time as) —more abstract psychological or relationship issues are targeted. Assessments of mental health functioning and associated treatment recommendations should be present-focused, practical, and relevant to the everyday life of minority youth and their caretakers. Minority juveniles and their families/caretakers always should know why certain information is being gathered and how it will be used in the future.

As much as possible, personnel providing mental health services to juvenile offenders from minority backgrounds should reflect the makeup of the youth they serve. Minority individuals often prefer to work with professionals of their own race and background. And there is some evidence that individuals are less likely to terminate treatment prematurely when working with an ethnically matched clinician (Yeh, Takeuchi, & Sue, 1994). However, this type of matching is not always possible. There is a shortage of formally trained, degreed and licensed mental health professionals from various racial and ethnic backgrounds. Therefore, when agencies attempt to provide minority youth with counselors of a similar race, some minority youth may be assigned to paraprofessionals with minimal training and experience. Matching minority juveniles with clinicians similar to themselves is important, but the level of training, knowledge and experience are also important.

Female Juvenile Offenders

Although males engage in delinquent behaviors at much higher rates than females, criminal behavior among adolescent girls is increasing (Snyder & Sickmund, 1999). This increase has resulted in more girls becoming involved with the juvenile justice system, including an increase in the number of female offenders entering juvenile justice facilities. Girls are much less likely to commit serious offenses such as murder, robbery, arson, weapon offenses and motor vehicle theft in comparison to their male counterparts. However, girls are much more likely than males to come into contact with juvenile justice for:

- Running away from home
- Not attending school
- Drinking while underage
- Violating curfew
- Defying parental/caretaker control

Some states have attempted to decriminalize these *status offenses* (behaviors considered law violations only if committed by an individual under the age of 18). In those particular states, the child welfare system is often the first to respond to youth participating in these types of behaviors. If the child welfare system is unsuccessful or additional intervention is needed, however, many of these female status offenders are eventually referred to the juvenile justice system. In other states, the juvenile justice system may be the first to respond to status offenders. Formal probation is typically the most restrictive disposition for these nonviolent types of behaviors. But, if youth violate their probation/court order, secure detention can result. Therefore, many young female offenders receive sanctions out of proportion to the seriousness of their offense. In fact, these girls could possibly be detained for a longer period than boys who were initially arrested for a *criminal* offense.

Not all girls in the juvenile justice system commit status offenses. A growing number of females are committing serious criminal acts. Females comprise about 23 percent of all juvenile arrests for delinquent behavior, and the rate of criminal behavior has increased more for girls than for boys in recent years (Poe-Yamagata & Butts, 1996; Snyder & Sickmund, 1999).

Although most gang members are males, an increasing number of females are becoming involved with gangs, with recent estimates around 10 percent. Although there has been an increase in the number of females engaging in serious—and sometimes violent—criminal behavior, some differences exist regarding the specific nature of their offenses. For example, drug-related offenses among female offenders are often associated with *using* drugs versus selling drugs. Prostitution and theft are often related to economics. Girls who live on the street often need money to support themselves and/or their substance using behavior.

Female murderers are more likely to kill someone they know, including family members or a romantic partner, and less likely to kill a stranger. In some cases, their victims have physically or sexually assaulted them. Males, however, are more likely to kill a stranger or acquaintance and less likely to kill someone in

294

Juvenile Offenders with Mental Health Disorders: Who Are They and What Do We Do With Them?

their family—making males a somewhat greater threat to the public at large. Very few girls are transferred to the adult criminal justice system.

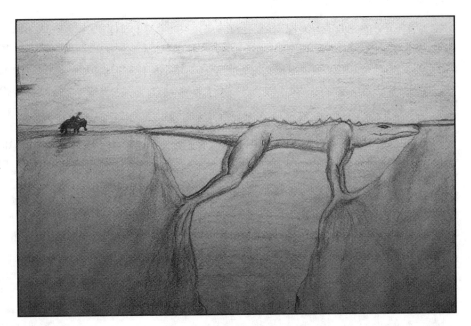

Most female offenders have a significant amount of contact with the court system before being incarcerated. Juvenile court judges are often cautious about removing girls from their home, and particularly so in relation to placing young women in juvenile justice facilities. Girls are often released under the supervision of a responsible adult and placed on informal or formal probation. Or girls may be given dispositional alternatives to juvenile justice facilities, such as placement in residential mental health or substance abuse treatment facilities. Female offenders who eventually end up in long-term public juvenile justice facilities typically have already been through numerous (outpatient and/or inpatient) rehabilitation programs. These other programs may have been unsuccessful in ameliorating the youths' difficulties. Or the young women may have been expelled from programs due to lack of participation, noncompliance, and/or aggressive behavior. Juvenile justice facilities are often the "last stop" for female juveniles with a significant number of emotional and behavioral difficulties.

Being a victim of physical or sexual abuse is one of the most common characteristics shared by females involved with the juvenile justice system. One study found that 92 percent of a group of female juvenile offenders reported being emotionally, physically and/or sexually abused. One quarter of the group said they had been stabbed or shot (Acoca & Dedel, 1998). The families of female offenders are often full of conflict between the youth and their parents/caregivers, as well as between the parents/caregivers themselves. This level of conflict appears to be even higher than the conflict observed among families of young male offenders.

Most young girls who come into contact with juvenile justice due to running away from home are attempting to escape abusive environments. Unfortunately, when these girls are arrested, many are returned to the exact situation they were trying to escape without any intervention services. Not surprisingly, these girls typically run away again.

A significant number of female juvenile offenders have been sexually victimized for years and have never told anyone about it. For those who did report their abuse, family members often did not believe the girls or significantly minimized their abusive experiences. Abuse can carry over into romantic relationships: these girls often become involved with boys/young men who emotionally, physically or sexually exploit them. These males are often a great deal older than the young girls.

In addition, many girls arrested for prostitution have histories of physical and sexual abuse. While working as a prostitute, they may continue to experience this type of violence at the hands of pimps and clients, as well as others with whom they interact on the street. Due to their past experiences and role models, many girls in the juvenile justice system have distorted views regarding relationships between males and females. Some girls who have been sexually abused do not know how to relate to males (including male juvenile justice professionals) without being sexual. They may flirt inappropriately or behave in ways that are seductive. Other girls are fearful of males, assuming that all men are going to take advantage of them and hurt them—emotionally and physically. These girls may withdraw and shut down when interacting with men, or may act aggressively in order to protect themselves.

Females in the juvenile justice system often have significant mental health needs, typically to a higher degree than their male counterparts (Stewart, Boesky, & Trupin, 1999; Timmons-Mitchell, *et al.*, 1997). When boys are distressed, they often turn their emotions outward, resulting in aggressive and delinquent behavior. Girls, however, often turn their emotions inward, resulting in higher rates of depression, anxiety and low self-esteem. Many females in juvenile justice believe they are flawed, defective and undeserving of love. Thoughts of suicide and suicidal threats are not unusual among this population of youth, with some female juvenile offenders engaging in serious suicidal behavior.

Self-injury/self-mutilation—such as cutting, carving and burning their own skin—is increasing among girls in juvenile justice. This behavior is often used as a method for the girls to cope with their distressing emotions. *(Please see Chapters 11 and 12 for additional information about Suicide and Self-injury.)* Because females typically turn their distress inward, it is possible that girls who express their emotions outwardly in aggressive and delinquent behavior are a particularly disturbed population of youth—with a variety of emotional and behavioral problems.

Drug use is also a significant problem among females involved with juvenile justice. A survey of state training schools found that more than 60 percent of girls in these facilities were identified as needing substance abuse treatment. More than half of the girls were abusing more than one substance (American Correctional Association, 1990). Experts suggest that many of these young women use substances as a way to self-medicate their mental health disorders and/or manage the effects of the trauma they have experienced. Girls with co-occurring mental health and substance abuse disorders pose significant challenges with regard to assessment and treatment of these problems.

The physical health needs of female offenders also differ from those of males. Some girls enter the juvenile justice system with sexually transmitted diseases, including HIV. Others may be pregnant. Girls who have been living on the streets and/or engaging in prostitution are at high risk for a variety of illnesses. Because of their high rate of internalizing negative emotions, many girls manifest their feelings of depression and anxiety in bodily symptoms such as headaches, stomachaches and extreme fatigue. Girls in distress may make numerous requests to visit a doctor or nurse for a variety of physical complaints.

A significant number of girls involved with juvenile justice also have academic difficulties and many have dropped out of school. Potential reasons for this include:

- Having a learning disability
- Difficulty concentrating due to negative events at home
- Being required to provide much of the caretaking for siblings
- Becoming pregnant and wanting to raise their children
- Wanting to spend time with a boyfriend who may not be attending school

In addition, a subset of girls have been suspended or expelled from school due to non-compliant or aggressive behavior.

Girls who are incarcerated can become very distressed when separated from those they care

296

Juvenile Offenders with Mental Health Disorders: Who Are They and What Do We Do With Them?

about, particularly if they are locked up for a considerable amount of time. Being unable to see their friends and family is difficult, and many of these girls are overly dependent on their romantic partners (even if they have only been involved with them for a short period of time).

For girls who have a child or children of their own, separation from their child/children during incarceration can be particularly upsetting. They not only miss their offspring but also feel guilty for not being able to be with them. Some young girls may have had to relinquish custody of their child/children upon being sentenced to juvenile justice facilities. To compensate for a lack of connection with loved ones, young female offenders often develop strong bonds with the other girls in residential facilities—as well as with the staff. The girls may even look to these individuals as a surrogate family during their period of incarceration. These girls can become "best friends" with female peers in a matter of days, sometimes hours. Many female offenders are desperate to connect with others, yet they do not always have the skills with which to do so.

Therefore, interpersonal relationships within juvenile justice facilities can be fulfilling, nurturing, confusing, overly dependent, frustrating, disappointing, and even tumultuous for young women. These girls may go through periods of conflict with peers, several experiences of hurt feelings, and episodic times of social withdrawal, even over minor incidents. At other times, the girls can feel supported and empowered in ways they have never experienced before. Some incarcerated girls may confuse their feelings of closeness toward peers with romantic love and become sexual with peers.

Most juvenile justice facilities and programs were initially designed for young male offenders. The physical layout of juvenile justice facilities, as well as the types of treatment groups, school-based programs and vocational training offered, are typically tailored to the needs of boys. This focus on males is due to their large representation among the juvenile justice population. Only in recent years has attention been paid to the unique programming needs of females in juvenile justice. The development of gender-specific programs within the juvenile justice system is so new that little information exists regarding the long-term effectiveness of these services (Covington, 1998). However, the most promising approaches focus on a holistic view of female juvenile offenders and the specific difficulties from which girls suffer.

Gender-specific services for girls in juvenile justice typically address issues such as:

- Education/Academic Skills
- Health Care/Pregnancy
- Mental Health
- Substance Abuse
- Parenting Skills
- Family Counseling
- Spirituality
- Vocational training/career skills
- Anger management/conflict resolution
- Violence/conflict in dating relationships
- Self-esteem/self-empowerment
- Grief and loss
- Healthy boundaries in interpersonal relationships
- Sexuality and intimacy

A small number of facilities are developing entirely new models of programming and treatment for female juvenile offenders. However, making modifications within current male-based programs to make programming more relevant for the females is more common for facilities. Most juvenile justice facilities have a token economy program (e.g., point system, level system) to provide incentives for youth to comply with facility requirements, participate in programming, and engage in prosocial behavior. Although this type of reinforcement system

Special Issues I: Minority Youth, Female Offenders, Homosexual Youth can be helpful for all juvenile offenders, it may be more effective for girls when rewards are tailored to the needs of females. For example, privileges such as a trip to the canteen to buy snack food, a later bedtime, or extra time playing video games may be strong incentives for male offenders. However, females may find extra time on the telephone, additional time with peers, or private time with staff more rewarding activities.

> Girls also tend to be more communicative than boys and are often quite verbal with staff. Individuals working with females must learn how to respond constructively and supportively to youth who disclose personal information.

Girls are more *relational* in nature and usually find interaction with others particularly reinforcing. Girls should have access to the standard treatment groups offered within most juvenile justice facilities (*e.g.*, anger management, social skills, victim empathy). But they should also have access to specific groups related to trauma, abuse, pregnancy/parenting, health issues and sexuality that are specifically designed for females. Due to the high percentage of female juvenile offenders from minority racial and ethnic backgrounds, all interventions should be culturally relevant. Mentors and prosocial role models from diverse cultural backgrounds can be particularly beneficial.

Juvenile justice programs for girls should be explicitly developed with the unique needs of females at the forefront. Girls in juvenile justice tend to feel safer residing in living units with same-sex peers. In addition, girls are often more comfortable expressing themselves in treatment groups without the presence of male offenders. Programs should be strength-based to counter the negative beliefs that many of these young

women hold about themselves and their abilities. The emphasis should be on recognizing how these girls have successfully coped in the past, as well as identifying adults in their lives who can serve as responsible and healthy supports. Girls should not only *talk* about their issues but also be taught specific *skills* so that they can make healthier choices in the future.

When they are empowered and provided with particular coping strategies to use in difficult situations, girls are less likely to become overly dependent on individuals who exploit them. Assessment and treatment specifically related to mental health disorders should be an integral part of gender-specific programming. Interventions should address trauma issues, as well as relationships with families/caretakers. If young women are not returning home, locating a safe and supportive place for them to live upon release is critical. As with boys, girls need to be linked with a variety of community services *prior* to their release from juvenile justice facilities in order to maintain academic, vocational, and/or treatment gains made during incarceration.

It is optimal for girls' living units to be staffed with personnel who want to work with female offenders and who are adequately trained to work with this population of youth. All juvenile justice professionals who work with girls should be trained on typical female development, as well as the various issues that plague young women in juvenile justice (*e.g.*, trauma, mental illness, health care, substance abuse). Without this type of training, staff members can inadvertently re-traumatize girls while they are incarcerated.

The manner in which room searches or strip searches are conducted can be extremely invasive and intrusive for females, particularly if they have been sexually abused. These searches can result in significant anxiety and anger for this population. Some sexual abuse victims panic when male staff conduct room checks in the middle of the night—particularly if staff need to knock on the young women's doors or

298

Juvenile Offenders with Mental Health Disorders: Who Are They and What Do We Do With Them?

peer into their windows before they enter. These actions can remind girls of when abusers came into the girls' bedroom at night. The physical restraint of girls, or any situation in which staff need to touch females, may bring back traumatic memories of physical or sexual abuse. This does not mean that these practices should be discontinued. But staff need to be taught the most effective ways of managing females' behavior without re-traumatizing the youth and making a situation worse. Girls also tend to be more communicative than boys and are often quite verbal with staff. Individuals working with females must learn how to respond constructively and supportively to youth who disclose personal information. Staff also need to know to whom they can refer young women if critical information is reported (*e.g.*, suicidal thoughts, previous abuse, psychiatric symptoms, sexual activity within the facility).

Some staff members find female offenders more difficult to work with than males due to their increased psychological, emotional and physical needs. Girls within juvenile justice often desire a great deal of attention, and staff members can experience the girls as emotionally needy and draining. However, girls also have characteristics that usually make them easier to work with including:

- Less potential for physical violence
- Less physically demanding to manage
- Greater reliance on peers for support and accountability
- Greater likelihood of engaging and participating in treatment programs

Females in juvenile justice should be viewed as a *different* group of youth within the system, not necessarily a more *difficult* group of youth (Miller, 1998). In fact, female offenders can be some of the most rewarding juveniles with whom staff can interact. This situation is particularly true when the girls transform into strong, prosocial young women who learn to take increased control over the decisions in their lives.

Homosexual Youth

Adolescence is a time of tremendous growth and change for all youth. Biological changes of the body, development of new friendships and intimate relationships, separation from one's family, and experimentation with different roles and belief systems typically occur during the teenage years. Adolescence can be not only an exciting but also a difficult time. For homosexual youth, this developmental stage can be particularly challenging and isolating, especially for gay and lesbian youth involved with the juvenile justice system. Although this section of the current chapter is focused on gay and lesbian juveniles, the issues also apply to bisexual and transgendered youth (youth who perceive themselves as being different than their biological sex).

Homosexual adolescents are exposed to a great deal of discrimination and stigmatization from society. Negative beliefs about homosexuality are embedded in laws, social policy and religious teachings. Gay and lesbian youth are often exposed to:

- Verbal harassment
- Threats of violence
- Physical assaults

Bias against homosexuality exists in schools, and many gay and lesbian teens are repeatedly taunted, ridiculed and physically attacked on school property. One study found that adolescents react more negatively to homosexuals than to any other minority group and that some teenagers feel legitimized in openly attacking gay individuals (Radowsky & Siegel, 1997). Not surprisingly, many gay and lesbian youth are frightened to go to school, or find it difficult to focus on their work when they are there. A considerable number of homosexual teenagers drop out of school, often due to the significant amount of harassment they receive.

Gay and lesbian adolescents frequently have difficulty forming and maintaining significant interpersonal relationships during the teen years, a critical part of adolescence. As their attraction to individuals of the same sex emerges, gay and lesbian youth may be confused, upset or scared. They are typically afraid to talk to anyone about their homosexual orientation for fear of rejection by others.

Same-sex friendships often suffer because homosexual youth may withdraw socially in order to avoid developing romantic feelings toward their friends. If they remain in social circles with heterosexual youth, homosexual youth often spend much of their time hiding their homosexual thoughts and feelings. These youth are often forced to conceal who they really are from others. Many gay and lesbian youth have reported losing friends once they disclosed their same-sex orientation. Due to their struggles with emerging homosexual feelings, homosexual juveniles may not be comfortable engaging in same-sex romantic relationships, but heterosexual romantic relationships are unfulfilling for them. The result is that the teen years are often tremendously isolating for homosexual youth.

Whereas many juveniles look to family members for emotional support during difficult times, homosexual youth often do not have this option. Many gay and lesbian teens are afraid to tell their parents about their homosexual feelings for fear of disapproval and rejection. This fear is often not unfounded. If they disclose their homosexuality, many gay and lesbian youth receive negative responses from their parents/caretakers. Verbal assaults and emotional abandonment are not uncommon. Some family members have physically attacked their teenage children once their same-sex orientation had been discovered. Lesbian youth tend to face more verbal and emotional abuse from parents/caretakers, while gay male youth are more likely to be expelled from their homes (Radowsky & Siegel, 1997).

Gay and lesbian youth may leave home at an early age. This premature departure can be due to:

- Parental rejection
- Verbal and/or physical abuse

- Being thrown out of the house

Alternative living options are often limited for these juveniles. Other family members may not want to take in gay or lesbian youth. And living with friends is often not viable because many of these youth have not disclosed their sexual orientation to even their closest friends. Gay and lesbian adolescents make up 40-60 percent of the street population of youth (Kunreuther, 1991). Most of these youth have nowhere else to go. On the street, these juveniles can be exposed to muggings, assaults and rape. The youth may engage in prostitution, theft or other illegal activities in order to obtain money, food, shelter and drugs.

The disapproval and rejection that homosexual youth receive from family, peers and society as a whole can lead to profound feelings of:

- Loneliness
- Guilt
- Shame
- Self-hatred

A significant number of homosexual youth conceal their secret and avoid engaging in activities that would arouse suspicion in those around them. Therefore, many gay and lesbian teens are not exposed to positive homosexual role models or healthy same-sex relationships. Much of these youths' beliefs about being gay is based on myths and negative stereotypes of homosexuality, which further reinforces their sense of defectiveness and inferiority. Homosexual juveniles often suffer from feelings of depression and anxiety. The future may appear hopeless and full of nothing but more pain, rejection and discrimination. Many homosexual youth deal with their emotional pain by using drugs and alcohol. Gay and lesbian youth have much higher rates of substance abuse in comparison to their heterosexual peers.

Given their intense feelings of isolation and lack of social support, it is not surprising that homosexual youth have high rates of suicidal behavior. Gay and lesbian adolescents make up

Juvenile Offenders with Mental Health Disorders: Who Are They and What Do We Do With Them?

30 percent of all youth suicides. and suicide is the leading cause of death among homosexual teens. Although homosexual adolescents experience a great deal of stress in general, their suicide attempts appear to be particularly related to stress associated with their sexual orientation (*e.g.*, questioning their sexuality, not yet disclosing their homosexuality, facing rejection when disclosing their sexual orientation; Rotheram-Borus, Hunter, & Rosario, 1994).

Homosexuality is no longer considered a mental health disorder (American Psychiatric Association, 1973). The American Psychiatric Association removed homosexuality from the *Diagnostic and Statistical Manual of Mental Disorders* in 1973—because research indicated that there were no differences between heterosexuals and homosexuals with regard to stability, judgment, capabilities and the like. Homosexuality is considered a normal variation of sexual expression. When provided with supportive and loving environments, homosexual youth have no more mental health problems than other adolescents. Much of the distress experienced by gay and lesbian juveniles appears to be related to the constant rejection, discrimination and stigmatization from those around them. Individuals who eventually accept their sexual orientation (and integrate it into their identity) tend to be more psychologically healthy than those who continue to deny or hide their homosexual thoughts and feelings. Despite the position of the American Psychiatric Association, some clinicians still have a biased or inadequate understanding of issues related to gay and lesbian individuals.

Homosexual youth come into contact with the juvenile justice system for a variety of reasons. Although they may be arrested for similar behaviors as many heterosexual youth, the motivating factors underlying these behaviors may be different from those of their non-gay peers. For example, status-offending homosexual youth may have run away from home due to parental rejection, emotional abuse or violence. Repeated truancy may be a result of continuous harassment or physical attacks at school. If they choose to fight back against perpetrators, homosexual youth can be detained on assault charges. Survival behaviors on the street such as prostitution, theft and drug dealing can result in arrest.

Being incarcerated can be a stressful experience for any youth, but it can be particularly difficult for gay and lesbian youth. In environments where being tough, maintaining status and fitting in are critical, homosexual youth are often at a significant disadvantage. This disadvantage is particularly evident for gay males. Juvenile justice staff and peers alike often hold negative biases against homosexual youth and many are quite verbal about their views. Incarcerated gay and lesbian youth often face tremendous amounts of ridicule and harassment, and physical victimization is not uncommon. The more youth diverge from sex-role stereotypes, the more difficulties the youth typically have in juvenile justice.

Homosexual youth have a particularly difficult time in facilities where groups of juveniles are required to shower together and/or sleep in dorm-style settings (where large numbers of juveniles sleep in one room). Many homosexual youth are afraid to fall asleep while locked up, for fear of what may happen to them when they are not awake and on guard. Gay and lesbian youth in juvenile justice facilities often spend a great deal of time concealing their same-sex orientation from others in order to avoid possible victimization. Mental health issues are most likely to occur among homosexual youth when they reside in environments where homosexuality is viewed negatively, and there is a great deal of stigma related to being gay (Ross, 1989). Most juvenile justice facilities fit this description.

Juvenile justice professionals should pay close attention to warning signs of mental health disorders among gay and lesbian youth. Homosexual youth are at high risk for significant distress and self-destructive behavior due to high rates of:

- Depression
- Anxiety

- Substance abuse
- Suicidal behavior

This risk is particularly high in stigmatizing settings such as juvenile justice facilities. However, stigmatizing experiences can differ among male and female populations. Gay males tend to be at high risk of victimization from peers in living units if the gay youth exhibit effeminate and/or "flamboyant" behavior. For the most part, lesbian youth are shunned and rejected by their female peers. In recent years, however, declaring oneself a lesbian has actually raised the status of some girls in residential facilities. Juvenile justice professionals should always model respect and tolerance for all youth, and harassment/victimization by peers in a living unit should never be tolerated.

A number of adolescents (homosexual and heterosexual) consent to various medical tests during incarceration, sometimes including a test for the Human Immunodeficiency Virus (HIV). Youth testing positive on this type of blood test are at particularly high risk for suicide and should be evaluated and monitored.

Disposition planning should always consider gay or lesbian youths' living situation in the community, as well as the support systems (or lack thereof) available to the youth upon release.

302

Juvenile Offenders with Mental Health Disorders: Who Are They and What Do We Do With Them?

CHAPTER 16

Special Issues II:
Head Trauma/Neuropsychiatric Factors, Violence and Mental Illness, Seclusion and Restraint, Malingering, Staff Training

"Juvenile offenders have so many issues, how can we address them all?"

Juvenile Justice Administrator

There is a subset of unmanageable youth within juvenile justice that does not seem to fit into any of the diagnoses contained in the *Diagnostic and Statistical Manual of Mental Disorders (DSM)*. These young men and women stand out to most juvenile justice professionals because of the youths' impulsivity, irritability and repeated aggression, including violent outbursts. These youth have great difficulty controlling their emotions. They are often easily upset (*e.g.*, angry, sad, frustrated) and once distressed, they are difficult to calm or soothe. These juveniles tend to be very self-centered and show little concern for those around them. They have little to no insight regarding how their negative behavior affects others, even though they may cause significant damage to staff, peers and physical property.

Some of these juveniles may genuinely feel bad after causing pain to another, but these feelings tend to be short-lived and fairly superficial. Typical juvenile justice programming and sanctions have little effect on their behavior, and these juveniles tend to repeat the same negative behaviors time and time again—even after receiving significant negative consequences.

In addition, psychotropic medication seems to be less effective for the behavior of these youth. Juvenile justice professionals often become frustrated when managing this subset of young offenders because they are often disruptive to everyone in their living environment and exhausting to supervise. When these youth are referred to mental health/medical professionals, the juveniles often return with a diagnosis of Conduct Disorder—and little to no

303

Special Issues II: Head Trauma/Neuropsychiatric Factors, Violence and Mental Illness, Seclusion and Restraint, Malingering, Staff Training

additional information or recommendations for staff regarding effective management strategies.

The type of youth described above is not an anomaly in juvenile justice facilities. Common theories regarding the etiology of this type of behavior tend to be associated with family troubles, child abuse and neglect, poverty, substance abuse, the youth being born a "bad seed," and/or the youth choosing to act this way intentionally to get their needs met. Such explanations seem too simplistic to describe this extraordinary group of juveniles. On several occasions, juvenile justice professionals have described these youth as being constitutionally "different," stating, "Something is not right with these kids." Staff may not know what is wrong with the youth, but they know that they are disturbed on a level different from most. The difficulties with mood and behavior that these youth exhibit appear fundamentally distinct from those of their peers. Although various psychosocial issues may play a role, physiological factors should not be overlooked.

Research on animals has demonstrated a significant relationship between brain function and aggressive/violent behavior. When faced with a threatening situation, an animal may react with uncontrollable anger or passive submission depending on which area of the brain is being stimulated or destroyed. In addition, humans who have experienced traumatic brain injuries exhibit a variety of emotional and behavioral changes. For example, women who have been romantically involved with men who have sustained injuries to the head have reported that after the injury their partners became:

- Less communicative
- More angry
- More depressed
- More verbally abusive
- More physically abusive

These findings were in comparison with men who sustained injuries to another area of the body (Warnken, Rosenbaum, Fletcher, Hoge, & Adelman, 1994).

In the 1800s, a man named Phineas Gage sustained damage to the frontal lobes of his brain when an explosion drove a metal rod (which was an inch thick and three feet long) through the front of his head and skull. Miraculously, Phineas sustained no long-term physical damage, but his personality changed completely after the incident. Before his head injury, he was a discreet, responsible and respected member of his community. After the head injury, however, Phineas:

- Became rude and flippant
- No longer cared about anyone but himself
- Was not concerned about what others thought of him
- Began using profanity
- Lost his focus
- Became easily distracted
- Was motivated by immediate gratification instead of his previous long-term goals

The front part of the brain, known as the frontal lobes, controls the "executive" functions of the brain. The frontal lobes are responsible for:

- Planning ahead
- Making judgments about situations
- Regulating emotions
- Regulating behavior
- Prioritizing what to pay attention to
- Prioritizing what behaviors to engage in

Frontal lobes allow individuals to consider things in the abstract: to think about things hypothetically versus only thinking about things that can be seen, touched or felt. The functions of the frontal lobes are critical to:

- Controlling one's emotions
- Following rules or directives
- Delaying immediate gratification in favor of long-term rewards
- Maintaining socially appropriate behavior when faced with obstacles and challenges

Not surprisingly, damage to the frontal area of the brain can result in individuals:

Juvenile Offenders with Mental Health Disorders: Who Are They and What Do We Do With Them?

- Thinking concretely
- Having difficulty modulating their emotions
- Having difficulty modulating their behavior
- Being primarily motivated by immediate gratification of their needs
- Remaining focused on the here and now versus what might happen in the future
- Having low frustration tolerance
- Being egocentric
- Not adhering to rules
- Lacking insight
- Lacking remorse

Many of these descriptors have been used to describe juveniles who have been labeled antisocial or diagnosed with Conduct Disorder.

Similarities with Brain-injured Animals

Laboratory animals that have suffered injury to the frontal lobes appear to behave similarly to antisocial human adults and juveniles. For example, most animals discontinue approaching a food dish once they have received one or two shocks in response to their approach behavior. Animals who have sustained injury to the front part of the brain continue to approach the food dish numerous times despite receiving continual shocks; they seem much less affected by punishment (Gorenstein, 1990). Juvenile offenders often continue to engage in the same negative, dangerous, and/or illegal behaviors that have resulted in significant punishment for them in the past. This pattern of behavior is exhibited even more strongly when the behavior animals or youth engage in is related to something positive (*e.g.*, food, money, pleasurable sensations).

If a negative consequence lies in the future, animals and humans with brain injuries tend to experience less fear and anxiety regarding the impending consequence—versus those without brain injuries. In one study, young adults were

asked to observe the numbers 1-12 consecutively flash on screen. They were told they would receive a shock when the number 8 appeared. Antisocial individuals only became nervous right before the number 8 flashed, and some only when the number 8 was directly on the screen in front of them. Nonantisocial individuals became nervous much sooner in *anticipation* of the upcoming electric shock, and their nervousness increased the closer they grew to the number 8 (Hare, 1965). Many juvenile offenders show little to no fear or anxiety about upcoming punishments or sanctions as long as they appear to be somewhat remote. Only when negative consequences are about to happen do they seem to have any influence on these juveniles' behavior.

Animals with injuries to the frontal lobe also have difficulty holding onto internal representations of something in their mind—particularly with regard to something that is going to happen in the future. When performing tasks in which they need to avoid responding for a specified interval of time, brain-injured animals respond too quickly. Holding onto the abstract notion of time in their mind is difficult for them. However, when this type of animal is provided with some type of cue regarding how much time has elapsed, the cue helps them delay their response, and they perform just fine (Gorenstein, 1990).

Juvenile delinquents appear to have more of this "restrictive time perspective" than their nondelinquent peers. When asked to list possible future events, juvenile offenders state that future events will occur much sooner than their nonoffending peers think they will. Other studies have asked youth to estimate how much time has elapsed during a variety of intervals. Nonjuvenile offenders' guesses are fairly accurate, but juvenile offenders tend to significantly overestimate the passage of time (*e.g.*, signaling 15 seconds had elapsed when only 10 seconds had elapsed; Siegman, 1961). The passage of time may be experienced more slowly for juvenile offenders, just as it appears to be for

305

Special Issues II: Head Trauma/Neuropsychiatric Factors, Violence and Mental Illness, Seclusion and Restraint, Malingering, Staff Training

brain-injured animals. This might explain why some juvenile offenders continuously think they have been confined in their rooms for significantly longer than they really have—often leading youth to adamantly accuse staff of being unfair and mean.

In addition, many juvenile offenders are similar to animals with brain lesions in regard to reacting to positive reinforcement. If given the option, both brain-injured animals and juvenile offenders prefer a less valuable, but immediately available, reinforcement instead of a superior reinforcement that is delayed (Mischel, 1961).

Finally, both juvenile offenders and brain-injured animals appear to have a significantly greater need for stimulation in comparison to their "normal" counterparts. During laboratory experiments, brain-damaged animals engage in more exploration for its own sake, as well as engage in specific behaviors that they know will produce additional sensory stimuli (*e.g.*, pressing a bar to see a change in lights or hear different sounds; Gorenstein, 1990).

A popular theory of antisocial behavior is that the nervous system of antisocial individuals is chronically underaroused. Much of their negative behavior is supposedly an attempt to seek stimulation so that these individuals can achieve a relatively "normal" or optimum feeling of arousal. In laboratory experiments, antisocial individuals prefer new and interesting stimuli to a greater extent than individuals who are not antisocial. Further, antisocial juveniles lose interest more quickly during mundane tasks in comparison to their nonantisocial peers (Gorenstein, 1990).

Neuropsychiatric Findings Among Juvenile Offenders

Injury to the brain is not uncommon among adolescents. One study found that 40-50 percent of youth, delinquents and nondelinquents alike, suffered from at least one blow to the head during their childhood or teenage years (Hux, Bond, Skinner, Belau, & Sanger, 1998). Short-term

effects from blows to the head can include confusion, dizziness, headaches, blurred vision, loss of memory, and loss of consciousness. Fortunately, most brain injuries that occur in youth are mild and have little to no long-term consequences. However, even minor injuries can have lasting negative consequences. Mild brain injuries are often not apparent on traditional brain imaging devices such as CAT scans, PET scans, and MRIs. This type of trauma is typically subtle and diffuse. Although an injury to the brain may be too slight to be detected, it can have a profound influence on youths' functioning.

Disorders such as Attention-Deficit/Hyperactivity Disorder (ADHD), Learning Disorders, and seizure disorders can indicate some type of brain-related impairment, and are common among juvenile offenders.

Trauma to the brain can result from a variety of incidents. Juvenile offenders have reported hurting their head as a result of:

- Being in a car accident
- Participating in a sporting event
- Falling from a tree, building or roof
- Fighting
- Being beat up by peers, or jumped by gang members
- Being hit or shaken by an adult
- Being thrown down a flight of stairs
- Being shot
- Having their head smashed into the ground or a wall

Some juvenile offenders have experienced trauma to the brain when in utero because during pregnancy their mother:

- Used drugs and alcohol
- Did not receive appropriate prenatal care
- Was malnourished
- Was infected with an illness

In addition, a considerable number of juvenile offenders were born prematurely, before the brain was fully developed. Or they experienced complications during the birth

Juvenile Offenders with Mental Health Disorders: Who Are They and What Do We Do With Them?

itself, including decreased oxygen to the juveniles' brains. Poor postnatal care among the mothers of these youth, resulting in the children being malnourished after birth, is also not uncommon. Many juvenile offenders have damaged their brains from years of using alcohol and other drugs, and others have suffered minor brain damage due to failed suicide attempts (*e.g.*, hanging, overdosing). Some juvenile offenders tell horrendous stories of repeated abuse at the hands of family members, including:

- Being hit in the head with metal objects, wooden planks, glass vases or belt buckles
- Being kicked in the head by an adult wearing steel-toed boots

Studies that have specifically investigated brain functioning among incarcerated juvenile offenders have found significantly elevated rates of impairment among this population of youth. Incarcerated juveniles have considerably high rates of serious medical problems, including dangerous accidents, face and head injuries, difficulties related to their birth, and severe child abuse. These youth are more likely to suffer from cognitive problems, hallucinations, blackouts and difficulties with comprehension in comparison to nonincarcerated peers of similar ages and backgrounds (Lewis, Pincus, Lovely, Spitzer, & Moy, 1987; Lewis, Shanok, Pincus, & Giammarino, 1982; Lewis, Shanok, & Balla, 1979). Studies of the following juveniles found high rates of head injury and birth complications (Lewis, Shanok, Grant, & Ritvo, 1983; Lewis, *et al.*, 1985; Lewis, *et al.*, 1988):

- Youth on death row
- Juveniles who later became murderers
- Homicidally aggressive youth in a psychiatric hospital

The majority of these youths' brain-related injuries had been undetected and undiagnosed, even though many of the juveniles had been involved with various types of child-serving services (*e.g.*, child welfare, psychiatric hospitals, juvenile justice). In addition, child abuse among the juvenile offenders studied was grossly under-reported, even among doctors examining youth for medical problems related to the abuse.

Effects of Trauma to the Brain

A head injury during childhood or adolescence can have many more devastating effects than an injury in adulthood. As juveniles' brains mature, youth continue to develop cognitively, perceptually and socially. If parts of the brain are compromised, new information may not be incorporated and integrated appropriately—especially when the frontal part of youths' brains are injured. This area of the brain has a profound affect on a variety of other areas of functioning (*e.g.*, planning, judgment, regulation of mood and behavior, thinking flexibly). Sustaining damage to the brain as a youth can affect current mood and behavior, as well as the attainment of future and more advanced skills in these areas. If juveniles have not developed sufficient emotional and behavioral controls before sustaining brain impairment, developing these critical controls afterward will be extremely difficult. Unfortunately, this is not an unusual scenario among juvenile offenders because many of them sustain trauma to the brain during the early years of their lives.

If juveniles' brains are damaged, particularly the frontal lobes, one can expect a variety of negative consequences. The youth may have more difficulty controlling their emotions and behavior, even during times when they want to do so. Their frustration tolerance is typically lowered, so they become easily irritated and angry. Whereas most juveniles reflect about their decisions and weigh the advantages and disadvantages of their choices, youth with frontal lobe impairment typically react without reflection. Their judgment is compromised, as is their insight regarding the behaviors in which they engage. If brain-injured youth cannot hold an internal representation of their previous punishments and sanctions in their mind, these types of consequences are not likely to deter

307

Special Issues II: Head Trauma/Neuropsychiatric Factors, Violence and Mental Illness, Seclusion and Restraint, Malingering, Staff Training

future negative behavior. Not surprisingly, juvenile offenders with brain impairment often engage in the same negative behaviors repeatedly, usually in an unsophisticated and disorganized manner. Because of the damage to their brain, it is much harder for these youth to learn from their experiences than it is for their non-brain-injured peers. In addition, brain-injured juveniles are driven by the immediate gratification of their needs. Fear of apprehension or discipline does not seem to play a major role in deterring their antisocial behavior unless it is immediate and close at hand. Because of their difficulties regulating their moods, youth with brain impairment can become aggressive and violent over seemingly minor incidents.

It has also been suggested that brain impairment can result from persistent fear or neglect during the early years of youths' lives (Lewis, 1991). Juveniles who are raised in families or communities fraught with violence can experience physiological changes in the brain due to persistent fear as their body adapts to what is going on around them. Juvenile offenders who are likely to have experienced high levels of fear for much of their early years include (but are not limited to) those who:

- Were chronically physically abused

- Were coerced to engage repeatedly in sexual behavior

- Were forced to participate in satanic worship rituals

- Lived with an alcoholic parent/caregiver

- Lived with a violent/caregiver

Exposure to continual violence and/or trauma can actually alter youths' neurodevelopmental processes. When individuals are faced with threatening situations, the body automatically goes into the "fight or flight" mode and releases certain chemicals (*i.e.,* epinephrine, norepinephrine). If a specific chemical response in the brain is activated enough times (*e.g.,* some juveniles are in a constant state of arousal due to the unpredictable and danger-

ous nature of their environment), it can result in actual structural, molecular and functional changes in youths' brains (Perry, Pollard, Blakley, Baker, & Vigilante, 1995). Chronic stress can be particularly damaging to youths' brains if the stress is unpredictable. In addition, caregiver neglect—such as relatively little attention, touch, social interaction, and/or speech—during the first few years of life, appears to be just as detrimental to brain development as persistent fear, if not more so. It seems that harmful stimulation may be more beneficial than having no stimulation at all (Perry & Pollard, 1997). As would be expected, negative effects or changes within the brain during critical developmental periods can make it more difficult for youth to handle stressful events and challenges in the future. Neurochemicals and hormones such as dopamine, serotonin, endorphins, androgens and gluccocordicoids may also play a role in the type of emotional and behavioral reactions seen among juvenile offenders. But more research is needed in this area before any firm conclusions can be drawn.

Aggression, criminal behavior and violence are complex behaviors that are multi-determined. It is not being suggested that all juvenile offenders have some type of brain trauma which leads them to engage in antisocial behaviors. However, the role of neurological and neuropsychiatric factors among the juvenile justice population is probably much larger than has been previously acknowledged. One cannot dismiss the possible role of brain trauma in the lives of many youth behind bars given the similarities between:

- The behavior of brain-injured animals and antisocial adults/juvenile offenders

- The moods and behaviors of individuals suffering from observable brain injuries/ neurochemical imbalances and those of incarcerated juveniles

The similarities are particularly evident for those youth who engage in repeated, persistent aggressive behavior and who do not respond to

Juvenile Offenders with Mental Health Disorders: Who Are They and What Do We Do With Them?

typical juvenile justice sanctions and punishments. Brain-injured juveniles are likely to commit their crimes in an impulsive, poorly-thought-out manner and are unlikely to take basic precautions to avoid apprehension. Even after being caught and receiving significant sanctions, this type of youth is likely to return to the same type of negative behavior in an almost stereotypical fashion. Their moods tend to be labile (unstable), and they are difficult to calm once upset. Their angry outbursts are often out of proportion to whatever initially provoked them. This subset of youth is one of the most difficult to manage in a juvenile justice facility due to their:

- Unpredictability

- Apparent lack of concern for others

- Minimal response to psychotropic medication and negative consequences

Juvenile justice professionals often describe feeling helpless when working with these youth because "nothing seems to make much of a difference." Creative management strategies that have consistently worked with other offenders often have little to no effect on youth with trauma to the brain. In addition, mental health/medical professionals are often at a loss with regard to making effective recommendations for this complex and disruptive population of youth.

Brain trauma by itself is not likely to cause violence, aggression or criminal behavior. Large numbers of youth have experienced mild brain injuries and have never engaged in such behaviors. Although numerous studies have found a possible association between aggression/antisocial behavior and brain-related injuries (particularly in the frontal region of the brain), there is still some controversy in this area. This controversy is partly because many of the studies on this topic have methodological limitations. Additional research is necessary before we fully understand how trauma to the brain is related to the emotions and behaviors of juvenile offenders.

> CREATIVE MANAGEMENT STRATEGIES THAT HAVE CONSISTENTLY WORKED WITH OTHER OFFENDERS OFTEN HAVE LITTLE TO NO EFFECT ON YOUTH WITH TRAUMA TO THE BRAIN.

A Combination of Factors

When researchers investigate the role of brain impairment among juvenile offenders, particularly with regard to aggressive behavior, additional important factors should also be considered. Many juvenile offenders are raised in families/caretaking environments in which youth are not only witnesses to serious violence but also victims of it. Youth in this type of environment might learn that aggression is an acceptable way to deal with strong emotions or to get what they want. Juveniles who are physically and emotionally abused may also experience anger and rage toward the perpetrators and then displace this anger onto others. This is in addition to the fact that some of these youth sustain their head injuries from abuse suffered at the hands of caretakers.

A number of juvenile offenders have been found to exhibit transient psychotic symptomatology, typically in the form of paranoid ideation (Lewis *et al.*, 1987). These youth are typically not Schizophrenic and tend to appear normal much of the time. However, there are periods, particularly when youth are stressed, when these juveniles lose touch with reality, misperceive situations and become extremely paranoid about those around them. Their violence and aggression are often directly related to a misperception that they are in danger and in need of protecting themselves. These youth may have inherited a biological predisposition for this type of paranoid thinking and/or some other type of mental illness from a parent.

The youths' head trauma or injury itself is not necessarily the problem. A combination of factors probably increases the likelihood that these difficult-to-manage youth will become disruptive, aggressive or violent. Not all youth who receive a blow to the head are aggressive. Not all abused juveniles are disruptive. And not all paranoid youth become violent. But experiencing this combination of factors can place juvenile offenders at a much higher risk for disruptive, aggressive and violent behavior. Why some of these youth are overly aggressive and extremely difficult to manage is not exactly clear. However, trauma to the head is likely to be a key ingredient. Juveniles' head trauma is likely to reduce their ability to control their impulses and emotions. In turn, the youth are likely to react quickly when stressed or threatened, and aggress against others. Then they find it difficult to control themselves once they become upset or start to fight. (Lewis *et al.*, (1987) have used the term "Limbic-Psychotic-Aggressive Syndrome" to try to capture the subgroup of youth who evidence neurological impairment (head trauma/central nervous system problems), psychiatric impairment (transient psychosis/paranoid ideation) and aggression (inability to regulate/control emotions, particularly anger). These youth typically do not fit into clear mental health or neurological categories. More research is needed to classify these complicated, difficult-to-manage, and often-dangerous youth residing in juvenile justice facilities.

Standard classification systems such as the *DSM* do not capture the multifaceted nature of these particular youth, and typical juvenile justice and mental health interventions are minimally successful with them. Consequently, many of these seriously disturbed youth spend much of their time in juvenile justice facilities, confined to a small room, with access to minimal resources—due to continued sanctions and loss of privileges in response to negative behavior. For some, the situation is bleaker, with much of their time spent in restraint chairs and isolation cells, or an eventual transfer to the adult criminal justice system. What makes the situation even more unfortunate is that decisions about the youths' placement and programming are typically reactions to viewing the

youth as a "bad" kid making "bad" choices. Decision-makers are often completely unaware of the youths' organic damage.

Because a significant number of youth involved with juvenile justice may be suffering from some type of brain/central nervous system impairment, neuropsychological screening should be available to these juveniles. Currently, comprehensive neuropsychological assessments are rarely obtained for juvenile offenders, partly due to the high cost and length of time involved in this type of evaluation (usually four to six hours). A relatively brief neuropsychological screening should be conducted with youth who exhibit persistent aggressive and/or violent behavior. This type of screening should also be considered for impulsive, emotionally unstable youth when progress is not seen with standard juvenile justice and mental health interventions. These types of screenings should consist of more than one or two subtests. *(Please see Gorenstein, 1990 for details on neuropsychololgical screening batteries.)* If positive findings are detected during neuropsychological screening, youth should be referred for a comprehensive neuropsychological battery. The cost of this type of assessment may be high. But this cost it is likely to be relatively less than the numerous physical and financial resources allotted to continue managing these youth unsuccessfully.

Determining that youth have brain impairment can have significant implications for juvenile justice programming and disposition decisions. Many of these youth receive significant sanctions within the juvenile justice system for not "choosing" to do the right thing. Some juvenile justice professionals believe that if this type of youth receives enough punishment/negative consequences, the youth will eventually "straighten up." This approach has been used with some brain-injured youth for years, resulting in unnecessary and sometimes unethical treatment—as well as little positive change in the juvenile offenders' behavior. Ironically, when treated in this manner, brain-

Juvenile Offenders with Mental Health Disorders: Who Are They and What Do We Do With Them?

injured youth often become more angry, paranoid and aggressive because they feel frustrated and unjustly treated. When this vicious cycle continues for an extended period of time, these juvenile offenders may end up in the adult criminal justice system—where the cycle is likely to begin again.

When juvenile justice professionals become aware that part of youths' difficulties stem from brain-related impairment, this knowledge can help the staff set realistic expectations for the youth. Realistic expectations typically result in less frustration for the juveniles and the staff who monitor them. Juvenile offenders with brain impairment typically need additional structure and supervision. Directives need to be particularly firm, concise and consistent.

Any evidence of brain injury is critical information that should be taken into account in both facility programming and community supervision plans. Because youth with frontal lobe injuries have difficulty representing something in their head, they need multiple reminders and cues regarding prosocial behavior. They tend to be driven by habit and immediate needs, and require assistance in breaking engrained patterns of behavior. Left to their own devices, these juveniles are likely to return to the same type of behavior that got them in trouble in the first place. Threats of punishment (*e.g.*, return to a juvenile justice facility) have little impact because these youth have difficulty conceptualizing abstract and future events/consequences.

In addition, youth with brain injuries are more susceptible to the effects of drugs and alcohol, which may disinhibit these juveniles further—increasing their risk of violence. Juvenile offenders who have sustained brain damage need interventions that focus on:

- Decreasing/discontinuing substance use
- Thinking before they act
- Managing their anger
- Interacting in a prosocial manner with others
- Reducing stress

- Correctly perceiving social cues (versus paranoid misperceptions)
- Empathizing with others/victim empathy
- Communicating their desires and emotions through words versus actions

Mental health/medical professionals who prescribe psychotropic medication also need to be informed if youth have brain impairment, as the youths' response to this type of medication is likely to be affected. The prognosis for brain-injured youth is not good, particularly if they have a history of serious physical abuse and/or paranoid ideation. But awareness of juveniles' brain-related problems makes effective supervision and management possible, and serious violence and aggression may be prevented.

 ## Violence and Mental Illness

Juvenile justice professionals without much knowledge about mental illness often believe juveniles with mental health disorders are more dangerous than nonmentally ill juveniles. The staff may be concerned about the assault potential of mentally ill youth (toward staff and/or other youth) during interpersonal interactions with them. Such a belief is not surprising, as many members of the general population also have misguided views of individuals with mental illness. A significant portion of society is frightened of persons who are mentally ill, believing that they are dangerous and violent.

The juvenile justice system (and now the adult criminal justice system as well) houses some of the most violent youth in the nation. Violence in and of itself is not a mental health disorder. Violence also does not necessarily signify that symptoms of mental illness are present. However, some youth with mental health disorders do engage in violent and/or assaultive behavior. The question most juvenile justice professionals want answered is, "Are juveniles with mental health disorders more likely to be violent and assaultive than juveniles without these disorders?" The answer is, *it depends*.

In general, mentally ill individuals are not more violent and assaultive than those without mental illness. However, there is a small subgroup of mentally ill individuals who are significantly more likely to engage in violent and assaultive behavior. These youth typically cannot be distinguished by their mental health diagnosis, but they may be distinguished by the particular mental health symptoms the youth experience and exhibit. For example, youth experiencing specific types of psychotic symptoms are significantly more likely to engage in interpersonal assaults than youth without these symptoms. This risk is even higher when symptoms are combined with alcohol and drug use.

Hallucinations and delusions are common symptoms experienced by individuals suffering from psychotic disorders. Hallucinations are false sensory perceptions that are not associated with real external stimuli (*e.g.*, hearing things that other people do not hear, seeing things that other people do not see). Delusions are false personal beliefs that youth hold despite obvious proof that they are false and/or irrational (*e.g.*, believing they are pregnant although they have not been sexually active, believing the CIA has implanted computer chips in their brains). In general, experiencing hallucinations or delusions does not appear to increase youths' assault risk. However, experiencing delusions that fall into the *threat/control-override* (TCO) category does increase risk (Swanson, Borum, Swartz, & Monahan, 1996). The types of beliefs associated with threat/control-override (TCO) include:

- Believing others can control how they think or move, even against their will
- Believing others are plotting against them or trying to hurt or poison them
- Believing someone can insert thoughts directly into their mind or steal thoughts from out of their mind
- Believing other people are following them

Hallucinations and delusions are not based on reality. However, psychotic individuals experience these symptoms and react to them as if they were real. Therefore, psychotic individuals' assaultive actions are often a *rational* response occurring within an *irrational* way of viewing the world (Link & Stueve, 1994). This explanation is not meant to condone psychotic youths' violent behavior but to help juvenile justice professionals understand how it often comes about. Individuals experiencing TCO symptoms often feel threatened, and their aggressive behavior can be justified in their own minds—because of the dangerous and harmful actions they believe are being directed against them. Risk of assault is heightened even more when these juveniles also believe their self-control has been compromised (*e.g.*, external forces are putting thoughts into their head or removing their thoughts against their will).

Although these specific TCO types of symptoms are associated with an increased risk of assault, other psychotic symptoms are not (*e.g.*, hearing voices others do not hear, believing one has special powers, believing the radio is sending special messages, believing parts of one's body are rotting away). Therefore, staff should not infer that just because youth are mentally ill, even psychotic, that they are more likely to be assaultive. *(Please see Chapter 8 for additional information about Schizophrenia and other Psychotic Disorders.)*

The combination of TCO symptoms and current substance use puts juveniles at particularly high risk for assaultive behavior. In addition to their unusual thoughts, the use of drugs can impair youths' perception of a situation even further. This impairment can result in the youth paying closer attention to certain social cues but minimizing or ignoring others. Intoxication can also affect the judgments and interpretations juveniles make during interpersonal interactions with staff or peers. Also, youth who are intoxicated may be less inhibited and more likely to act upon aggressive impulses. Youth arriving at juvenile detention facilities directly from the community who are drunk or high when arrested and detained are an especially high assault risk if they are psychotic and experiencing TCO symptoms. Juveniles can also be intoxicated within longer-term juvenile justice facilities if they are directly admitted from the community (*e.g.*, youth who are allowed to leave on pass, parole/probation violators).

TCO symptoms do not commonly occur among the majority of youth with mental health disorders. These symptoms are most commonly seen among individuals with Schizophrenia. Schizophrenia is not a frequently occurring mental health disorder among youth in juvenile justice, but it does exist among this population of youth at a higher rate than youth in the general population. Individuals with other types of mental illness (*e.g.*, substance abuse, severe traumatic experiences, cognitive disorders, delusional disorders, severe situational disorders) can also experience TCO symptoms. However, among mentally ill juvenile offenders, the risk of violence is likely to be highest among youth with a major mental health disorder (*e.g.*, Schizophrenia, Major Depression, Bipolar Disorder) who also have TCO symptoms and a co-occurring substance abuse disorder (Swanson, *et al.*, 1996). These youth form a very small subgroup of juvenile offenders. Proper mental health intervention (*e.g.*, psychotropic medication, psychological treatment) can help decrease the symptoms of this group of mentally ill youth, making assaultive behavior less likely.

Even if particular juveniles fit the description above, it does not necessarily indicate that they will become assaultive. It only suggests that they are at higher risk than youth (mentally ill or not) without similar symptoms. The following factors also play an important role in assaultive behavior:

- Youths' individual characteristics
- Youths' social environment
- The peers and staff with whom youth are interacting

The majority of individuals with mental health disorders are not assaultive. In fact, mentally ill individuals are often the victims of violence versus the ones perpetrating it.

Aggression Among Juvenile Offenders

Aggression is a common occurrence within juvenile justice facilities, and incarcerated youth can become verbally and physically aggressive toward staff or peers. Juvenile offenders who engage in aggressive behavior do not necessarily have a mental health disorder. Even if juveniles are mentally ill, their illness may not play a role in their aggression.

Predicting which juvenile offenders within juvenile justice facilities are going to exhibit verbal or physical aggression is difficult. Many of these individuals would be considered a high risk for aggressive behavior based on:

- Their families (*e.g.*, witnessing domestic violence)
- Their childhood experiences (*e.g.*, experiencing child abuse)
- The communities/neighborhoods where they have spent much of their lives (*e.g.*, witnessing violence)

One of the best predictors of aggressive behavior among youth (with and without mental health disorders) is recent and past aggression—a characteristic of many incarcerated juvenile offenders. However, most incarcerated youth do not become aggressive with juvenile justice staff or other young offenders. The social and physical environment of particular juvenile justice facilities (or even particular living units) can play a significant role in the aggressive behaviors of juveniles—as can the interpersonal dynamics between particular staff and the youth they supervise (Harrington, 1972).

In comparison to their nonaggressive peers, aggressive adolescents often exhibit deficiencies when processing information regarding social interactions and interpersonal situations. These youth tend to be biased in how they interpret social situations, perceiving ambiguous interactions as more hostile than they really are (Dodge, 1982). This interpretation often leads to youth feeling as if they need to defend themselves or "save face." Aggressive juvenile offenders, in particular, show significantly more problems related to social problem-solving when compared to youth in the community—even when compared to other highly aggressive but nonoffending youth (Slaby & Guerra, 1998). When interacting with others, these juvenile offenders tend to:

- Define interpersonal problems in hostile ways

- Choose goals that are more hostile in nature

- Come to quick judgments about situations without seeking additional facts

- Generate few alternative solutions when attempting to solve problems between themselves and others

- Anticipate fewer negative consequences of aggression

Juvenile justice professionals are often taken aback by some juveniles' aggressive reactions or "over-reactions" to minor interpersonal conflicts or benign requests from staff. Given their tendency to misinterpret social situations, these aggressive youth may perceive staff members as being purposefully disrespectful, antagonistic or argumentative even when they are not.

In addition, aggressive juvenile offenders tend to have positive beliefs about aggression in general. In comparison to nonaggressive youth, aggressive juveniles frequently believe that aggression:

- Is a legitimate response to interpersonal difficulties

- Increases self-esteem

- Makes them appear more positively in the eyes of peers

- Does not lead to suffering by victims

Incidents of verbal and physical aggression within juvenile justice facilities are not surprising given the combination of youth:

- Misperceiving social situations

- Attributing hostile intentions to others even when such intentions are not present

- Being deficient in effective social problem-solving

- Holding positive beliefs about the use of aggression

Juvenile justice facilities typically house many adolescents who think in the ways described above. The most effective anger management programs for aggressive youth—including juvenile offenders—focus on teaching the youth specific social problem-solving skills and attempting to modify their positive beliefs about the use of aggression (Goldstein and Glick, 1987; Guerra & Slaby, 1990).

 SECLUSION AND RESTRAINT

Some juvenile offenders with mental health disorders become violent and destructive to themselves, peers, staff and facility property. In these circumstances, many juvenile justice facilities rely on *seclusion* or *restraint* strategies to manage youths' behavior. *Seclusion, segregation, isolation and solitary confinement* all typically refer to removing youth from their living environment to an individual cell/room for the purpose of behavioral control. An isolation cell/room may be located in youths' primary living unit, in a medical infirmary, or in a special disciplinary or treatment unit (*e.g.*, segregation unit, intensive management unit). Disciplinary units are usually designed to separate the most assaultive and/or disruptive youth from the rest of the juveniles within a facility. Most, or all, rooms in these units are typically designated for isolation purposes. Most juveniles housed within these segregation units are secluded for disciplinary reasons (*e.g.*, threatening behavior,

Juvenile Offenders with Mental Health Disorders: Who Are They and What Do We Do With Them?

escape attempts, extreme agitation, assaultive behavior). But some facilities also segregate youth in these units if they are in need of protective custody or if they are a significant danger to themselves (*e.g.*, engaging in suicidal or self-injurious/self-mutilating behavior). Youths housed in segregation units are typically placed in a special room for 23-hours-per-day and allowed one hour outside of their room for meals and/or exercise.

Juvenile justice facilities vary in their use of seclusion rooms and/or seclusion units. Some mentally ill juvenile offenders may be involved in incidents of seclusion because they:

- Have significant difficulty regulating their emotions (including anger)

- Engage in extremely bizarre behaviors

- Are destructive to themselves or others

The primary goal of seclusion is to isolate juvenile offenders from the general population of youth. However, secluded juveniles should still have access to the same living conditions (*e.g.*, clothing, food, room space, exercise, and other services and privileges) as their peers in the general population (American Correctional Association, 1991a; 2002). Unfortunately, many youth in seclusion are placed in rooms with little to nothing to do and do not have access to schoolwork or any other types of activities.

The American Correctional Association has specific standards related to the use of seclusion in juvenile justice facilities (ACA, 1991a, b; 2002) All agencies using seclusion as a management strategy should consult these standards for information related to this critical area. ACA standards specify that using room restriction as a response to minor misbehavior should be used only as a "cooling off" period and should be of short duration (*i.e.*, 15–60 minutes). Staff should discuss with youth the specific time parameters associated with the confinement as soon as the room assignment begins. Many juvenile offenders impulsively act out or lose control of their emotions but are then able to quickly regain their composure. Oftentimes, several minutes of room restriction is all that is needed to remedy the situation. These juveniles should then be permitted to rejoin the rest of the youth and continuing engaging in normal activities.

The amount of time youth spend in confinement should be directly proportionate to the youths' behavior. The juveniles' prior behavior, their individual program needs, and other relevant factors should be considered (ACA, 1991; 2002). Youths may be confined for a major rule violation for a period of "up to 24 hours for the safety of the juvenile, other juveniles, or to ensure the security of the facility. Confinement for periods of over 24 hours is reviewed every 24 hours by the administrator or designee who was not involved in the incident" (ACA, 1991; 2002).

Upper limits of time spent in seclusion for an offense should be consistent with case law and statutes of the jurisdiction.

Depending on juveniles' emotional state, staff should interact with juveniles every 15 minutes to solve any problems and determine a release time. **Confined juveniles who become suicidal require more intensive staff monitoring.** Secluded juveniles should receive daily visits from mental health, religious, administrative and medical professionals during confinement. These visits should be face-to-face and should not occur through the window or door of juveniles' rooms. These visits do not need to be extensive, but it is important that qualified health and mental health professionals assess confined youths' physical and psychological functioning on a daily basis. Physical or psychological deterioration during incidents of isolation is very possible.

Juvenile offenders can experience significant negative effects from long periods of isolation. Effects of sensory deprivation seen among individuals in solitary confinement include (Grassian & Friedman, 1986):

- Significant anxiety

- Perceptual distortions and hallucinations

- Over-reactions to what is going on around them

- Feeling as if things were not "real"
- Memory and concentration difficulties
- Confusion
- Aggressive fantasies
- Paranoid thoughts (which can become delusional)
- Excess energy (which can result in outbursts of violent, destructive, or self-mutilating behavior)

Juvenile offenders with mental health disorders may be particularly vulnerable to the negative effects of isolation (Mitchell & Varley, 1990). Fortunately, youths' symptoms often quickly disappear once the juveniles are released from seclusion.

There are numerous case examples of youth with no history of suicidal or self-injurious/self-mutilating behavior who have engaged in these self-destructive acts after long periods of isolation. This situation is especially true for youth with mental health disorders. Regressive behavior such as rocking, uncontrollable crying and feces smearing can also result.

Some youth are so dangerous and/or difficult to manage in juvenile justice facilities that they spend weeks or months in a segregation unit. This practice should be avoided at all costs. When this type of situation does arise, a variety of staff involved with youths' care (e.g., line staff, administration, medical, mental health, school, recreation) should work together to devise a strategy emphasizing the juveniles' return to a generic living unit. Creative problem-solving, individually tailored treatment plans, and re-evaluation of current behavioral expectations are typically required. Any improper use of seclusion or restraint should be reported immediately to administration.

Some juvenile justice facilities automatically isolate youth who are suicidal and/or engage in self-injurious/self-mutilating behavior. This practice is not a recommended treatment strategy because separating self-destructive youth from their peers increases their sense of aloneness and isolation. Feelings of depression

and anxiety can also increase (Lendemeijer & Shortridge-Baggett, 1997). When placed in a seclusion cell, most suicidal and self-injurious/self-mutilating youth have nothing to occupy their time—except thinking about how upset they are and what creative strategies they can use to injure themselves. Placing self-harming youth in seclusion can also make it more difficult for staff to supervise them because they are separated from the rest of the group. Taking into account safety concerns, staff should manage suicidal and self-injurious/self-mutilating youth in the least restrictive environment possible. Many of these juveniles can be effectively managed within the general population, as long as they have additional monitoring by staff (e.g., every five minutes, every 10 minutes). If youth need extra monitoring overnight, they can sleep in a special treatment unit, in the medical infirmary, or in a suicide-safe room in a generic living unit.

IF LESS EXTREME MANAGEMENT MEASURES HAVE BEEN UNSUCCESSFUL AND MENTALLY ILL JUVENILE OFFENDERS MUST BE SECLUDED OR RESTRAINED, MENTAL HEALTH AND JUVENILE JUSTICE STAFF SHOULD DEVELOP INDIVIDUALIZED TREATMENT PLANS FOR THESE YOUTH.

If less extreme management measures have been unsuccessful and mentally ill juvenile offenders must be secluded or restrained, mental health and juvenile justice staff should develop individualized treatment plans for these youth. These plans should specifically indicate which of the youths' behavior(s) resulted in seclusion/restraint and specifically list what the youth need to do to return to the general population. All behaviors and expectations should be stated in objective, observable and easy-to-understand terms. Juveniles experiencing seclusion/restraint should always be given an incentive to engage in prosocial behavior and *earn* their way back to the general population. However, behavioral expectations must be realistically attainable. Some facilities require secluded youth to "refrain from any angry outbursts, profanity and yelling for five consecutive days " to move out of a segregation unit. Not surprisingly, most of these difficult-to-manage juveniles are unable to abstain from these behaviors 24-hours-a-day for five days in a row. Given this type of expectation, some youth can remain in segregation units for weeks or months at a time.

Reduced time in seclusion in exchange for meeting behavioral expectations can be a powerful motivator for secluded youth. For example, some youth are scheduled to be housed in segregation units for three days (23 hours in their room and one hour out) as a sanction for engaging in serious negative behavior. Allowing these youth to earn two hours out of a room in exchange for compliant behavior can have positive effects. If youths' behavior continues to improve, they can work toward three hours out, then four hours out, and so forth. The goal is to motivate juveniles to engage in increasingly more positive and prosocial behaviors. When juvenile offenders know that they will remain in a segregation unit for three days (23 hours in their room), no matter what, they typically have no motivation to engage in positive behavior. Why would they—because positive behavior change does not result in increased freedom or privileges.

Going from the intense structure of a segregation unit back into a general living unit can be overwhelming and stressful for some juveniles—particularly if the youth spent a significant period of time in isolation. Allowing secluded youth incrementally increased time out of their room before returning to general population can ease their transition back into the general population. Additional time out of a seclusion room helps these youth practice the skills necessary to function in the general population. Without practice of these skills,

many of these youth will return to segregation shortly after departing, due to not being able to successfully function in the general population.

Whenever youth are placed in seclusion, the focus should be on helping the juveniles identify:

- What behavior resulted in their restricted placement?
- What do they need to do differently in order to avoid similar negative consequences in the future?

Seclusion is not a time for youth to sleep. It is a time to reflect on what triggered their negative behavior and what different, prosocial choices the youth will make the next time they are in a similar situation. A simple way to help youth figure this out is to have them focus on their *A,B, C's*. The B stands for the specific *behavior* the youth engaged in that resulted in seclusion. Juveniles should be very clear about exactly what they did (*e.g.*, assaulted someone, threw a chair, flooded their room, attempted to escape) versus having a vague notion of being "disrespectful," "inappropriate," "dangerous," "violent," or "angry." The A represents the *antecedent* that came before their negative behavior (*e.g.*, what triggered their behavior/ reaction/response). The C represents the more *constructive choice* they will make the next time they are in a similar situation. All interactions between staff and youth in seclusion should be centered on conversations about the ABC's—as well as behavioral expectations that the juveniles must fulfill to return to the general population. Time in seclusion should be time spent learning new skills and ways of behaving. Just separating youth from their peers (and allowing them to sleep), with little focus on the behavior they need to modify, is not likely to result in behavior change.

In general, seclusion with the sole aim of punishment is contraindicated (Lendemeijer & Shortridge-Baggett, 1997). Instead, short time-out periods, with staff periodically interacting with juveniles to problem-solve current difficul-

317

Special Issues II: Head Trauma/Neuropsychiatric Factors, Violence and Mental Illness, Seclusion and Restraint, Malingering, Staff Training

ties, appears to be more effective. Mitchell and Varley (1990) have even recommended eliminating separate isolation units altogether. They note that these types of specialized disciplinary units:

- Are expensive to run
- Decrease the likelihood that creative behavior management programs will be developed and implemented with difficult-to-manage youth
- Provide an environment where there will likely be an over-reliance on isolation as the primary behavior management strategy

---

Mechanical/therapeutic restraints typically refer to devices that are designed to confine juveniles' bodily movements and restrict their physical activity. Restraint strategies are typically used to help calm youth down or prevent injury to the youth or others. Using restraints with mentally ill juvenile offenders should be a last-resort management strategy. It should be used only in emergency situations, when there is imminent danger to the youth or others. Restraints should never be implemented as discipline/punishment (ACA, 1991a, b; 2002) and should be discontinued at the earliest point possible.

Some facilities use fleece-lined leather, canvas, or rubber hand and leg restraints. Others use special restraint chairs or straitjackets to restrain youth whose behavior is out of control. Experts recommend that hard plastic or metal devices—such as handcuffs and leg shackles not be used for therapeutically restraining youth. In addition, juveniles should not be restrained in unnatural positions such as face down, hog-tied, or spread-eagled.

Placing youth in restraints should require approval from administration (*i.e.*, superintendent/director or designee) and a qualified health care authority. Due to the potential negative physical effects of restraints, experts recommend that restrained youth be medically monitored (*e.g.*, circulation, nerve damage, airway obstruction, psychological trauma) at least every 15 minutes by a health care professional. A mental health professional should assess restrained youths' psychological functioning. In addition, the juveniles should be under constant visual observation by appropriately trained juvenile justice staff. Any staff member applying restraints to juveniles should be properly trained to do so—because serious injuries and even deaths have occurred during restraint procedures, as well as during the period the youth are restrained. Nerve or artery constriction can occur, as can air restriction (*e.g.*, gagging, choking on youths' own vomit, covering the mouth or nose of the youth).

Medical and mental health authorities should also advise whether restrained youth should be transferred to a medical/mental health facility for emergency treatment. If restrained youth remain in a juvenile justice facility, specific and individualized plans should be developed for each youth in relation to releasing them from restraints as soon as possible.

Staff should problem-solve (*e.g.*, ABC approach) with youth who require restraints about:

- What behavior led to the youth being restrained?
- What can the youth can do differently the next time they are in a similarly difficult situation?

A primary goal is to help these juveniles develop more effective internal controls regarding their emotions and behavior, rather than relying on external controls (*e.g.*, restraints) to calm down. Some juvenile justice facilities have been successful in avoiding the use of restraints as a strategy to manage juveniles' behavior. These facilities instead rely on effective behavior management programs, verbal de-escalation and seclusion. Because of this success, experts have suggested that the use of restraints be eliminated in juvenile justice settings (Mitchell & Varley, 1990).

318

Juvenile Offenders with Mental Health Disorders: Who Are They and What Do We Do With Them?

Not all juvenile offenders find seclusion a negative experience. Mentally ill juvenile offenders may find seclusion a pleasant reprieve because they are:

- Being overly stimulated by the activity in general living units
- Experiencing auditory hallucinations
- Being annoyed by close contact with peers
- Suffering from depression and want to withdraw from others
- Fearing for their safety around the other offenders
- Attempting to avoid school and other programming expectations

If particular youth are repeatedly secluded, mental health and juvenile justice staff should explore what need these juveniles are meeting by being segregated from others. Intervention strategies should focus on these underlying issues (*e.g.*, hallucinations, fear, overstimulation, avoidance). To prevent youth from trying to be secluded as a means of avoiding aversive activities, juveniles in seclusion should not be able to "escape" from their daily responsibilities. These youth should still be required to clean their room, maintain proper hygiene, complete school assignments, and so forth. Seclusion should not be perceived by juveniles as a way to "get out of doing things."

Along the same lines, some juvenile offenders do not perceive being restrained as a negative experience. A number of youth have reported that they feel safe and protected after being restrained. Other youth have said they sometimes provoke staff to restrain them when they are afraid or need attention from adults. If they suspect these dynamics, juvenile justice professionals should discuss them with their supervisor and the entire team. Staff should focus on helping these youth express their needs in a more socially adaptive manner. Whenever juveniles are repeatedly restrained, mental health and juvenile justice staff should try to discover whether there is something about the experience that is reinforcing for the youth.

Written policies and procedures should exist and be closely followed regarding the seclusion and restraint of youth, including:

- How determinations about seclusion/restraint are made
- How determinations about seclusion/restraint are reviewed
- How long and in what manner youth can be secluded/restrained
- The type of documentation required for each seclusion/restraint incident

These management strategies can result in significant physical injury, and possibly death. Therefore, medical personnel should be involved in the development and review of all seclusion and restraint policies.

(Note: The American Correctional Association's *Performance-Based Standards for Correctional Health Care for Juvenile Correctional Facilities* is pending approval from the Standards Committee.)

 ## Malingering

Malingering is defined as "pretending to be ill or otherwise incapacitated in order to escape duty or work" (Neufeldt & Guralink, 1988). Some individuals malinger or fake mental health symptoms to avoid certain responsibilities. Because lying is common among juvenile offenders, juvenile justice professionals often think that youth are malingering when they exhibit symptoms of mental illness or tell staff about their disorder. Staffs' perception of youth malingering is usually strengthened when juveniles boldly state, "I can't do that. I have ADHD," "It is because of my Bipolar Disorder that I don't follow the rules," or some similar type of statement. Unfortunately, this perception can lead to staff making sweeping generali-

319

Special Issues II: Head Trauma/Neuropsychiatric Factors, Violence and Mental Illness, Seclusion and Restraint, Malingering, Staff Training

zations about all mentally ill youth. Staff may assume that all juveniles who exhibit unusual behavior or openly discuss their mental health disorder are:

- Avoiding taking responsibility for their actions
- Attempting to get staff to pay attention to them
- Just trying to get medication (drugs) from the doctor

Although there is likely a small subset of juveniles primarily motivated by these goals, most mentally ill youth are not. This does not mean that mentally ill youth do not avoid taking responsibility for negative behavior, that they do not want staff attention, or that they would refuse mind-altering chemicals from a doctor. The youth may even want these things. However, many juvenile offenders *without* mental health disorders want these things as well. Pretending to have a mental health disorder to achieve these goals is a more difficult task for youth than it appears. Malingering tends to occur much less often than most juvenile justice professionals believe. Or malingering dissipates when direct results are not obtained.

There are a variety of reasons why incarcerated youth might want to pretend that they are experiencing mental health symptoms (*e.g.*, hearing voices, wanting to kill themselves, reporting they cannot sleep). Juveniles may want to:

- Be transferred from a juvenile justice setting to a mental health setting (*e.g.*, co-ed, less restrictive)
- Ensure numerous interactions with mental health/medical staff
- Avoid being held accountable for negative behavior
- Receive a prescription for mind-altering medications
- Receive special programming allowances
- Obtain individualized attention from juvenile justice staff

However, there are just as many—if not more—reasons why incarcerated youth would *not* want anyone to think they have a mental health disorder. In fact, some juvenile offenders who are truly mentally ill minimize their mental health symptoms. Mental illness often carries significant stigma in juvenile justice facilities. Juvenile offenders typically want to portray tough exteriors, and having a mental illness can result in youth being viewed as weak or vulnerable. Respect and youths' standing among peers can be critical within juvenile justice settings. Therefore, a reputation for being "crazy" or "strange" can considerably reduce youths' status. Whereas some incarcerated juveniles will do anything (literally) to elicit attention from adult figures, other youth find extra attention from adults an unpleasant and negative experience. For some juvenile offenders, the following can be incredibly uncomfortable, and something they wish to avoid at all costs:

- Being required to talk to mental health/medical staff about personal issues
- Being required to talk to juvenile justice staff and supervisors on an individual basis
- Having to participate in various mental health evaluations
- Having to take psychotropic medication (*e.g.*, negative side effects)
- Being transferred to a psychiatric hospital

In addition, being placed in special precautionary programming for their safety (*e.g.*, suicide watch, mental health watch) can be embarrassing, intrusive and annoying for some youth.

Juvenile justice professionals may observe the "contagion" effect in some of the living units within juvenile residential facilities. For example, when one youth is diagnosed with Attention-Deficit/Hyperactivity Disorder (ADHD) and prescribed stimulant medication, all of a sudden the other youth in a unit complain of attention problems. All youth begin requesting to see the doctor to obtain stimulant

320

Juvenile Offenders with Mental Health Disorders: Who Are They and What Do We Do With Them?

medication. Or, if a living unit houses a juvenile who engages in self-injurious/self-mutilating behavior, several of the youth's peers may begin cutting or carving their skin. This behavior can occur even when the youths' peers have no history of such behavior. This situation is most likely to occur when peers observe the juvenile's self-harm behavior resulting in positive consequences that the peers too would like to obtain.

The goal for juvenile justice and mental health professionals is to avoid *reinforcing* juvenile offenders for exhibiting symptoms of mental illness. Although mentally ill youth should receive appropriate evaluations and treatment, they should not receive rewards for having a mental health disorder. When they perceive that benefits are associated with mental health symptoms (*e.g.*, threatening suicide, cutting themselves, exhibiting bizarre behavior), nonmentally ill offenders are more likely to malinger in order to obtain these benefits for themselves.

To qualify for a mental health diagnosis, juveniles must demonstrate specific mental health symptoms for a specified period of time. "Faking" mental health symptoms for the period of time and level of severity required to be considered mentally ill is difficult. Youth who are not true self-injurers/self-mutilators have difficulty engaging in this type of behavior for a significant period of time because it hurts. Youth feigning appetite and sleep disturbances often get too hungry and tired after a few days to sustain the charade. Pretending to be psychotic by acting bizarrely (and/or as if hearing voices) can be exhausting to youth and a challenge to maintain over time.

There are no cut-and-dried rules for determining whether or not juveniles are malingering with regard to mental illness. However, some of the most important things for juvenile justice professionals to do when working with youth suspected of possibly faking or exaggerating mental health symptoms are to:

- Observe

- Document
- Refer

Observing juveniles' behavior is critical to determining whether youth are exhibiting symptoms of mental illness for personal gain or whether they are truly suffering from a mental health disorder. For example, if youth complain of having appetite disturbances, staff should observe the juveniles during mealtimes. If they have appetite disturbances, youth should be eating very little or nothing at all. Staff should pay attention to whether the juveniles continue to eat desserts at mealtimes, eat chips or cookies at snack time, and whether candy wrappers are found hidden in the youths' room.

When juvenile offenders complain of not being able to sleep, staff should observe youths' sleeping pattern for several nights in a row. Staff working the overnight shift are typically required to monitor incarcerated youth as they sleep (usually every 15–30 minutes). Facilities can create a "sleep log" so that staff can document whether particular youth were sleeping throughout the night during each of the 15–30 minute checks (*i.e.*, staff initial the time blocks). These nighttime checks can help provide information about whether the youth are:

- Truly not sleeping
- Feel like they are not sleeping because they awaken regularly
- Sleeping fine and possibly trying to obtain sleep medication for its mind-altering effects

If juveniles behave bizarrely, particularly when specific staff are around (*e.g.*, mental health professionals, medical professionals), observing the youth when they are unaware that anyone is watching them can be helpful. Staff observation of juvenile behavior is critical, and all observations should be documented in a matter-of-fact, objective manner (*e.g.*, "Youth is complaining of sleep difficulties, but after three nights of staff observing their sleep behavior every 20 minutes, it appears the youth is sleeping from 11:00 p.m.–5:30 a.m.").

In addition to observing and documenting youth behavior indicative of possible mental illness, juvenile justice professionals should refer potentially mentally ill youth to a supervisor and/or mental health/medical professional (depending on local policies and procedures). Staff observations and documentation of juveniles' behavior should be communicated during the referral process. For example, youth may complain of hearing voices. But staff may think that a youth is malingering because the voices are exactly the same (with the exact same words) as the youth's psychotic roommate. Staff should document the youth's complaints and note that the juvenile's possible hallucinations are an exact replica of his roommate's hallucinations.

Juvenile justice professionals should refrain from making an assessment or forming an opinion about whether the youth's hallucinations are indicative of mental illness or an attempt at malingering. The juvenile should be referred to a professional with knowledge, training and experience in these matters. If a mental health/medical professional is not immediately available, supervisors can typically make a decision as to who should best evaluate the youth.

A similar response should occur when juvenile offenders make a suicidal threat, and staff do not believe that the youth are serious. Staff should objectively document what the youth say, as well as how the youth behave, without inferring the juveniles' underlying motivation and goal (e.g., "Youth is stating she is are going to hang herself if staff do not allow her to call her boyfriend tonight"). Appropriate actions should be taken according to policies and procedures, which often includes an evaluation of the youth by a mental health/medical professional. Making determinations as to whether youth are truly suicidal, are really suffering from auditory hallucinations, and the like, should not be the responsibility of juvenile

justice professionals. However, referring youth who display these behaviors (or verbalizes these complaints) to a professional who is trained in making these types of judgments *is* the responsibility of staff.

Unfortunately, it is often difficult to determine whether or not a juvenile offender is faking or exaggerating symptoms of mental illness. Because they tend to have difficulties in a variety of areas (*e.g.*, mental health, substance abuse, school, family, peers), juvenile offenders often present with complex and complicated clinical pictures. Even mental health professionals with years of training and experience may struggle to tease apart the various issues affecting the lives of these youth.

JUVENILE JUSTICE PROFESSIONALS, AS WELL AS OTHER PROFESSIONALS WHO WORK WITH JUVENILE OFFENDERS, SHOULD RECEIVE TRAINING IN HOW TO *identify* JUVENILE OFFENDERS WITH MENTAL HEALTH DISORDERS.

In addition, juvenile offenders who malinger and those with valid mental health disorders are not mutually exclusive groups. For example, youth with a true, diagnosable mental illness may also want extra attention, mind-altering drugs, or transfer to a different facility, so may exaggerate or "use" their illness to obtain these objectives. This does not mean that the youth are faking all of their mental health symptoms, but there may be some malingering aspects to their behavior. Staff should observe, document and refer all potentially mentally ill youth to someone qualified to analyze these dynamics; staff should err on the side of caution and refer a youth even if they only have a "hunch" that something is not right with a particular juvenile. After a mental health/medical professional or supervisor evaluates a youth, feedback should be provided to the juvenile, as well as to the

Juvenile Offenders with Mental Health Disorders: Who Are They and What Do We Do With Them?

staff who made the referral about the presence (or apparent lack) of mental health symptoms. Regardless of whether it is established that a youth is mentally ill or malingering, resulting feedback should be integrated into the youth's programming and treatment plan.

 ## Staff Training on the Identification and Management of Juvenile Offenders with Mental Health Disorders

All staff working with juvenile offenders (*e.g.*, line staff, case managers, supervisors, probation/parole staff, teachers, clergy, vocational supervisors, law enforcement, nurses) come into contact with youth who have mental health disorders. These individuals may be required to supervise, interact with, and/or involve themselves in the rehabilitation of mentally ill juveniles. However, most professionals involved with juvenile offenders have never received any formal training in mental illness or psychiatric symptoms.

Juvenile justice professionals, as well as other professionals who work with juvenile offenders, should receive training in how to *identify* juvenile offenders with mental health disorders. Signs and symptoms of the most common psychiatric disorders (*e.g.*, Attention-Deficit/Hyperactivity Disorder, Posttraumatic Stress Disorder, Major Depression, Bipolar Disorder, Dysthymic Disorder, Psychotic Disorders, Mental Retardation, Fetal Alcohol Syndrome, Learning Disorders, Co-Occurring Mental Health and Substance Use Disorders), as well as suicide and self-injury/self-mutilation, should be included in this type of training. Staff training should focus specifically on how these disorders are exhibited throughout the adolescent years, particularly among youth involved with the juvenile justice system. Basic information about psychotropic medications commonly prescribed to juvenile offenders should also be reviewed, as should the side effects associated with these medicines. In addition, the following topics should be covered:

- Effective strategies for inquiring about youths' mental health symptoms
- Objectively reporting youth behavior
- Screening youth for suicide risk

When they are able to recognize that youth are experiencing mental health symptoms (*e.g.*, depressed mood, auditory hallucinations, suicidal ideation), juvenile justice professionals can make appropriate referrals to mental health/medical professionals. Juvenile justice staff also can provide valuable information to treatment providers about juvenile offenders' behavior, including any visible effects of psychotropic medication.

Juvenile justice professionals are in an ideal position to detect a change in youths' behavior. Because they observe and monitor offenders, juvenile justice staff may be the first to notice if juveniles start to behave differently and/or engage in unusual or bizarre behavior. In addition, staff who work within juvenile justice facilities are able to get a glimpse of youths' behavior when the juveniles are not using drugs and alcohol. These observations can provide valuable information about the source of juveniles' symptoms (mental health versus substance related).

Mental health screening tools are increasingly being used at various points throughout the juvenile justice continuum. Juvenile justice professionals should be able to recognize signs and symptoms of mental illness to help validate, contradict or supplement youths' self-report on these mental health instruments. This information is vital for ensuring appropriate placement, management and treatment of young offenders.

If they have not been trained in how to identify mental health symptoms among adolescents, juvenile justice professionals may view the behavior of mentally ill juveniles as purposeful and manipulative. This misperception can result in the reliance on severe sanctions and other negative consequences to alter youths' mental health symptoms. Sanctions are not an effective strategy to control mental illness, and some sanctions can exacerbate the youths' symptoms. Sole reliance on sanctions can also delay an appropriate mental health evaluation, as well as necessary treatment.

In addition to learning how to identify juvenile offenders with mental health disorders, juvenile justice professionals should be trained in how to effectively *manage* this complex group of youth. Even when juvenile offenders are referred for a mental health evaluation or treatment, they typically interact with mental health professionals on a limited basis. The youth are still supervised/managed by juvenile justice professionals.

For example, incarcerated youth may meet with a mental health professional several times while residing in a juvenile justice facility. But the youth are still housed in a living unit, and they participate in juvenile justice programming. The line staff and correctional educators typically spend the most time interacting with mentally ill juveniles on a daily basis. Juvenile offenders with mental health disorders who reside in the community typically meet with a mental health provider once a week or less—if and when the youth actually attend their scheduled treatment sessions.

Further, some juvenile offenders feel more comfortable telling juvenile justice facility staff, community supervision staff, or correctional educators personal information about their lives, families, and mental health symptoms versus treatment providers. Juvenile justice professionals need to know how to react to this information, as well as how to respond most effectively to mentally ill youth.

When a crisis occurs with incarcerated juveniles who are mentally ill, line staff must immediately respond to the youths' behavior. If they do not understand juveniles' mental health symptoms, juvenile justice staff may unintentionally escalate the situation, resulting in a worsening of the youths' behavior. This situation can be dangerous for both the youth and staff. In addition, certain intervention and treatment strategies are more effective than

others when working with youth who have specific mental health disorders. Some strategies can actually be harmful for these youth. When they are knowledgeable about mental health issues, staff's choice of intervention approaches can be more strategic and effective.

Every interaction between juvenile offenders and juvenile justice professionals can have a positive or negative effect on youths' behavior. Juvenile justice, mental health and medical professionals often unintentionally reinforce youths' self-injurious behavior, angry outbursts, or reports of hearing voices. Staff can learn how to avoid inadvertently rewarding this behavior and instead reinforce juveniles' adaptive and prosocial ways of coping. The result is typically a safer and more secure environment for staff and youth alike.

Additionally, the relationship between juvenile offenders and the professionals who work with them can serve as a protective factor against youths' future negative behavior. Many juvenile offenders look to staff members (*e.g.*, juvenile justice professionals, probation/parole staff, teachers, mentors, recreation staff) as role models. Some youth also become emotionally attached to these individuals. Understanding juveniles' mental health symptoms can help this type of relationship develop and remain strong. This relationship, in turn, can lessen some of the effects of the negative factors present in the lives of many of these young offenders (Werner & Smith, 1992).

Because juvenile offenders with mental health disorders can be particularly challenging to supervise and manage, many juvenile justice professionals have requested training on mental health issues. A study of correction officers who work with mentally ill adult offenders found that 90 percent of the staff reported that working with mentally ill offenders adds to the stress of the job. Eighty-six percent said the training for their current job did not prepare them to work with offenders who have mental health disorders. And 95 percent reported that they would like to have more training to deal with mentally ill offenders

Juvenile Offenders with Mental Health Disorders: Who Are They and What Do We Do With Them?

(Kropp, Cox, Roesch, & Eaves, 1989). Although this study involved a group of correction officers who work with adults, the same sentiments are consistently found among staff in the juvenile justice system.

Training staff how to identify and manage juvenile offenders with mental health disorders can also help reduce the likelihood of liability related to the care of mentally ill youth. This reduction is particularly likely if there is a claim that a juvenile justice agency failed to protect mentally ill juveniles or failed to recognize and treat youths' mental health disorders.

Which Staff Should Attend?

Mental health training can be beneficial for a variety of personnel working within the juvenile justice system. Because all professionals who work with juvenile offenders are likely to interact with youth who have mental health disorders, *anyone* working with juvenile offenders is a prime candidate for mental health training. The following is a list (though not exhaustive and in no particular order) of professionals who can benefit from training on how to identify and manage juvenile offenders with mental health disorders:

- Juvenile justice facility staff
- Probation officers
- Parole officers
- Supervisors
- Program Managers
- Diversion staff
- Educators
- Vocational supervisors
- Health care providers
- Mental health providers
- Substance abuse counselors
- Child welfare personnel

- Chaplains
- Recreational specialists
- Art therapists
- Administrators
- Law enforcement
- Policy makers
- Attorneys
- Judges

The effective management and treatment of juvenile offenders with mental health disorders typically requires coordination and collaboration among a variety of professionals and systems. Providing mental health training to a *diverse* group of participants can be a first step in bringing together these various disciplines. The training itself can help the staff of each system learn more about how the other systems work and can serve as a starting point for making professional contacts and exchanging ideas.

The effective management and treatment of juvenile offenders with mental health disorders also requires the coordination and collaboration of professionals *within* the same system. Staff

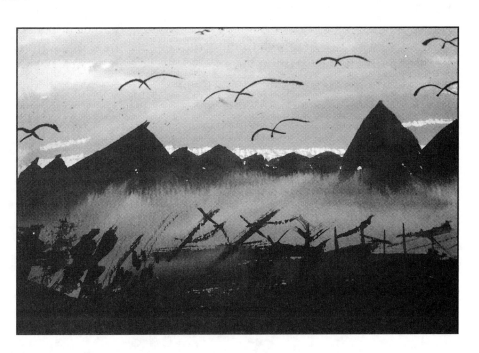

325

Special Issues II: Head Trauma/Neuropsychiatric Factors, Violence and Mental Illness, Seclusion and Restraint, Malingering, Staff Training

teams must work together—whether in short-term detention facilities, training schools, boot camps, work camps, ranches or group homes—to effectively manage mentally ill juveniles. Staff teams, as well as entire units or facilities, can lose their focus and end up in chaos over the management of juveniles with a serious mental health disorder(s). Different staff members commonly have diverse beliefs and philosophies about managing mentally ill juveniles. Half of a staff team may think the youth are "faking" their mental illness and should receive more restrictions and consequences for their unusual or negative behavior.

The other half of the staff team may believe that the youth need more support and understanding, with less stringent expectations for their behavior. Such division can be detrimental to the mentally ill youth, the staff team and a living unit as a whole. Because of this common dynamic, sending entire staff teams to mental health training can be beneficial so that they are all exposed to the same information at the same time. Admission/orientation units, living units with higher percentages of youth with mental health disorders, and security/disciplinary units should be given first priority in attending mental health training—due to the characteristics of the juveniles being supervised.

After attending an intensive training on mental health disorders and implementing new management/supervision strategies, juvenile justice professionals frequently report the following about the young offenders:

- Fewer episodes of self-injury/self-mutilation
- Less frequent threats of suicide
- Increased medication compliance
- Fewer aggressive outbursts

In addition, staff often report that they make more appropriate referrals to mental health/medical professionals for mental health evaluations and treatment. After receiving intensive mental health training, both residential and community supervision staff have also said that they are more likely to integrate issues related to youths' mental health into juvenile justice treatment/supervision plans.

The above issues reflect only a small portion of what can and should be done in relation to providing mental health training to juvenile justice professionals. For each mental health disorder, there is a wide array of information and management recommendations to help staff better serve this clinically complicated population of juvenile offenders. Providing mental health training within the juvenile justice system can be complex and challenging. However, given the increasing number of youth with mental health disorders involved with all aspects of the juvenile justice system, mental health training for staff has become a necessity.

Juvenile Offenders with Mental Health Disorders: Who Are They and What Do We Do With Them?

REFERENCES

Preface

Myers, W.C., Burket, R.C., & Otto, T.A. (1993). Conduct disorder and personality disorders in hospitalized adolescents. *Journal of Clinical Psychiatry, 54,* 21–26.

Chapter 1: Juvenile Offenders with Mental Health Disorders

American Psychiatric Association (2000). *Diagnostic and Statistical Manual of Mental Disorders,* (4th ed., Text Revision). Washington, DC: American Psychiatric Association.

Burrell, S., & Warboys, L. (2000). Special education and the juvenile justice system. *Juvenile Justice Bulletin.* Washington, DC: Office of Juvenile Justice and Delinquency Prevention.

Casey, P.A., & Keilitz, I. (1990). Estimating the prevalence of learning disabled and mentally retarded juvenile offenders. In P.E. Leone (Ed.), *Understanding Troubled and Troubling Youth* (pp. 82–101). Newbury Park, CA: Sage.

Cauffman, E., Feldman, S.S., Waterman, J., & Steiner, H. (1998). Posttraumatic stress disorder among female juvenile offenders. *Journal of the American Academy of Child and Adolescent Psychiatry, 37,* 1209–1216.

Cohen, R., Parmelee, D.X., Irwin, L., Weisz, J.R., Howard, P., Purcell, P., & Best, A.M. (1990). Characteristics of children and adolescents in a psychiatric hospital and a corrections facility. *Journal of the American Academy of Child and Adolescent Psychiatry, 29,* 909–913.

Davis, D.L., Bean Jr., G.J., Schumacher, J.E., & Stringer, T.L. (1991). Prevalence of emotional disorders in a juvenile justice institutional population. *American Journal of Forensic Psychology, 9* (1), 5–17.

Fergusson, D.M., Horwood, L.J., & Lynskey, M.T. (1993). Prevalence and comorbidity of DSM-III-R diagnoses in a birth cohort of 15 year olds. *Journal of the American Academy of Child and Adolescent Psychiatry, 32,* 1127–1134.

Giaconia, R., Reinherz, H., Silverman, A., Bilge, P., Frost, A., & Cohen, E. (1995). Traumas and posttraumatic stress disorder in a community population of older adolescents. *Journal of the American Academy of Child and Adolescent Psychiatry, 34,* 1369–1380.

Hakim-Larson, J., & Essau, C.A. (1999). Protective factors and depressive disorders. In C.A. Essau & F. Peterman (eds.), *Depressive Disorders in Children and Adolescents: Epidemiology, Risk Factors and Treatment.* Northvale, New Jersey: Jason Aronson, Inc.

Kashani, J.H., Beck, N.C., Hoeper, E.W., Fallahi, C., Corcoran, C.M., McAllister, J.A., Rosenberg, T.K., & Reid, J.C. (1987). *American Journal of Psychiatry, 144,* 584–589.

Regier, D.A., Myers, J.K., Kramer, M., Robins, L.N., Blazer, D.G., Hough, R.L., Eaton, W.W., & Locke, B.Z. (1984). The NIMH Epidemiologic Catchment Area Program. Historical context, major objectives, and study population characteristics. *Archives of General Psychiatry, 41,* 934–941.

Smykla, J.O., & Willis, T.W. (1981). The incidence of learning disabilities and mental retardation in youth under the jurisdiction of the juvenile court. *Journal of Criminal Justice, 9,* 219–225.

Snyder, H.N., & Sickmund, M. (1999). *Juvenile offenders and victims: 1999 national report.* Washington, DC: Office of Juvenile Justice and Delinquency Prevention.

Steiner, H., Garcia, I.G., & Matthews, Z. (1997). Posttraumatic stress disorder in incarcerated juvenile delinquents. *Journal of the American Academy of Child and Adolescent Psychiatry, 36,* 357–365.

Timmons-Mitchell, J., Brown, C., Schulz, C., Webster, S.E., Underwood, L.A., & Semple, W.E. (1997). Comparing the mental health needs of female and male incarcerated juvenile delinquents. *Behavioral Sciences and the Law, 15,* 195–202.

Ulloa, R.E., Birmaher, B., Axelson, D., Williamson, D.E., Brent, D.A., Ryan, N.D., Bridge, J., & Baugher, M. (2000). Psychosis in a pediatric mood and anxiety disorders clinic: Phenomenology and correlates. *Journal of the American Academy of Child and Adolescent Psychiatry, 39,* 337–345.

Wasserman, G.A., McReynolds, L.S., Lucas, C.P., Fisher, P., & Santos, L. (2002). The Voice DISC-IV with incarcerated male youths: Prevalence of disorder. *Journal of the American Academy of Child and Adolescent Psychiatry*, 41, 314–321.

Chapter 2: The Diagnosis of Mental Health Disorders

American Psychiatric Association (2000). *Diagnostic and Statistical Manual of Mental Disorders,* (4th ed., Text Revision). Washington, DC: American Psychiatric Association.

Arnett, J.J. (1999). Adolescent storm and stress, reconsidered. *American Psychologist*, 54, 317–326.

Dryborg, J., Larsen, W.F., Nielsen, S, Byman, J. Buhl-Nielsen, B., & Gautre-Delay, F. (2000). The children's global assessment scale (CGAS) and global assessment of psychosocial disability (GAPD) in clinical practice—substance and reliability as judged by interclass correlations. *European Child and Adolescent Psychiatry*, 9, 195–201.

Ferdinand, R.F., & Verhulst, F.C. (1995). Psychopathology from adolescence into young adulthood: An 8-year follow-up study. *American Journal of Psychiatry*, 152, 1586–1594.

Flaskerud, J.H., & Hu, L. (1992). Relationship of ethnicity to psychiatric diagnosis. *Journal of Nervous and Mental Disease*, 180, 296–303.

Kilgus, M.D., Pumariega, A.J., & Cuffe, S.P. (1995). Influence of race on diagnosis in adolescent psychiatric inpatients. *Journal of the American Academy of Child and Adolescent Psychiatry*, 34, 67–72.

Lewis, D.O., Balla, D.A., & Shanok, S.S. (1979). Some evidence of race bias in the diagnosis and treatment of the juvenile offender. *American Journal of Orthopsychiatry*, 49, 53–61.

Lewis, D.O., Shanok, S.S., Cohen, R.J., Kligfeld, M., & Frisone, G. (1980). Race bias in the diagnosis and disposition of violent adolescents. *American Journal of Psychiatry*, 137, 1211–1216.

McClellan, J., & Werry, J. (2000). Introduction—research psychiatric diagnostic interviews for children and adolescents. *Journal of the American Academy of Child and Adolescent Psychiatry*, 39, 19–27.

Miller, R.D., & Metzner, J.L. (1994). Psychiatric stigma in correctional facilities. *Bulletin of the American Academy of Psychiatry*, 22, 621–628.

Reeves, J.C., Werry, J.S., Elkind, G.S., & Zametkin, A. (1987). Attention-deficit, conduct, oppositional, and anxiety disorders in children. II. Clinical characteristics. *Journal of the American Academy of Child and Adolescent Psychiatry*, 26, 144–155.

Weiner, I.B. (1990). Distinguishing healthy from disturbed adolescent development. *Developmental and Behavioral Pediatrics*, 11, 151–154.

Chapter 3: Oppositional Defiant Disorder and Conduct Disorder

Alexander, J.F., & Barton, C. (1995). Family therapy research. In R.H. Mikesell, D.D. Lusterman, & S. McDaniel (Eds.), *Family Psychology and Systems Therapy: A Handbook*. Washington, DC: American Psychological Association.

Alexander, J.F., & Pugh, C.A. (1996). Oppositional and conduct disorders of children and youth. In F.W. Kaslow (Ed.), *Handbook of Relational Diagnosis and Dysfunctional Family Patterns*, (pp. 210–224). New York, NY: John Wiley & Sons.

American Correctional Association. (1991). *Standards for Juvenile Training Schools*. Lanham, MD: American Correctional Association.

American Correctional Association. (2002). *2002 Standards Supplement*. Lanham, MD: American Correctional Association.

American Psychiatric Association (2000). *Diagnostic and Statistical Manual of Mental Disorders*, (4th ed., Text Revision). Washington, DC: American Psychiatric Association.

Anderson, J.C., Williams, S., McGee, R., & Silva, P.A. (1987). DSM-III disorders in preadolescent children: Prevalence in a large sample from the general population. *Archives of General Psychiatry*, 44, 69–76.

Atkins, M.S., & Ricciuti, A. (1992). The disproportionate use of seclusion in a children's psychiatric state hospital. *Residential Treatment for Children and Youth*, 10, 23–33.

Boesky, L.M., Toro, P.A., Wright, K.L., & Wolfe, S.M.(1997). *Maltreatment among homeless adolescents: A subgroup comparison*. Manuscript submitted for publication.

Cairns, R.B., Peterson, G., & Neckerman, H.J. (1988). Suicidal behavior in aggressive adolescents. *Journal of Clinical Child Psychology*, 17, 298–309.

328

Juvenile Offenders with Mental Health Disorders: Who Are They and What Do We Do With Them?

Cullen, M.C., & Wright, J. (1996). *Cage Your Rage for Teens.* Lanham, MD: American Correctional Association.

Davis, D.L., Bean Jr., G.J., Schumacher, J.E., & Stringer, T.L. (1991). Prevalence of emotional disorders in a juvenile justice institutional population. *American Journal of Forensic Psychology*, 9 (1), 5–17.

Dishion, T.J., McCord, J., & Poulin, F. (1999). When interventions harm: Peer group and problem behavior. *American Psychologist*, 5, 755–764.

Dodge, K.A. (1985). Attributional bias in aggressive children. In P.C. Kendall (Ed.), *Advances in Cognitive-Behavioral Research and Therapy* (Vol. 4). Orlando, FL: Academic.

Feldman, R.A., Caplinger, T.E., & Wodarski, S.S. (1981). *The St. Louis conumdrum: Prosocial and antisocial boys together.* Unpublished manuscript.

Glueck, S., & Gleuck, E. (1968). *Delinquents and nondelinquents in perspective.* Cambridge, MA: Harvard University Press.

Goldstein, A.P., & Glick, B. (1994). Aggression replacement training: Curriculum and evaluation. *Simulation and Gaming*, 25, 9–26.

Goldstein, A.P., Glick, B., Reiner, S., Zimmerman, D., & Coultry, T. (1986). *Aggression Replacement Training.* Champaign, IL: Research Press.

Halikas, J.A., Meller, J., Morse, C., & Lyttle, M.D. (1990). Predicting substance abuse in juvenile offenders: Attention deficit disorder vs. aggressivity. *Child Psychiatric and Human Development,* 21, 49–55.

Henggeler, S.W., Melton, G.B., & Smith, L.A. (1992). Family preservation using multisystemic therapy: An effective alternative to incarcerating serious juvenile offenders. *Journal of Consulting and Clinical Psychology*, 60, 953–961.

Henggeler, S.W., Schoenwald, S., Borduin, C.M., Rowland, M.D., & Cunningham, P.B. (1998). *Multisystemic treatment of antisocial behavior in children and adolescents.* New York: Guilford.

Kashani, J.H., Beck, N.C., Hoeper, E.W., Fallahi, C., Corcoran, C.M., McAllister, J.A., Rosenberg, T.K., & Reid, J.C. (1987). Psychiatric disorders in a community sample of adolescents. *American Journal of Psychiatry*, 144, 584–589.

Kazdin, A.E. (1989). Conduct and oppositional disorders. In C. Last, & M. Hersen (Eds.), *Handbook of Child Psychiatric Diagnosis* (pp. 129–155). New York, NY: John Wiley & Sons.

Kazdin, A.E. (1994). Interventions for aggressive and antisocial children. In L.D. Eron, J.H. Gentry, & P. Schlegel (Eds.), *Reason To Hope: A Psychological Perspective on Violence and Youth* (pp. 341–382). Washington, DC: American Psychological Association.

Kazdin, A.E., Siegel, T.C., & Bass, D. (1992). Cognitive problem-solving skills training and parent management training in the treatment of antisocial behavior in children. *Journal of Consulting and Clinical Psychology*, 60, 733–747.

Lewis, D.O., Lewis, M., Unger, L., & Goldman, C. (1984). Conduct disorder and its synonyms: Diagnoses of dubious validity and usefulness. *American Journal of Psychiatry*, 141, 514–519.

Lewis, D.O., Shanok, S.S., & Balla, D.A. (1979). Perinatal difficulties, head and face trauma, and child abuse in the medical histories of seriously delinquent children. *American Journal of Psychiatry*, 136, 419–423.

Lipsey, M.W., & Derzon, J.H. (1998). Predictors of violent or serious delinquency in adolescence and early adulthood. In R. Loeber & D.P. Farrington, (Eds.), *Serious and Violent Juvenile Offenders* (pp. 86–105). Thousand Oaks, CA: Sage.

Loeber, R. (1991). Antisocial behavior: More enduring than changeable? *Journal of the American Academy of Child and Adolescent Psychiatry*, 30, 393–397.

Mitchell, J., & Varley, C. (1990). Isolation and restraint in juvenile correctional facilities. *Journal of the American Academy of Child and Adolescent Psychiatry*, 29, 251–255.

Moffitt, T.E. (1990). Juvenile delinquency and attention deficit disorder: Boys' developmental trajectories from age 2 to age 15. *Child Development*, 61, 893–910.

Moretti, M.M., Emmrys, C., Grizenko, N., Holland, R., Moore, K., Shamsie, J., & Hamilton, H. (1997). The treatment of conduct disorder: Perspectives from across Canada. *Canadian Journal of Psychiatry*, 637–648.

Moss, G.R. (1994). A biobehavioral perspective on the hospital treatment of adolescents. In P.W. Corrigan & R.P. Liberman (Eds.), *Behavior Therapy in Psychiatric Hospitals*. New York, NY: Springer Publishing Co.

Murray, J. (1980). *Television and youth: 25 Years of Research and Controversy.* Boys Town, NE: Boys Town Center for the Study of Youth Development.

Offord, D.R. (1989). Risk factors and prevention [OSAP Prevention Monograph-2]. *Prevention of Mental Disorders, Alcohol and Other Drug Use in Children and Adolescents*, Chapter 8, 273–307.

Olweus, D. (1979). Stability of aggressive reaction patterns in males: a review. *Psychological Bulletin*, 86, 852–875.

Patterson, G.R., DeBaryshe, B.D., & Ramsey, E. (1989). A developmental perspective on Antisocial Behavior. *American Psychologist*, 44, 329–335.

Sarason, I.G., & Ganzer, V.J. (1969). Developing appropriate social behaviors of juvenile delinquents. In J. Krumboltz & C. Thoresen (Eds.), *Behavior Counseling Cases and Techniques* (pp. 178–1993). New York: Holt, Rinehart & Winston.

Student, D., & Myhill, J. (1986). *Mental Health Needs at the Montrose and Hickey Schools: Models for Treatment*. Unplublished manuscript.

Weisinger, H. (1985). *Dr. Weisinger's Anger Work-Out Book*. New York, NY: William Morrow & Co.

West, D.J., & Farrington, D.P. (1977). *The Delinquent Way of Life*. London: Heinemann.

Chapter 4: Mood Disorders: Major Depression, Dysthymic Disorder, and Bipolar Disorder

Akiskal, H.S., & Weise, R.E. (1992). The clinical spectrum of so-called "minor" depressions. *American Journal of Psychotherapy*, 46,9–22.

American Psychiatric Association (2000). *The Diagnostic Statistical Manual of Mental Disorders*, (4th ed., Text Revision). *American Psychiatric Association*: Washington, DC.

Arnett, J.J. (1999). Adolescent storm and stress, reconsidered. *American Psychologist*, 54, 317–326.

Brook, J.S., Cohen, P., & Brook, DW (1998). Longitudinal study of co-occurring psychiatric disorders and substance use. *Journal of the American Academy of Child and Adolescent Psychiatry*, 37, 322–330.

Carlson, G.A. (1990). Annotation: Child and adolescent mania—diagnostic considerations. *Journal of Child Psychology and Psychiatry*, 31, 331–341.

Compas, B.E., Ey, S., & Grant, K.E. (1993). Taxonomy, assessment, and diagnosis of depression during adolescence. *Psychological Bulletin*, 114, 323–344.

Davis, D.L., Bean, G.J., Schumacher, J.E., & Stringer, T.L. (1991). Prevalence of emotional disorders in a juvenile justice institutional population. *American Journal of Forensic Psychology*, 9, 5–17.

Faber, A., & Mazlish, E. (1980). *How to Talk So Kids Will Listen and Listen So Kids Will Talk*. New York: Avon Books.

Gershon, E.S., Hamovit, J., Girpff. K., Dibble, E., Leckman J.F., Sceery, W., Targum, S.D., Nurnberger, J.I., Goldin, L.R., & Bunney, W.E. (1982). A family study of schizoaffective, bipolar I, bipolar II, unipolar probands and normal controls. *Archives of General Psychiatry*, 39, 1157–1167.

Hovens, J.G., Cantwell, D.P., & Kiriakos, R. (1994). Psychiatric comorbidity in hospitalized adolescent substance abusers. *Journal of the American Academy of Child and Adolescent Psychiatry*, 33, 476–483.

Ingersoll, B.D., & Goldstein, S. (1995). *Lonely, Sad and Angry: A Parent's Guide to Depression in Children and Adults*. New York: Doubleday.

Kandel, D.B. (1988). Substance use, depressive mood, and suicidal ideation in adolescence and young adulthood. In A.R. Stiffman & R.A. Feldman (Eds.), *Advances in adolescent mental health. A research-practice annual: Depression and suicide* (Vol. 3, pp. 127–143). Greenwich, CT: JAI Press.

Kandel, D.B., & Davies, M. (1986). Adult sequelae of adolescent depressive symptoms. *Archives of General Psychiatry*, 43, 255–262.

Kovacs, J., Akiskal, H.S., Gatsonis, C., & Parrone, P.L. (1994). *Archives of General Psychiatry*, 51, 365–374.

Kovacs, M., Feinberg, T.L., Crouse-Novak, M., Paulauskas, S.L., Pollock, M., & Finkelstein, R. (1984). Depressive disorders in childhood. II. A longitudinal study of the risk for a subsequent major depression. *Archives of General Psychiatry*, 41, 643–649.

Kovacs, M., Goldston, D., & Gatsonis, C. (1993). Suicidal behaviors and childhood-onset depressive disorders: A longitudinal investigation. *Journal of the American Academy of Child and Adolescent Psychiatry*, 32, 8–20.

McCauley, E., Myers, K., Mitchell, J., Calderon, R., Schloredt, K., & Treder, R. (1993). Depression in young people: Initial presentation and clinical course. *Journal of the American Academy of Child and Adolescent Psychiatry*, 32, 714–722.

McClellan, J., & Werry, J.S. (1993). Practice parameters for the assessment and treatment of children and adolescents with bipolar disorder. *Journal of the American Academy of Child and Adolescent Psychiatry*, 36 (10 Supplement), 157S–176S.

Puig-Antich, J., Lukens, E., Davies, M., Goetz, D., Brennan-Quattrock, J., & Todak, G. (1985). Psychosocial functioning in prepubertal major depressive disorders: II. Interpersonal relationships after sustained recovery from affective episodes. *Archives of General Psychiatry*, 42, 511–517.

Reynolds, W.M. (1994) Depression in adolescence: Contemporary issues and perspectives. In T.H. Ollendick & R.J. Prinz (Eds.), *Advances in Clinical Child Psychology* (Vol 16, pp. 261–315). New York: Plenum Press.

Rice, J., Reich, T., Andreasen, N.C., *et al.* (1987). The familial transmission of bipolar disorder. *Archives of General Psychiatry*, 44, 441–447.

Timmons-Mitchell, J., Brown, C., Schultz, S.C., Webster, S.E., Underwood, L.A., & Semple, W.E. (1997). Comparing the mental health needs of female and male incarcerated juvenile delinquents. *Behavioral Sciences and the Law*, 15, 195–202.

Chapter 5: Attention-Deficit/Hyperactivity Disorder

American Psychiatric Association (2000). *The Diagnostic Statistical Manual of Mental Disorders*, (4th ed., Text Revision). American Psychiatric Association: Washington, DC.

Barkley, R.A. (1995). *Taking Charge of ADHD: The complete, authoritative guide for parents*. Guilford Press: New York.

Biederman, J., & Steingard, R. (1989). Attention-deficit hyperactivity disorder in adolescents. *Psychiatric Annals*, 19, 587–596.

Boris, M., & Mandel, F.S. (1994). Foods and additives are common causes of the attention deficit hyperactive disorder in children. *Annals of Allergy*, 72, 462–468.

Davis, D.L., Bean, G.J., Schumacher, J.E., & Stringer, T.L. (1991). Prevalence of emotional disorders in a juvenile justice institutional population. *American Journal of Forensic Psychology*, 9, 5–17.

Edwards, M.C., Schulz, E.G., & Long, N. (1995). The role of the family in the assessment of attention deficit hyperactivity disorder. *Clinical Psychology Review*, 15, 375–394.

Gillis, J.J., Gilger, J.W., Pennington, B.F., & Defries, J.C. (1992). Attention-deficit disorder in reading-disabled twins: Evidence for a genetic etiology. *Journal of Abnormal Child Psychology*, 20, 303–315.

Halikas, J.A., Meller, J., Morse, C., & Lyttle, M.D. (1990). Predicting substance abuse in juvenile offenders: Attention deficit disorder vs. aggressivity. *Child Psychiatry and Human Development*, 21, 49–55.

Hartsough, C.S., & Lambert, N.M. (1985). Medical factors in hyperactive and control children: Prenatal, developmental, and health history findings. *American Journal of Orthopsychiatry*, 55, 190–201.

Kavale, K.A., & Forness, S.R. (1983). Hyperactivity and diet treatment: A meta-analysis of the Feingold hypothesis. *Journal of Learning Disabilities*, 16, 324–330.

Lowe, C. (1999, September). Paying attention. *Energy Times*, pp. 24–28.

National Institute of Health (November, 1998). Diagnosis and treatment of attention deficit hyperactivity disorder. *NIH Consensus Statement*, 16(2), 1–37.

Riggs, P.D., Leon, S.L., Mikulich, M.S., & Pottle, L.C. (1998). An open trial of Bupropion for ADHD in adolescents with substance use disorders and conduct disorder. *Journal of the American Academy of Child and Adolescent Psychiatry*, 37, 1271–1278.

Rosen, L.A., Booth, S.R., Bender, M.E., McGrath, M.L., Sorrell, S., & Drabman, R.S. (1988). Effects of sugar (sucrose) on children's behavior. *Journal of Consulting and Clinical Psychology*, 56, 583–589.

Timmons-Mitchell, J., Brown, C., Schultz, S.C., Webster, S.E., Underwood, L.A., & Semple, W.E. (1997). Comparing the mental health needs of female and male incarcerated juvenile delinquents. *Behavioral Sciences and the Law*, 15, 195–202

Weiss, B. (1982). Food additives and environmental chemicals as sources of childhood behavior disorders. *Journal of the American Academy of Child Psychiatry*, 21, 144–152.

Chapter 6: Posttraumatic Stress Disorder

American Psychiatric Association (2000). *Diagnostic and Statistical Manual of Mental Disorders*, (4th ed., Text Revision). Washington, DC: American Psychiatric Association.

Berliner, L. (2000, January). *Treating Psychosocial Trauma in Children*. Grand Rounds, Division of Child and Adolescent Psychiatry, Children's Hospital and Regional Medical Center, Seattle.

Cauffman, E., Feldman, S.S., Waterman, J., & Steiner, H. (1998). Posttraumatic stress disorder among female juvenile offenders. *Journal of the American Academy of Child and Adolescent Psychiatry*, 37, 1209–1216.

Davidson, J.R., Hughes, D., Blazer, D.G, & George, L.K. (1991). Posttraumatic stress disorder in the community: An epidemiological study. *Psychological Medicine*, 21, 713–721.

Fitzpatrick, K.M., & Boldizar, J.P. (1993). The prevalence and consequences of exposure to violence among African-American youth. *Journal of the American Academy of Child and Adolescent Psychiatry*, 32, 424–430.

Giaconia, R.M, Reinherz, H.Z., Silverman, A.B., Pakiz, B., Frost, A.K., & Cohen, E. (1995). Traumas and posttraumatic stress disorder in a community population of older adolescents. *Journal of the American Academy of Child and Adolescent Psychiatry*, 34, 1369–1380.

Horowitz, K., Weine, S., & Jekel, J. (1995). PTSD symptoms in urban adolescent girls: Compounded community trauma. *Journal of the American Academy of Child and Adolescent Psychiatry*, 34, 1353–1361.

Lipovsky, J.A. (1991). Posttraumatic stress disorder in children. *Family Community Health*, 14, 42–51.

Marmar, C.R. (1991). Brief dynamic psychotherapy of posttraumatic stress disorder. *Psychiatric Annuals*, 21, 405–414.

Martinez, P., & Richters, J.E. (1993). The NIMH Community Violence Project: II. Children's distress symptoms associated with violence exposure. *Psychiatry*, 56, 22–35.

Putnam, F.W. (1997). *Dissociation in Children and Adolescents* (p. 279). New York, NY: The Guilford Press.

Pynoos, R.S. (1992). Grief and trauma in children and adolescents. *Bereavement Care*, 11, 2–11.

Pynoos, R.S., & Eth, S. (1984). The child as witness to homicide. *Journal of Social Issues*, 87–108.

Saywitz, K.J., Mannarino, A.P., Berliner, L., & Cohen, J.A. (2000). Treatment for sexually abused children and adolescents. *American Psychologist*, 55, 1040–1049.

Steiner, H., Garcia, I.G., & Matthews, Z. (1997). Posttraumatic stress disorder in incarcerated juvenile delinquents. *Journal of the American Academy of Child and Adolescent Psychiatry*, 36, 357–365.

Terr, L.C. (1991). Childhood traumas: An outline and overview. *American Journal of Psychiatry*, 148, 10–20.

Warner, B.S., & Weist, M.D. (1996). Urban youth as witnesses to violence: Beginning assessment and treatment efforts. *Journal of Youth and Adolescence*, 25, 361–377.

Chapter 7: Developmental Disorders: Mental Retardation, Learning Disorders, and Fetal Alcohol Syndrome (FAS)

Aase, J.M., Jones, K.L., & Clarren, S.K. (1995). Do we need the term "FAE"? *Pediatrics*, 95, 428–430.

American Psychiatric Association (2000). *Diagnostic and Statistical Manual of Mental Disorders*, (4th ed., Text Revision). Washington, DC: American Psychological Association.

Astley, S.J., & Clarren, S.K. (1999). *Diagnostic Guide for Fetal Alcohol Syndrome and Related Conditions: The 4-Digit Diagnostic Code*, (2nd ed.). University of Washington Publication Services. Seattle, WA: University of Washington.

Casey, P.A., & Keilitz, I. (1990). Estimating the prevalence of learning disabled and mentally retarded juvenile offenders. In P.E. Leone (Ed.), *Understanding Troubled and Troubling Youth* (pp. 82–101). Newbury Park, CA: Sage.

Gardner, H. (1993). *Multiple Intelligences*. New York: Basic Books.

Goleman, D. (1995). *Emotional Intelligence*. New York: Bantam Books.

Leone, P.E., & Meisel, S. (1997). Improving education services for students in detention and confinement facilities. *Children's Legal Rights Journal*, 17, 1–12.

National Institute of Mental Health (1993). *Learning Disabilities* (NIH Publication No. 93-3611). Bethesda, MD: U.S. Department of Health and Human Services, Public Health Service, National Institutes of Health.

332

Juvenile Offenders with Mental Health Disorders: Who Are They and What Do We Do With Them?

Chapter 8: Schizophrenia and Other Psychotic Disorders

American Academy of Child and Adolescent Psychiatry (AACAP): Primary Authors: McClellan, J., & Werry, J. Practice parameters for the assessment and treatment of children and adolescents with schizophrenia, revised (2001). *Journal of the American Academy of Child and Adolescent Psychiatry*.

American Psychiatric Association (APA) (2000). *Diagnostic and Statistical Manual of Mental Disorders*, (4th ed., Text Revision). Washington, DC: American Psychiatric Association.

Del Beccaro, M.A., Burke, P., & McCauley, E. (1988). Hallucinations in children: A follow-up study. *Journal of the American Academy of Child and Adolescent Psychiatry*, 27, 462–465.

Garralda, M.E. (1984). Hallucinations in children with conduct and emotional disorders: I. The clinical phenomena. *Psychological Medicine*, 14, 589–596.

Kumra, S., Jacobsen, L.K., Lenane, M., Zahn, T.P., Wiggs, E., Alaghband-Rad, J., Castellanos, F.X., Frazier, J.A., McKenna, K., Gordon, C.T., Smith, A., Hamburger, S., & Rapoport, J.L. (1998). "Multidimensionally Impaired Disorder": Is it a variant of very early-onset schizophrenia? *Journal of the American Academy of Child and Adolescent Psychiatry*, 37, 91–99.

Lewis, D.O., Pincus, J.H., Lovely, R., Spitzer, E., & Moy, E. (1987). Biopsychosocial characteristics of matched samples of delinquents and nondelinquents. *Journal of the American Academy of Child and Adolescent Psychiatry*, 26, 744–752.

Timmons-Mitchell, J., Brown, C., Schultz, S.C., Webster, S.E., Underwood, L.A., & Semple, W.E. (1997). Comparing the mental health needs of female and male incarcerated juvenile delinquents. *Behavioral Sciences and the Law*, 15, 195–202.

Ulloa, R.E., Birmaher, B., Axelson, D., Williamson, D.E., Brent, D.A., Ryan, N.D., Bridge, J., & Baugher, M. (2000). Psychosis in a pediatric mood and anxiety disorders clinic: Phenomenology and correlates. *Journal of the American Academy of Child and Adolescent Psychiatry*, 39, 337–345.

Werry, J.S., & Taylor, E. (1994). Schizophrenia and allied disorders. In *Child and Adolescent Psychiatry: Modern Approaches*, (3rd ed.). Rutter, M., Hersov, L., & Taylor, E. (Eds.), (pp 594–615). Oxford: Blackwell Scientific.

Werry, J.S., McClellan, J.M., & Chard, L. (1991). Childhood and adolescent schizophrenic, bipolar, and schizoaffective disorders: a clinical and outcome study. *Journal of the American Academy of Child and Adolescent Psychiatry*, 30, 457–465.

Chapter 9: Substance Use Disorders

American Psychiatric Association (APA) (2000). *Diagnostic and Statistical Manual of Mental Disorders*, (4th ed., Text Revision). Washington, DC: American Psychiatric Association.

Davis, D.L., Bean Jr., G.J., Schumacher, J.E., & Stringer, T.L. (1991). Prevalence of emotional disorders in a juvenile justice institutional population. *American Journal of Forensic Psychology*, 9, 5–17.

Deschenes, E., & Greenwood, P. (1994). Treating the juvenile drug offender. In D. MacKenzie & C. Uchida (Eds.), *Drugs and Crime: Evaluating Public Policy Initiatives*. Thousand Oaks, CA: Sage.

Hawkins, J.D., Lishner, D.M., Catalano, R.F., & Howard, M.O. (1985). Childhood predictors of adolescent substance abuse: Toward an empirically grounded theory. *Journal of Children in Contemporary Society*, 18, 11–48.

McLellan, T., & Dembo, R. (1995). Screening and assessment of alcohol and other drug-abusing adolescents. *Treatment Improvement Protocol (TIPS) Series #3*. Rockville, MD: Center for Substance Abuse Treatment, U.S. Department of Health and Human Services.

National Institute of Justice (1994). Drug use forecasting: 1993 annual report on juvenile arrestees/detainees. *Research in Brief*. Washington, DC: National Institute of Justice.

Oetting, E.R., & Beauvais, F. (1990). Adolescent drug use: Findings of national and local surveys. *Journal of Consulting and Clinical Psychology*, 58, 385–394.

Tarter, R.E., & Hegedus, A.M. (1991). The Drug Use Screening Inventory: Its application in the evaluation and treatment of alcohol and other drug use. *Alcohol Health and Research World*, 15, 65–75.

Winters, K. (1999). Screening and assessing adolescents for substance use disorders. *Treatment Improvement Protocol (TIPS) Series #31*. Rockville, MD: Center for Substance Abuse Treatment, U.S. Department of Health and Human Services.

Winters, K.C. (1992). Development of an adolescent alcohol and other drug abuse screening scale: Personal Experience Screening Questionnaire. *Addictive Behaviors*, 17, 479–490.

Winters, K.C., & Henly, G.A. (1989). *Personal Experience Inventory Test and Manual*. Los Angeles: Western Psychological Association.

Winters, K.C., & Henly, G.A. (1993). *Adolescent Diagnostic Interview Schedule and Manual*. Los Angeles: Western Psychological Association.

Chapter 10: Co-Occurring Mental Health and Substance Use Disorders

American Psychiatric Association (APA) (2000). *Diagnostic and Statistical Manual of Mental Disorders*, (4th ed., Text Revision). Washington, DC: American Psychiatric Association.

Brent, D.A., Perper, J.A., Moritz, G., Allman, C., Friend, A., Roth, C., Schweers, J., Balach, L., & Baugher, M. (1993). Psychiatric risk factors for adolescent suicide: A case-control study. *Journal of the American Academy of Child and Adolescent Psychiatry*, 32, 521–529.

Drake, R.E., Mercer-McFadden, C., Mueser, K.T., McHugo, G.J., & Bond, G.R. (1998). Review of integrated mental health and substance abuse treatment for patients with dual disorders. *Schizophrenia Bulletin*, 24, 589–608.

Hawkins, J.D., Catalano, R.F., & Miller, J.Y. (1992). Risk and protective factors for alcohol and other drug problems in adolescence and early adulthood: Implications for substance abuse prevention. *Psychological Bulletin*, 112, 64–105.

Kaminer, Y., Tarter, R.E., Bukstein, O.G., & Kabene, M. (1992). Comparison between treatment completers and noncompleters among dually diagnosed substance-abusing adolescents. *Journal of the American Academy of Child and Adolescent Psychiatry*, 31, 1046–1049.

Milin, R., Halikas, J.A., Meller, J.E., & Morse, C. (1991). Psychopathology among substance abusing juvenile offenders. *Journal of the American Academy of Child and Adolescent Psychiatry*, 30, 569–574.

Miller, W.R., & Rollnick, S. (1991). *Motivational Interviewing: Preparing People for Change*. New York: Guilford Press.

Peters, R.H., & Bartoi, M.G. (1997). *Screening and Assessment of Co-Occurring Disorders in the Justice System*. Department of Mental Health Law and Policy, Louis de la Parte Florida Mental Health Institute University of South Florida. The GAINS Center.

Peters, R.H., & Hills, H.A. (1993). Inmates with co-occurring substance abuse and mental health disorders. In H.J. Steadman & J.J. Cocozza (Eds.), *Mental Illness in America's Prisons*. Seattle, WA: National Coalition for the Mentally Ill in the Criminal Justice System.

Ries, R. (1995). Assessment and treatment of patients with coexisting mental illness and alcohol and other drug abuse. *Treatment Improvement Protocol (TIPS) Series #9*. Rockville, MD: Center for Substance Abuse Treatment, U.S. Department of Health and Human Services.

Chapter 11: Suicidal Behavior Among Juvenile Offenders

Alessi, N.E., McManus, M., Brickman, A., & Grapentine, L. (1984). Suicidal behavior among serious juvenile offenders. *American Journal of Psychiatry*, 141, 286–287.

Berman, A.L. & Jobes, D.A. (1994). *Adolescent Suicide: Assessment and Intervention*. Washington, D.C.: American Psychological Association.

Brent, D.A., & Perper, J.A. (1995). Research in adolescent suicide: Implications for training, service delivery, and public policy. *Suicide and Life Threatening Behavior*, 25, 222–230.

Brent, D.A., Perper, J.A., & Allman, C. (1987). *Alcohol, firearms and suicide among youth: Temporal trends in Allegheny County, PA, 1960–1983*. Journal of American Medical Association (JAMA), 257, 3369–3372.

Brent, D.A., Perper, J.A., Goldstein, C.E., *et al.* (1988). Risk factors for adolescent suicide: A comparison of adolescent suicide victims with suicidal inpatients. *Archives of General Psychiatry*, 45, 581–588.

Brent, D.A., Perper, J.A., Moritz, G., Allman, C., Friend, A., Roth, C., Schweers, J., Balach, L., & Baugher, M. (1993). Psychiatric risk factors for adolescent suicide: A case control study. *Journal of the American Academy of Child and Adolescent Psychiatry*, 32, 521–529.

Centers for Disease Control and Prevention (1997). *Deaths and death rates: All races, both sexes, 15–24 years old*. Hyattsville, MD: U.S. Department of Health and Human Services.

Davis, D.D., Bean, G.J., Schumacher, J.E., & Stringer (1991). Prevalence of emotional disorders in a juvenile justice institutional population. *American Journal of Forensic Psychology*, 9, 5–17.

Dembo, R., Williams, L., Wish, E.D., Berry, E., Getreu, A., Washburn, M., & Schmeidler, J. (1990). Examination of the relationships among drug use, emotional/psychological problems, and crime among youths entering a juvenile detention center. *The International Journal of the Addictions*, 25, 1301–40.

Hayes, L.M. (1995). *Prison Suicide: An Overview and Guide to Prevention*. Washington, DC: U.S. Justice Department, National Institute of Corrections.

Hayes, L.M. (1999). *Suicide Prevention in Juvenile Correction and Detention Facilities*. Office of Juvenile Justice and Delinquency Prevention, Office of Justice Programs, U.S. Department of Justice.

Hayes, L.M., & Rowan, J.R. (1988). *National Study of Jail Suicides: Seven Years Later*. Washington, DC: U.S. Department of Justice, National Institute of Corrections.

Hughes, D.H. (1995). Can the clinician predict suicide? *Psychiatric Services*, 46, 449–451.

Ladely, S.J., & Puskar, K.R. (1994). Adolescent suicide: Behaviors, risk factors, and psychiatric nursing interventions. *Issues in Mental Health Nursing*, 15, 497–504.

Marttunen, M. (1994). Psychosocial maladjustment, mental disorders and stressful life events precede adolescent suicide. *Psychiatria Fennica*, 25, 39–51.

Parent, D.G., Leiter, V., Kennedy, S., Livens, L., Wentworth, D., & Wilcox, S. (1994). *Conditions of Confinement: Juvenile Detention and Correction Facilities*. Washington, D.C.: U.S. Department of Justice, Office of Justice Programs, Office of Juvenile Justice and Delinquency Prevention.

Rhode, P., Seeley, J.R., & Mace, D.E. (1997). Correlates of suicidal behavior in a juvenile detention population. *Suicide and Life-Threatening Behavior*, 27, 164–175.

Shaffer, D., Gould, M.S., Fisher, P., Trautman, P., Moreau, D., Kleinman, M., & Flory, M. (1996). Psychiatric diagnosis in child and adolescent suicide. *Archives of General Psychiatry*, 53, 339–348.

Shafii, M., Carrigan, S., Whittinghill, J.R., & Derrick, A. (1985). Psychological autopsy of completed suicides in children and adolescents. *American Journal of Psychiatry*, 142, 1061–1064.

Chapter 12: Self-Injurious Behavior Among Juvenile Offenders

Favazza, A.R., & Favazza, B. (1987). *Bodies Under Siege: Self-Mutilation in Culture and Psychiatry*. The John Hopkins University Press: Baltimore, MD.

Kahan, J., & Pattison, E.M. (1984). Proposal for a distinctive diagnosis: the Deliberate Self-Harm Syndrome. *Suicide and Life Threatening Behavior*, 14, 17–35.

Rosen, P.M., Walsh, B.W., & Rode, S.A. (1990). Interpersonal loss and self-mutilation. *Suicide and Life Threatening Behavior*, 20, 177–184.

Walsh, B.W., & Rosen, P.M. (1988). *Self-Mutilation: Theory, Research and Treatment*. The Guilford Press: New York.

Chapter 13: Screening and Assessment of Juvenile Offenders with Mental Health Disorders

Abikoff, H.A., Courtney, M., Pelham, W.E., & Koplewicz, H.D. (1993). Teachers' ratings of disruptive behaviors: The influence of halo effects. *Journal of Abnormal Child Psychology*, 21, 519–533.

Achenbach, T.M. (1991). *Manual for the child behavior checklist*. Burlington, VT: The University of Vermont, Department of Psychiatry.

American Correctional Association (1991a). *Standards for Juvenile Training Schools*. Lanham, MD: American Correctional Association.

American Correctional Association (1991b). *Standards for Juvenile Detention Facilities*. Lanham, MD: American Correctional Association.

American Correctional Association. (2002). *2002 Standards Supplement*. Lanham, MD: American Correctional Association.

Bernstein, D.P., Ahluvalia, T., Pogge, D., & Handelsman, L. (1997). Validity of the childhood trauma questionnaire in an adolescent psychiatric population. *Journal of the American Academy of Child and Adolescent Psychiatry*, 36, 340–348.

Briere, J. (1996). *Trauma Symptom Checklist for Children*. Odessa, FL: Psychological Assessment Resources, Inc.

Butcher, J.N., Williams, C.L., Graham, J.R., Archer, R.P., Tellegren, A., Ben-Porath, Y.S., & Kaemmer, B. (1992). *Minnesota Multiphasic Personality Inventory-Adolescent (MMPI-A): Manual for administration, scoring, and interpretation.* Minneapolis: University of Minnesota Press.

Comtois, K.A., Ries, R., & Armstrong, H.E. (1994). Case manager ratings of the clinical status of dually diagnosed outpatients. *Hospital and Community Psychiatry, 45,* 568–573.

Conners, C.K., Sitarenios, G., Parker, J.D., & Epstein, J.N. (1998a). The revised Conners Parent Rating Scale (CPRS-R): Factor structure, reliability, and criterion validity. *Journal of Abnormal Child Psychology, 26,* 257–268.

Conners, C.K., Sitarenios, G., Parker, J.D., & Epstein, J.N. (1998b). Revision and Restandardization of the Conners Reacher Rating Scale (CTRS-R): Factor structure, reliability, and criterion validity. *Journal of Abnormal Child Psychology, 26,* 279–291.

Derogatis, L.R. (1983). *The SCL-90-R: Administration, Scoring, and Procedures Manual-II.* Towson, MD: Clinical Psychometric Research.

Derogatis, L.R., & Melisaratos, N. (1983). The brief symptom inventory: An introductory report. *Psychological Medicine, 13,* 595–605.

Epstein, M.H. (1999). The development and validation of a scale to assess the emotional and behavioral strengths of children and adolescents. *Remedial and Special Education, 20,* 258–263.

Grisso, T., & Barnum, R. (2000). *Massachusetts Youth Screening Instrument-2: User's Manual and Technical Report.* Worcester, MA: University of Massachusetts Medical School.

Herjanic, B., & Reich, W. (1982). Development of a structured psychiatric interview for children: Agreement between child and parent on individual symptoms. *Journal of Abnormal Child Psychology, 10,* 307–324.

Hodges, K., & Wong, M.M. (1996). Psychometric characteristics of a multidimensional measure to assess impairment: The Child and Adolescent Functional Assessment Scale. *Journal of Child and Family Studies, 5,* 445–467.

Kaminer, Y., Bukstein, O., & Tarter, R.E. (1991). The teen-addiction severity index: rationale and reliability. *International Journal of Addiction, 26,* 219–226.

Latimer, W.M., Winters, K.C., & Stinchfield, R.D. (1997). Screening for drug abuse among adolescents in clinical and correctional settings using the problem-oriented screening instrument for teenagers. *American Journal of Drug and Alcohol Abuse, 23,* 79–98.

Meyers, K., McLellan, A.T., & Jaeger, J.L., & Pettinati, H.M. (1995). The development of the Comprehensive Addiction Severity Index for adolescents (CASI-A). An interview for assessing multiple problems of adolescents. *Journal of Substance Abuse Treatment, 12,* 181–193.

Millon, T.M. (1983). *Millon Adolescent Clinical Inventory (MACI) manual.* Minneapolis, MN: National Computer Systems, Inc.

Office of Juvenile Justice and Delinquency Prevention (OJJDP) (1995). *Guide for implementing the comprehensive strategy for serious, violent, and chronic juvenile offenders.* Washington, DC: U.S. Department of Justice.

Oldenettel, D., & Wordes, M. (2000). *The community assessment center concept.* Office of Juvenile Justice and Delinquency Prevention (OJJDP) Juvenile Justice Bulletin. US Department of Justice.

Peters, R.H., & Bartoi, M.G. (1997). *Screening and Assessment of Co-Occurring Disorders in the Justice System.* Department of Mental Health Law and Policy, Louis de la Parte Florida Mental Health Institute, University of South Florida. The GAINS Center.

Ramirez, S.Z., Wassef, A., Paniagua, F.A., & Linskey, A.O. (1996). Mental health providers' perceptions of cultural variables in evaluating ethnically diverse clients. *Professional Psychology: Research and Practice, 27,* 284–288.

Reynolds, W.M. (1987). *Reynolds Adolescent Depression Scale (RADS): Professional Manual.* Odessa, FL: Psychological Assessment Resources.

Reynolds, C.R., & Paget, K.D. (1983). National normative and reliability data for the revised children's manifest anxiety scale. *Journal of Consulting and Clinical Psychology, 49,* 352–359.

Sattler, J.M. (1988). *Assessment of Children,* 3rd ed. San Diego, CA: Jerome M. Sattler.

336

Juvenile Offenders with Mental Health Disorders: Who Are They and What Do We Do With Them?

Shaffer, D., Fisher, P., Lucas, C.P., Dulcan, M.K., & Schwab-Stone, M.E. (2000). NIMH diagnostic interview schedule for children version IV (NIMH DISC-IV): Description, differences from previous versions, and reliability of some common diagnoses. *Journal of the American Academy of Child and Adolescent Psychiatry*, 39, 28–38.

Sitarenios, G., & Kovacs, M. (1999). Use of the children's depression inventory. In M.E. Maruish (Ed.), *The Use of Psychological Testing for Treatment Planning and Outcomes Assessment*, 2nd ed., (pp. 267–298). Mahwah, NJ: Lawrence Erlbaum Associates, Inc.

Steer, R.A., Kumar, G., Ranieri, W.F., & Beck, A.T. (1998). *Journal of Psychopathology and Behavioral Assessment*, 20, 127–137.

Suzuki, L.A., & Kugler, J.E. (1995). Intelligence and personality assessment: Multicultural perspectives. In J.G. Ponterotto, J.M. Casas, L.A. Suzuki, & C.M. Alexander (Eds.), *Handbook of Multicultural Counseling*. Thousand Oaks, CA: Sage Publications, Inc.

Verhulst, F.C., & Van der Ende, J. (1992). Agreement between parents' reports and adolescents' self-reports of problem behavior. *Journal of Child Psychology and Psychiatry*, 33, 1011–1023.

Washington State Detention Managers Association & Boesky, L.M. (2000). *The Mental Health Juvenile Detention Admission Tool (MH-JDAT)*. Seattle, WA: Washington State Detention Managers Association and L.M. Boesky.

Winters, K.C., Stinchfield, R.D. & Henly, G.A. (1993). Further validation of new scales measuring adolescent alcohol and other drug abuse. *Journal of Studies on Alcohol*, 54, 534–541.

Chapter 14: Treatment of Juvenile Offenders with Mental Health Disorders

Alexander, J., Barton, C., Gordon, D., Grotpeter, J., Hansson, K., Harrison, R., Mears, S., Mihalic, S., Parsons, B., Pugh, C., Schulman, S., Waldron, H., & Sexton, T. (1998). *Blueprints for Violence Prevention, Book Three: Functional Family Therapy*. Boulder, CO: Center for the Study and Prevention of Violence.

Altschuler, D.M., & Armstrong, T.L. (1996). Aftercare not afterthought: Testing the IAP model. *Juvenile Justice*, 3, 15–22.

Altschuler, D.M., & Armstrong, T.L. (1997). Reintegrating high-risk juvenile offenders from secure correctional facilities into the community: Report on a four state demonstration. *Corrections Management Quarterly*, 1, 75–83.

American Correctional Association (1991a). *Standards for Juvenile Training Schools*, 3rd ed. Lanham, MD: American Correctional Association.

American Correctional Association (1991b). *Standards for Juvenile Detention Facilities*, 3rd ed. Lanham, MD: American Correctional Association.

American Correctional Association (1991c). *Standards for Small Juvenile Detention Facilities*. Lanham, MD: American Correctional Association.

American Correctional Association. (2002). *2002 Standards Supplement*. Lanham, MD: American Correctional Association.

Bedlington, M.M., Braukmann, C.J., Ramp, K.A., & Wolf, M.M. (1988). A comparison of treatment environments in community-based group homes for adolescent offenders. *Criminal Justice and Behavior*, 15, 349–363.

Borduin, C.M., Mann, B.J., Cone, L.T., Henggeler, S.W., Fucci, B.R., Blaske, D.M., & Williams, R.A. (1995). Multisystemic treatment of serious juvenile offenders: Long-term prevention of criminality and violence. *Journal of Consulting and Clinical Psychology*, 569–578.

Bowler, S.M. (April, 2001). *Project Hope*. Mental Health Issues and Juvenile Justice Teleconference. Washington, DC: Office of Juvenile Justice and Delinquency Prevention.

Braukmann, C.J., & Wolf, M.M. (1987). Behaviorally-based group homes for juvenile offenders. In E.K. Morris & C.J. Braukmann (Eds.), *Behavioral Approaches to Crime and Delinquency: A Handbook of Application, Research, and Concepts*, (pp. 135–159). New York, NY: Plenum Press.

Burns, B.J., Costello, J., Angold, A., Tweed, D., Stangl, D., Farmer, E., & Erkanli, A. (1995). Children's mental health service use across service sectors. *Health Affairs*, 14, 147–159.

Cohen, R., Parmelee, D.X., Irwin, L., Weisz, J.R., Howard, P., Purcell, P., & Best, A.M. (1990). Characteristics of children and adolescents in a psychiatric hospital and a corrections facility. *Journal of the American Academy of Child and Adolescent Psychiatry*, 29, 909–913.

Covington, S.S. (2000). Helping Women to Recover: Creating Gender-Specific Treatment for Substance Abusing Women and Girls in Community Corrections. In M. McMahon (Ed.), *What Works: Assessment to Assistance: Programs for Women in Community Corrections.* Lanham, MD: American Correctional Association and International Community Corrections Association.

Dishion, T.J., McCord, J., & Poulin, F. (1999) When interventions harm: Peer groups and problem behavior. *American Psychologist, 54*, 755–764.

Dodge, K.A., Price, J.M., Bachorowski, J., & Newman, J.P. (1990). Hostile attributional biases in severely aggressive adolescents. *Journal of Abnormal Psychology, 99*, 385–392.

Field, G. (1998). Continuity of offender treatment for substance use disorders from institution to community. *Treatment Improvement Protocol (TIP) Series #30, DHHS Publication No. (SMA) 98-3245.* Rockville, MD: Center for Substance Abuse Treatment, US Department of Health and Human Services.

Gendreau, P. (September, 1994). *What works in community corrections: Promising approaches in reducing criminal behavior.* Speech given at IARCA's Research Conference, Seattle, WA.

Goldstein, A.P., & Glick, B. (1987). Aggression replacement training. *Journal of Counseling and Development, 65*, 356–362.

Griffin, P.A., Hills, H.A., & Peters, R.H. (1996). Mental illness and substance abuse in offenders: Overcoming barriers to successful collaboration between substance abuse, mental health, and criminal justice staff. In S.H. Schnoll & S.M. Reiner (Eds.), *Criminal Justice Substance Abuse Cross Training: Working Together For Change.* Richmond, VA: Virginia Addiction Technology Transfer Center, Virginia Commonwealth University.

Guerra, N.G., & Slaby, R.G. (1990). Cognitive mediators of aggression in adolescent offenders: 2. Intervention. *Developmental Psychology, 26*, 269–277.

Henggeler, S.W., Melton, G.B., & Smith, L.A. (1992). Family preservation using multisystemic therapy: An effective alternative to incarcerating serious juvenile offenders. *Journal of Consulting and Clinical Psychology, 60*, 953–961.

Henggeler, S.W., Rowland, M.D., Randall, J., Ward, D.M., Pickrel, S.G., Cunningham, P.B., Miller, S.L., Edwards, J., Zealberg, J.J., Hand, L.D., & Santos, A.B. (1999). Home-based multisystemic therapy as an alternative to the hospitalization of youths in psychiatric crisis: Clinical outcomes. *Journal of the American Academy of Child and Adolescent Psychiatry, 38*, 1331–1339.

Herrera, J.M., Lawson, W.B., & Sramek, J.J. (1999). *Cross-Cultural Psychiatry.* Chichester, England: John Wiley and Sons.

Kamradt, B. (April, 2000). Wraparound Milwaukee: Aiding youth with mental health needs. *Journal of the Office of Juvenile Justice and Delinquency Prevention, 7*, 14–23.

Linehan, M. (1993). *Skills training manual for treating borderline personality disorder.* New York, NY: Guilford Press.

Lipsey, M.W. (1992). The effect of treatment on juvenile delinquents: results from meta-analysis. In F. Losel, T. Bliesener, & D. Bender (Eds.), *Psychology and Law: International Perspectives.* Berlin: de Gruyter.

Lipsey, M.W., & Wilson, D.B. (1998). Effective intervention for serious juvenile offenders. In R. Loeber & D.P. Farrington (Eds.), *Serious and Violent Juvenile Offenders: Risk Factors and Successful Interventions*, pp. 313–345. Thousand Oaks, CA: Sage Publications.

MacMahon, J.R. (1990). The psychological benefits of exercise and the treatment of delinquent adolescents. *Sports Medicine, 9*, 344–351.

McGuire, J., & Priestley, P. (1995). Reviewing "what works": Past, present and future. In J. McGuire (Ed.), *What Works: Reducing Reoffending—Guidelines from Research and Practice.* Sussex, England: John Wiley & Sons Ltd.

Pickrel, S.G., & Henggeler, S.W. (1996). Multisystemic therapy for adolescent substance abuse and dependence. *Child and Adolescent Psychiatric Clinics of North America, 5*, 201–211.

Rollnick, S., & Miller, W.R. (1995). What is motivational interviewing? *Behavioural and Cognitive Psychotherapy, 23*, 325–334.

Schoenthaler, S. (1985). Nutritional policies and institutional antisocial behavior. *Nutrition Today, 20*, 16–25.

Juvenile Offenders with Mental Health Disorders: Who Are They and What Do We Do With Them?

Schoenthaler, S.J. (1987). Malnutrution and maladaptive behavior: Two correlational analyses and a double-blind placebo-controlled challenge in five states. In W.B. Essman (Ed.), *Nutrients and Brain Function*. Basil, Switzerland: Karger.

Steadman, H.J. (1992). Boundary spanners: A key component for the effective interactions of the justice and mental health systems. *Law and Human Behavior*, 16, 75–87.

Swanson, A.J., Pantalon, M.V., & Cohen, K.R. (1999). Motivational interviewing and treatment adherence among psychiatric and dually diagnosed patients. *Journal of Nervous and Mental Disease*, 187, 630–635.

Zito, J.M., Safer, D.J., dosReis, S., Gardner, J.F., Boles, M., & Lynch, F. (2000). Trends in the prescribing of psychotropic medications to preschoolers. *Journal of the American Medical Association*, 283, 1025–1030.

Zito, J.M., Safer, D.J., dosReis, S., & Riddle, M.A. (1998). Racial disparity in psychotropic medications prescribed for youths with Medicaid insurance in Maryland. *Journal of the American Academy of Child and Adolescent Psychiatry*, 37, 179–184.

Chapter 15: Special Issues I: Minority Youth, Female Offenders, Homosexual Youth

Acoca, L., & Dedel, K. (1998). *No Place to Hide: Understanding and Meeting the Needs of Girls in the California Juvenile Justice System*. San Francisco, CA: National Council on Crime and Delinquency.

American Correctional Association (1990). *The Female Offender: What Does the Future Hold?* Laurel, MD: American Correctional Association.

American Psychiatric Association (1973). *DSMIVR*. Position statement on homosexuality and civil rights. *American Journal of Psychiatry*, 131, 497.

American Psychiatric Association (APA) (2000). *Diagnostic and Statistical Manual of Mental Disorders*, (4th ed., Text Revision). Washington, DC: American Psychiatric Association.

Blair, R.G. (1996). Risk and protective factors in the mental health status of Cambodian refugees in Utah. *Dissertation Abstracts*, 57, 2208.

Cohen, R., Parmalee, D.X., Irwin, L., Weisz, J.R., Howard, P., Purcell, P., & Best, A.M. (1990). Characteristics of children and adolescents in a psychiatric hospital and a corrections facility. *Journal of the American Academy of Child and Adolescent Psychiatry*, 29, 909–913.

Community Research Associates (1997). *Disproportionate Minority Confinement of Minority Juveniles in Secure Facilities: 1996 National Report*. Washington, DC: Office of Juvenile Justice and Delinquency Prevention.

Corley, C.J., Bynum, T.S., Prewitt, A., & Schram, P. (1996). The impact of race on juvenile court processes: Quantitative analyses with qualitative insights. *Caribbean Journal of Criminology & Social Psychology*, 1, 1–23.

Covington, S.S. (2000). Helping Women to Recover: Creating Gender-Specific Treatment for Substance Abusing Women and Girls in Community Corrections. In M. McMahon (Ed.), *What Works: Assessment to Assistance: Programs for Women in Community Corrections*. Lanham, MD: American Correctional Association and International Community Corrections Association.

Diala, C., Muntaner, C., Walrath, C., Nickerson, K.J., LaVeist, T.A., & Leaf, P.J. (2000). Racial differences in attitudes toward professional mental health care and in the use of services. *American Orthopsychiatric Association*, 70, 455–464.

Duclos, C.W., Beals, J., Novins, D.K., Martin, C., Jewett, C.S., & Manson, S.M. (1998). Prevalence of common psychiatric disorders among American Indian adolescent detainees. *Journal of the American Academy of Child and Adolescent Psychiatry*, 37, 866–873.

Fabrega, H., Ulrich, R., & Mezzich, J.E. (1993). Do Caucasian and black adolescents differ at psychiatric intake? *Journal of American Academy of Child and Adolescent Psychiatry*, 32, 407–413.

Flaskerud, J.H., & Hu, L. (1992). Relationship of ethnicity to psychiatric diagnosis. *The Journal of Nervous and Mental Disease*, 180, 296–303.

Garland, A.F., Hough, R.L., Landsverk, J.A., McCabe, K.M., Yeh, M., Ganger, W.C., & Reynolds, B.J. (2000). Racial and ethnic variations in mental health care utilization among children in foster care. *Children's Services: Social Policy, Research, and Practice*, 3, 133–146.

Kilgus, M.D., Pumariega, A.J., & Cuffe, S.P. (1995). Influence of race on diagnosis in adolescent psychiatric inpatients. *Journal of the American Academy of Child and Adolescent Psychiatry*, 34, 67–72.

Kunreuther, F. (1991). The Hetrick-Martin Institute: Services for youth. *Focal Point*, 5, 10–11.

Lewis, D.O., Balla, D.A., & Shanok, S.S. (1979). Some evidence of race bias in the diagnosis and treatment of the juvenile offender. *American Journal of Orthopsychiatry*, 49, 53–61.

Lewis, D.O., Shanok, S.S., Cohen, R.J., Kligfeld, M., & Frisone, G. (1980). Race bias in the diagnosis and disposition of violent adolescents. *American Journal of Psychiatry*, 137, 1211–1216.

Lewis, D.O., Shanok, S.S., & Pincus, J.H. (1982). A comparison of the neuropsychiatric status of female and male incarcerated delinquents: Some evidence of sex and race bias. *Journal of the American Academy of Child Psychiatry*, 21, 190–196.

Martin, T.W., & Grubb, H.J. (1990). Race bias in the diagnosis and treatment of juvenile offenders: Findings and suggestions. *Journal of Contemporary Psychotherapy*, 20, 259–272.

McMiller, M.P., & Weisz, J.R. (1996). Help-seeking preceding mental health clinic intake among African American, Latino, and Caucasian youth. *Journal of the American Academy of Child and Adolescent Psychiatry*, 35, 1086–1094.

Miller, B. (1998). Different, not more difficult: Gender-specific training helps bridge the gap. *Corrections Today*, December, 142–144.

Poe-Yamagata, E., & Butts, J.A. (1996). *Female offenders in the juvenile justice system: Statistics summary*. Pittsburgh, PA: Office of Juvenile Justice and Delinquency Prevention.

Poe-Yamagata, E., & Jones, M.A. (2000). And justice for some: differential treatment of minority youth in the justice system. Washington, DC: Building Blocks for Youth.

Radowsky, M., & Siegel, L.J. (1997). The gay adolescent: Stressors, adaptations, and psychosocial interventions. *Clinical Psychology Review*, 17, 191–216.

Ross, M.W. (1989). Gay youth in four cultures: A comparative study. *Journal of Homosexuality*, 17, 299–314.

Rotheram-Borus, M., Hunter, J., & Rosario, M. (1994). Suicidal behavior and gay-related stress among gay and bisexual adolescents. *Journal of Adolescent Research*, 9, 498–508.

Snyder, H.N., & Sickmund, M. (1999). *Juvenile offenders and victims: 1999 national report*. Washington, D.C.: Office of Juvenile Justice and Delinquency Prevention.

Stewart, D., Boesky, L.M., & Trupin, E.T. (1999). *Mental health screening of youth in JRA with significant emotional and behavioral problems*. Unpublished report, Seattle, WA: University of Washington.

Timmons-Mitchell, J., Brown, C., Schulz, C., Webster, S.E., Underwood, L.A., & Semple, W.E. (1997). Comparing the mental health needs of female and male incarcerated juvenile delinquents. *Behavioral Sciences and the Law*, 15, 195–202.

Westendorp, F., Brink, K.L., Roberson, M.K., & Ortiz, I.E. (1986). Variables which differentiate placement of adolescents into juvenile justice or mental health services. *Adolescence*, 21, 23–37.

Wierson, M., & Forehand, R. (1995). Predicting recidivism in juvenile delinquents: the role of mental health diagnosis and the qualification of conclusion by race, *Behavior Research and Therapy*, 33, 63–67.

Wordes, M., Bynum, T.S., & Corley, C.J. (1994). Locking up youth: The impact of race on detention decisions. *Journal of Research in Crime and Delinquency*, 31, 149–165.

Yeh, M., Takeuchi, D.T., & Sue, S. (1994). Asian-American children treated in the mental health system: A comparison of parallel and mainstream outpatient service centers. *Journal of Clinical Child Psychology*, 23, 5–12.

Chapter 16: Special Issues II: Head Trauma/Neuropsychiatric Factors, Violence and Mental Illness, Seclusion and Restraint, Malingering, Staff Training

American Correctional Association (1991a). *Standards for Juvenile Training Schools, 3rd Edition.* Lanham, MD: American Correctional Association.

American Correctional Association (1991b). *Standards for Juvenile Detention Facilities, 3rd Edition.* Lanham, MD: American Correctional Association.

340

Juvenile Offenders with Mental Health Disorders: Who Are They and What Do We Do With Them?

American Correctional Association. (2002). *2002 Standards Supplement*. Lanham, MD: American Correctional Association.

American Psychiatric Association (1973). *DSMIVR.* Position statement on homosexuality and civil rights. *American Journal of Psychiatry*, 131, 497.

American Psychiatric Association (APA) (2000). *Diagnostic and Statistical Manual of Mental Disorders,* (4th ed., Text Revision). Washington, DC: American Psychiatric Association.

Dodge, K.A., & Frame, C.L. (1982). Social cognitive biases and deficits in aggressive boys. *Child Development*, 53, 629–635.

Goldstein, A.P., & Glick, B. (1987). Aggression replacement training. *Journal of Counseling and Development*, 65, 356–362.

Gorenstein, E.E (1990). Neuropsychology of juvenile delinquency. *Forensic Reports*, 3, 15–48.

Grassian, S., & Friedman, N. (1986). Effects of sensory deprivation in psychiatric seclusion and solitary confinement. *International Journal of Law and Psychiatry*, 8, 49–65.

Guerra, N.G., & Slaby, R.G. (1990). Cognitive mediators of aggression in adolescent offenders: 2. Intervention. *Developmental Psychology,* 26, 269–277.

Hare, R.D. (1965). Temporal gradient of fear arousal in psychopaths. *Journal of Abnormal Psychology*, 70, 442–445.

Harrington, J.A. (1972). Violence: A clinical viewpoint. *British Medical Journal*, 1, 228–231.

Hux, K., Bond, V., Skinner, S., Belau, D., & Sanger, D. (1998). Parental report of occurrences and consequences of traumatic brain injury among delinquent and non-delinquent youth. *Brain Injury*, 12, 667–681.

Kropp, P.R., Cox, D.N., Roesch, R., & Eaves, D. (1989). The perceptions of correctional officers toward mentally disordered offenders. *International Journal of Law and Psychiatry,* 12, 181–188.

Lendemeijer, B., & Shortridge-Baggett, L. (1997). The use of seclusion in psychiatry: A literature review. *Scholarly Inquiry for Nursing Practice: An International Journal*, 11, 299–315.

Lewis, D.O., Pincus, J.H., Lovely, R., Spitzer, E., & Moy, E. (1987). Biopsychosocial characteristics of matched samples of delinquents and nondelinquents. *Journal of the American Academy of Child and Adolescent Psychiatry*, 26, 744–752.

Lewis, D.O., Shanok, S.S., Pincus, J.H., & Giammarino, M. (1982). The medical assessment of seriously delinquent boys: A comparison of pediatric, psychiatric, neurologic and hospital record data. *Journal of Adolescent Health Care*, 3, 160–164.

Lewis, D.O., Shanok, S.S., & Balla, D.A. (1979). Perinatal difficulties, head and face trauma, and child abuse in the medical histories of seriously delinquent children. *American Journal of Psychiatry*, 136, 419–423.

Lewis, D.O., Lovely, R., Yeager, C., Ferguson, G., Friedman, M., Sloane, G., Friedman, H., & Pincus, J.H. (1988). Intrinsic and environmental characteristics of juvenile murderers. *Journal of the American Academy of Child and Adolescent Psychiatry*, 27, 582–587.

Lewis, D.O., Moy, E., Jackson, J.D., Aaronson, R., Restifo, N., Serra, S., & Simos, A. (1985). Biopsychosocial characteristics of children who later murder: A prospective study. *American Journal of Psychiatry*, 142, 1161–1167.

Lewis D.O., Shanok, S.S., Grant, M., & Ritvo, E. (1983). Homicidally aggressive young children: Neuropsychiatric and experiential correlates. *American Journal of Psychiatry,* 140, 148–153.

Link, B.G., & Stueve, A. (1994). Psychotic symptoms and the violent/illegal behavior of mental patients compared to community controls. In J. Monahan & H.J. Steadman (Eds.), *Violence and Mental Disorders: Developments in Risk Assessment*, pp. 137–159. Chicago: University of Chicago Press.

Mischel, W. (1961). Preference for delayed reinforcement and social responsibility. *Journal of Abnormal and Social Psychology*, 136, 1–7.

Mitchell, J., & Varley, C. (1990). Isolation and restraint in juvenile correctional facilities. *Journal of the American Academy of Child and Adolescent Psychiatry*, 29, 251–255.

Neufeldt, V., & Guralnik, D.B. (1988). *Webster's New World Dictionary: Third College Edition.* Webster's New World: New York, NY.

Perry, B.D., & Pollard, D. (1997). Altered brain development following global neglect in early childhood. *Society for Neuroscience: Proceedings from Annual Meeting*, New Orleans.

Perry, B.D., Pollard, R.A., Blakley, T.L., Baker, W.L., & Vigilante, D. (1995). Childhood trauma, the neurobiology of adaptation and use-dependent development of the brain: How states become traits. *Infant Mental Health Journal*, 16, 271–291.

Siegman, A.W. (1961). The relation between future time perspective, time estimation, and impulse control in a group of young offenders and a control group. *Journal of Consulting Psychology*, 25, 470–475.

Slaby R.G., & Guerra, N. (1988). Cognitive mediators of aggression in adolescent offenders: 1. Assessment. *Developmental Psychology*, 24, 580–588.

Swanson, J.W., Borum, R., Swartz, M.S., & Monahan, J. (1996). Psychotic symptoms and disorders and the risk of violent behaviour in the community. *Criminal Behavior and Mental Health*, 6, 309–329.

Warnken, W., Rosenbaum, A., Fletcher, K, Hoge, S., & Adelman, S. (1994). Head-injured males: A population at risk for relationship aggression? *Violence and Victims*, 9, 153–166.

Werner, E., & Smith, R. (1992). *Overcoming the Odds: High Risk Children From Birth to Adulthood*. New York: Cornell University Press.

Juvenile Offenders with Mental Health Disorders: Who Are They and What Do We Do With Them?

About the Author

The author has a rich background in working with juvenile offenders with mental health disorders, as well as helping others work more effectively with this complex population of youth.

Lisa Melanie Boesky, Ph.D., is a clinical psychologist specializing in adolescents. Dr. Boesky's focus is the identification and management/treatment of juvenile offenders with mental health disorders, including youth who are suicidal and/or who self-injure. She has designed several mental health training programs for correctional staff and trains juvenile justice personnel across the country. She has also trained judges, attorneys, teachers, foster care parents, child welfare personnel, mental health providers, substance abuse treatment providers, parents, and other professionals in issues related to mentally ill juvenile offenders. Dr. Boesky has consulted on mental health policy and programming to a variety of juvenile justice facilities and helped develop a mental health screening instrument for juvenile justice agencies to use with youth in their care. She regularly speaks at state, national, and international conferences on issues related to juvenile offenders with mental health disorders.

Dr. Boesky received her Bachelor of Arts degree in Psychology from the University of California, Santa Barbara. She received her Master of Arts degree and Doctor of Philosophy degree in Clinical Psychology from Wayne State University in Detroit, Michigan. Adolescents have always been the focus of her research and clinical interests, and Dr. Boesky's initial clinical work was in inpatient psychiatric settings. However, her interest in youth involved with the juvenile justice system grew and eventually became her primary focus. Dr. Boesky has worked directly with juvenile offenders within a correctional setting providing crisis intervention, psychological screening/assessment, and management services at a large juvenile detention center in Seattle, Washinton. She was also on the clinical faculty at the University of Washington, Department of Psychiatry and Behavioral Sciences. For several years she managed a project to enhance mental health services to state juvenile justice facilities in the state of Washington. During this time she served as the primary member of a mental health mobile team that traveled to a variety of juvenile justice facilities, providing consultation related to mentally ill youth. She also developed and provided several mental health training programs for juvenile justice facility staff and community supervision staff. Dr. Boesky has provided consultation to juvenile justice facilities undergoing lawsuits in relation to mental health matters. In addition to this book, she has also authored a number of chapters, articles, and training curricula on the topic of mentally ill youth in the juvenile justice system.

Dr. Boesky is one of the rare professionals who has expertise in both mental health and juvenile justice. She has found a way to take complex, clinical information, and make it interesting and easy to understand. This book is a compilation of research findings and years of clinical experience in both the mental health and juvenile justice arenas. It is hoped that you find the information interesting, as well as relevant to your interactions with juveniles.

Dr. Boesky can be reached through her website: www.drlisab.com.